mni

The Hale Clinic
GUIDE TO GOOD HEALTH

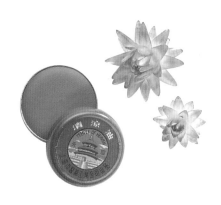

The Hale Clinic
GUIDE TO GOOD HEALTH

How to Choose the Right Complementary Therapy

TERESA HALE

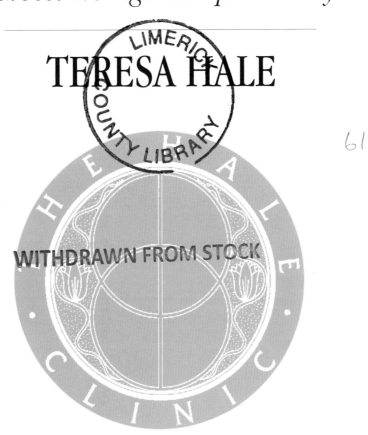

KYLE CATHIE LIMITED

I dedicate this book to my parents, William and Vee Hale,
for their unconditional love;
and to all the free spirits in medicine who have
the courage to continue the search for knowledge.

Kyle Cathie Limited
First published in Great Britain in 1996 by
Kyle Cathie Limited
20 Vauxhall Bridge Road
London SW1V 2SA

ISBN 1 85626 189 1

Photographs copyright © 1996 by Adrian Mott and Michelle Garrett
Contributing writers: Jerome Burne, Maggie Drummond,
Claire Gillman, Brigid McConville
See other photographic acknowledgements on page 7

A Cataloguing in Publication record for this book is available
from the British Library.

Edited by Caroline Taggart
Designed by Geoff Hayes
Printed in Spain by Cayfosa Industria Gráfica, Barcelona

Important Note

The information given in this book is intended for general guidance and is not a substitute for
individual diagnosis or treatment by a qualified practitioner and medical doctor. Always consult a
medical doctor and qualified practitionerbefore embarking on any treatment.
The reader is strongly advised not to attempt self-treatment for any serious or long-term
complaint without consulting a medical doctor and qualified practitioner. Neither the author,
the publishers nor the Hale Clinic can be held responsible for any adverse reaction to the
recommendations contained in this book, which are followed entirely at the reader's own risk.

Contents

Acknowledgements

I would like to thank Dianna Dusseault for co-ordinating the research for the book; Jane Martens for co-ordinating research and organizing the photography; Myriam Greene, Hale Clinic Manager, for managing the clinic and giving me time to focus on the book; Anna O'Meara for typing my original text, for her miraculous ability to read my illegible handwriting and for calmly managing my office so that I had time to concentrate on the book; Kyle Cathie for her belief and enthusiasm in the concept and for pushing me to write it; Caroline Taggart for her encouragement and patience with the complexity of all the material; Vee Hale for her encouragement, support and belief in the book, particularly when I mentioned to her I would never have the time to write it; and Lillo Militello of the Concordia restaurant in London for creating delicious Italian recipes for our patients based on the health principles outlined in the book.

Thanks also to Jerome Burne, Maggie Drummond, Claire Gillman and Brigid McConville, for their major contributions to the text.

Special thanks to Dr Harald Gaier who, through his knowledge of naturopathy, acupuncture, osteopathy and herbalism, as well as an extensive knowledge of research into complementary medicine, made a great contribution to this book. Dr Gaier is a registered naturopathic physician in South Africa. I am most grateful for all his time and for his fine judgement when approaching the treatment of illness with complementary medicine.

I am also very grateful to Dr Rajendra Sharma, who is a fully qualified doctor specializing in the use of complementary medicine. As a member of the Faculty of Homeopathy, London, and having studied and worked with specialists in most branches of complementary medicine, he has a broad knowledge of diagnostic techniques and therapies, enabling him to advise patients on the safest and quickest orthodox or complementary treatments for ill health. Dr Sharma has kindly used this knowledge and experience in this book to guide patients when to choose orthodox and/or complementary medicine for a particular illness. This information will greatly assist medical doctors, health care professionals and patients in gaining the maximum benefit from complementary medicine in the shortest period of time. His valuable contribution to the book will greatly enhance the co-operation between orthodox and complementary medicine.

Thanks are also due to all the Hale Clinic therapists who contributed their time and knowledge to this book:

Tracy Alderman – Auditory Integration Therapy

Peter Bartlett DO, MCO, MNTOS, MCrOA – osteopathy, naturopathy and nutritional therapy, with a special interest in computer-aided diagnosis and in the use of electro-magnetic devices such as Empulse in the field of migraine, chronic fatigue syndrome and pain control

Dr Lydia Boeken MD – integrative medicine, allergy treatment, ortho-molecular therapy, treatment of chronic fatigue/ME, Crohn's disease, fibromyalgia

Jing Hua Chen MD, MBAcA, MATCM, Professor of Chest Medicine – Chinese acupuncture, herbal medicine and *tuina*; runs an asthma clinic in complementary medicine for all ages

Peter Chin Kean Choy – Chi Kung, T'ai Chi, Taoist therapy (Trilogue process), director of the Rainbow T'ai Chi Centre and Foundation T'ai Chi Teachers' Training Centre

L M Crawford LCPH, MHMA (UK) – homeopathy, bioenergetics, psycho-therapy, NLP, hypnotherapy; runs the London Shyness Centre and the London Bio-Dynamics Centre

David Cunningham – spiritual healing

Dr David Curtin MB, BS, MFHom – homeopathy

Christopher P Drake, senior Buteyko practitioner, and **Alexander S**

Stalmatski, chief Buteyko practitioner

Tajinder K Deoora DO (Hons), MRO, MNIMH – osteopathy, medical herbalism; Senior Osteopath, Osteopathic Centre for Children; Senior Lecturer, Andrew Still College, Kingston University; author of *Fundamental Osteopathic Techniques*

Liza Elle Dip AT, RATh – Art-Psychotherapy

Angela Falaschi – nutritional medicine, iridology/allergy, homeopathy

Eileen Fairbane MIFAMHAF, CertEd – the Tangent method (holistic approach to body balance and mind balance) incorporating aromatherapy, Shiatsu, reflexology, exercise and movement

Belinda Freeman – clinical aromatherapy, reflexology, Chi Kung

Dr Maria Friedrich MD – acupuncture, homeopathy, hypnosis

Harald C Gaier ND, DO, DHomM, DipAc – naturopathy/nutrition; author of *Encyclopaedic Dictionary of Homoeopathy*

Scott Galloway BSc, MSc, CPsychol – clinical psychology and psychotherapy

Ursula Gateley – healing, colonic hydrotherapy, clinical nutrition, lymphatic drainage

Dr Marilyn Glenville BEd (Hons), MA, PhD (Camb), Dip EHP NLP – nutritional therapy, psychotherapy, hypnotherapy, NLP; chair of Foresight, the Association for Preconception Care and Natural Approach to Infertility; scientific adviser to the Society for the Promotion of Nutritional Therapy

Dr Shantha Godagama BA, MS, MALF, MBAcC, MF (Hom) – Ayurveda, acupuncture, homeopathy; specialist in *panchakarma* allergy testing, founder president of the Ayurvedic Medical Association UK

Dr Yun Guo MB (Beijing), BAcA – Chinese acupuncture, herbal medicine

Roger Golten BA (Hons) – Heller work

Salah ben Halim LCPHom, MCPHom, MHMA – homeopathy, Reiki

Lassara Hall MRSS – Shiatsu

Natalie Handley MBSR – reflexology, light therapy

Clare Harvey MAVMed, DipShen – flower essences, Shen Tao acupressure: runs professional courses in flower essences (vibrational medicine); director and founder of International Federation for Vibrational Medicine

Kiti Hitches ITEC Dip MFPhys, MIPTI – Moor therapy and Tri-Med treatment; member of the World Federation of Healing and the Faculty of Physiatrics

Angela Hope-Murray MA, SRCh, MChS – nutrition, Ayurveda, reflexology, chiropody, advanced remedial massage

Mary Chase Hopkins RCT, MCIA, MBTA – Bowen therapy, colon hydrotherapy, manual lymphatic drainage, microcurrent therapy

Virginie Host MCSP, SRP – chartered physiotherapist; GDS Method and Techniques

Sujata Jolly BSc – skincare and cosmetic scientist

Nish Joshi DO MRO – osteopathy, nutritional health

Kitty Kennedy BSc, MSc, IRTS, ITEC, PSCHI– yoga therapy, relaxation, breathing work, yoga and counselling meditation

Agnes Kernan SRN, BSc, DHomMed, HMA – homeopath; nurse practitioner specializing in alternative approach

Dr Malcolm Kirsh – psychotherapy and counselling for couples, individuals or businesses

Momo Kovacevic – bio-energy

Michael Landon MIT, ARIPHH – trichology; acts as an expert witness for the Law Society and as an independent consultant for a Singapore company

Alison Loftus DipION – nutritional therapy; member of the Professional Register of the Society for the Promotion of Nutritional Therapy; presently taking the post-graduate course at the Institute for Optimum Nutrition

Sir Thomas Lucas MA, MSMN – natural healing and health maintenance according to the NFSH, Usui Reiki and Krieger systems; full healer member of the National Federation of Spiritual Healers; Initiate of the Usui Reiki Universal Life Energy Technique

Kim Mendez MAR, IFA, ITEC, MBAcA, MRCHM – massage, reflexology, aromatherapy

Maria Mercati BA (Hons), ITEC, MTI, DS, C Tuina (Shanghai), **Gina Mercati** MA, ITEC, DipBH *tuina*/Thai and **Gisela**

Mercati ITEC, DipBH *tuina*/Thai – BodyHarmonics (*tuina* Chinese massage, Thai traditional massage and Indonesian massage), acupuncture

Georgina Milne MBRA – reflexology

Katherine Monbiot DThD, RCT (MCIA) – holistic nutrition, colonic hydrotherapy, Reiki; chaired the Colonic International Association for three years; teaches diet and nutrition on a degree course; runs nutrition, cookery and fertility awareness workshops and seminars

Marc Mortiboys BDS (Guys), MCAHyp, MABCH – holistic dentist

Samir Mostafa BScPhE, LicAc, DipTCM, MBAcC – Chinese medicine, 'acupuncture, herbs and diet'; adviser in the Egyptian army for physical fitness since 1968

Yuko Nakamura, member of the Society of Teachers of Alexander Technique – Alexander Technique, Shiatsu

Seka Nikolic – bio-energy healing

Robert Parsons MA, MNRHP – hypnotherapy, psychotherapy

Shauket Parvez MSc, MD, DAc, LicAcu, MBAcA, MAcF, DO, MRO, MRSH – osteopathy, cranial osteopathy, acupuncture, sports injury

Tanya Jane Patmore DipCouns, CHP (NC), CQSW – counselling, hypnotherapy

Dr Palle Pedersen DC, MPhil – chiropractic, specializing in occupational safety and health; co-author (contributing) of the WHO manual 'Chiropractic Methods in the Prevention and Management of Neuro-Musculoskeletal Disorders in Occupational Health'

Carina Petter DO, MRO – osteopathy

Rachel Piton MCIH – colonic hydrotherapy; certified Shiatsu therapist

Doja Purkit MD, BSc, DCH – Ayurveda, Marma, acupuncture, bio-chemic homeopathy, alternative medicine with self-care

Robert D Russell DHyp, FASM, RegHyp – stress management, hypnotherapy, psychotherapy, counselling, sports motivation, EMDR

Dr Rajendra Sharma MB, BCh, BAO, LRCP(I), LRCS(I), MRCH, MFHom – consultant in complementary medicine

Caroline Shaw – colonics, Chuaka massage

Aditi E Silverstein MA, CCC-SLP –

Sensory Integration Therapy for Communication; speech/language pathologist

Simone Simmons – energy healing

Gordon Spencer BA (Hons), DipEHy, PsyNLP (BHR) – hypnotherapy, psychotherapy, counselling

Dr Alan Stewart MB, BS, MFHom, MRCP(UK) – nutrition, homeopathy; also medical adviser to the Women's Nutritional Advisory Service

Kenneth Underhill DO, ND, MRN, MAcAMGOA – osteopathy, naturopathy, acupuncture, iridology, medical herbalism

Dr Gang Zhu RCMP, MMeSc – acupuncture, Chinese herbal medicine

Photographic Acknowledgements

Adrian Mott: pages 1, 8, 11, 13, 14 (top), 18 (both), 19, 21, 22, 23 (both) 25, 26, 27 (bottom), 28, 30, 32 (top), 33, 35 (both), 36, 37, 38, 39, 40, 41, 42 (bottom), 43 (bottom), 44, 47, 48, 49, 52 (both), 53, 55, 56, 58, 59, 60, 61, 62, 67, 68, 69, 70, 73 (top and bottom left), 75, 76 (bottom), 79, 80, 81, 83, 84 (top), 86, 88 (bottom), 90 (both), 91 (both), 92, 93, 94, 95, 97. 98 (all), 99 (top), 100, 102, 103 (both), 104, 105, 106, 108, 109 (right), 110, 111, 114, 115 (both), 116 (both), 118, 119 (right), 121 (top and bottom), 122, 123 (both), 125, 126, 128, 129, 130 (left), 131, 133, 136 (all), 137 (both), 138, 139, 140, 141, 144, 147, 150, 152 (all), 153 (bottom), 154 (bottom), 157 (top left and top right), 159 (both), 161 (bottom), 167, 169 (bottom), 171 (bottom), 172, 175 (both), 178, 179 (bottom), 180, 182, 184, 186, 188, 189 (both), 190, 191, 192, 194, 199, 201, 203, 207 (both), 210, 211 (both), 213 (top), 215, 216, 217 (all), 218, 220 (bottom), 221, 222, 224, 225, 226, 227, 228, 229, 230, 231, 235, 237, 238, 239, 240, 241, 242, 243, 244, 245, 246 (both), 249, 250

Michelle Garrett: pages 10, 14 (bottom), 15, 27 (top), 29 (both), 32 (bottom), 42 (top), 43 (top), 45, 57, 72, 73 (bottom right), 74, 76 (top), 77, 78, 84 (bottom), 87, 88 (top), 99 (bottom), 107, 109 (left), 113, 115 (bottom), 117, 119 (left), 121 (centre), 127,130 (right), 134 (both), 135, 145, 153 (top), 154 (top), 157 (bottom), 160 (both), 161 (top), 162, 163, 166, 169 (top), 171 (top), 173, 174, 177 (both), 179 (top), 181, 183, 185 (both), 193, 195, 197, 200, 202, 205, 209 (both), 213 (bottom), 220 (top), 232, 233, 234, 236, 247, 248

Science Photo Library: pages 16 (Scott Camazine), 24 (BSIP VEM), 124 (Wellcome Department of Cognitive Neurology) , 142 (Nancy Kedersha/Immunogen), 148 (CNRI), 165 (Department of Clinical Radiology, Salisbury District Hospital)

Nic Barlow: pages 85, 89, 198, 214

Biophoto Associates: pages 112, 212, 219

The publishers would also like to thank Francine Ismay for modelling for the Chi Kung photography

Introduction

There has been a phenomenal growth in the number of people using complementary medicine in the UK, Europe and the US over the past years. The reasons put forward for this have been diverse: the fear of iatrogenic illness (that is, one caused by the side effects of pharmaceutical drugs); finding orthodox treatment has not been effective (trying complementary medicine as a last resort); and growing awareness of the green movement with a greater emphasis on a more natural lifestyle.

Coupled with this growth of interest has come an explosion of books, media articles and even TV documentaries about complementary medicine. The public has been faced with information about some 50 or 60 complementary treatments. As a result, many people, with illnesses from migraine to cancer, are left wondering how to choose the most appropriate treatment for their particular illness. For example, someone suffering from back pain may not know whether to go for osteopathy, chiropractic, acupuncture, homeopathy or nutritional therapy. Unfortunately,

therefore, many people have tried several different treatments before they find the right one for their individual case. Even if a friend recommends a practitioner who has helped them, the treatment that practitioner offers may not be effective for someone else's problem.

Moreover, many members of the public – and even many doctors – are unaware of the range of problems for which some complementary medical treatments can be effective. For example, it is not widely recognized how helpful homeopathy and acupuncture can be for a person who has suffered a severe loss such as a bereavement.

For several years the Hale Clinic has been advising patients on the right treatment or combination of treatments for their particular illness. I was asked by my publisher, Kyle Cathie, if I would write a book which would act as a guide to people wanting help in choosing a complementary therapy, explaining the range of treatments available at the Hale Clinic, identifying some fifty common complaints that can benefit from these treatments and showing how we would use complementary medicine to help the patient back to good health.

It is part of the Hale Clinic practice that orthodox and complementary medicine should work together for the benefit of the patient. In some cases a combination of both approaches is the best course of action; with other illnesses there may be more emphasis on complementary medicine and less on orthodox treatment, or vice versa. For each complaint treated in the book there is a section called 'The Hale Approach'. Readers are particularly urged to read the words in bold type at the beginning of this section, which gives advice on whether orthodox treatment, complementary medicine or a combination of both should be considered first.

Orthodox and complementary medicine do not share the same philosophy when they approach an illness. Orthodox medicine will try to eradicate the symptoms of the illness with surgery or pharmaceutical drugs, which in certain cases may cause side effects. The orthodox approach accepts that in eradicating an illness, some damage may be done through the side effects of the drugs. For example, antibiotics may get rid of flu, but prolonged use will weaken the body's immune system. Chemotherapy may eradicate the cancer but leave the patient in a very weakened state as a result of the treatment.

Complementary medicine in general aims to strengthen the patient's organism so that an illness cannot take hold. For example, if a newborn baby suffers from sleeplessness or colic, cranial osteopathy will seek to strengthen and balance the rhythms of the cranium a means of removing these symptoms.

These two different approaches to medicine bring us to a key question: 'What is good health?' Orthodox medicine would see it as an absence of symptoms accompanied by positive results from a series of tests such as ECG, liver and kidney function, blood and urine tests, eye and ear tests, etc. The various complementary disciplines, on the other hand, would focus on the strength of the patient's general constitution, considering among other things diet, exercise and lifestyle. A patient's emotional, mental and spiritual life is often also enhanced by complementary treatment.

Good health is therefore not just an absence of symptoms where a patient hopes disease will not strike. It is an ongoing process in which the patient is fully involved; a lifelong discovery of how to strengthen their body, mind, emotions and spirit in order to achieve optimal health. Moreover, the participation and co-operation of the patient is of vital importance. He or she is not a passive recipient of a course of treatment. If the patient does not become actively involved in maintaining his or her own good health, there is often a limit to what the complementary practitioner can achieve.

There are frequently ups and downs in the pursuit of optimal health, with patients sometimes becoming worse before they get better. With homeopathic treatment, for example, a skin rash may temporarily get worse before it finally clears. In some cases an emotion or feeling that has been repressed may surface, making life rather uncomfortable in the short term, but in the long term enabling the person to achieve emotional and physical good health.

The journey towards optimal health is a unique one for each individual. The Hale Clinic cannot lay down an exact blueprint that will work for everyone. However, the purpose of this book is to give the reader various options and encourage them to choose the way forward that is best for them. Each individual also has to choose his or her own pace. Some

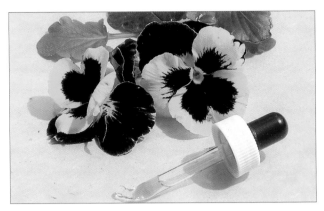

people will be more interested in improving their physical health, while others may put more emphasis on their spiritual development. It is up to the patient to determine the pace and nature of his or her own individual health programme.

There is far more medical research into complementary medicine than most people realize: a reference section at the back of the book lists some of the research available. The Hale Clinic has already been involved in several medical research projects and would fully support any future research. It is very important to measure the effects of these treatments. At the same time it is important to remember that human beings are very complex and that it is not always possible to measure everything.

Science is important, but the *art* of medicine must never cease to be practised. It is the art that guides the complementary medical practitioner when the way forward for that patient is not clear. Moreover, it is in the art of medicine that the co-operation between the patient and the practitioner is so crucial.

What does the future hold for complementary medicine? It seems likely that public demand will continue to grow. There will be increasing co-operation between orthodox and complementary practitioners. In the UK more and more general practitioners are referring patients to complementary medicine and some GP fundholders are even paying for the treatment. Medical insurance is also funding more treatment, due to public demand.

Complementary medicine can play an important role in hospitals, before and after surgery, as well as offering specific treatment programmes for serious cases. I sincerely hope that more government funds will be made available for research into complementary medicine. This will help create much more co-operation between the two disciplines. Worldwide, governments cannot sustain the increasing costs of orthodox medicine. Complementary medicine is low tech, so the cost of treatment is often much lower. Moreover, by improving the individual's all-round health, it can play an important role in the prevention of illness.

And what lies ahead for the Hale Clinic? It is our aim to open other clinics both in the UK and abroad; to continue to encourage research both in the more traditional complementary therapies such as acupuncture, homeopathy, osteopathy and chiropractic, and in more recent treatment developments such as Buteyko and light therapy; to encourage increased integration, understanding and communication between orthodox and complementary medicine. Furthermore, I sincerely hope this book will guide people in choosing their own personal integration between the two approaches. No one system has every answer to every medical problem and only by understanding the contribution the different medical systems can make can we improve the quality of our health care. I hope the trend of GPs paying for complementary medicine will develop considerably in the future, so that many more people will have access to the improvement in help that these therapies can bring.

Finally, never give up your own search for optimal health. You may not achieve it, but the journey itself will be truly enlightening.

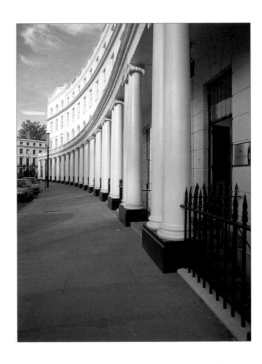

A Note on the Hale Clinic

The clinic was established in 1987 and officially opened by HRH The Prince of Wales in 1988. Its purpose is to combine and integrate the principles of conventional and complementary medicine, on the basis that no one system has the whole answer to every medical problem. Great emphasis is placed on preventative medicine as a way of maintaining good health after treatment. The Hale Clinic has pioneered research into the treatment of chronic fatigue syndrome, multiple sclerosis, autism, cerebral palsy and repetitive strain injury.

There are over 100 practitioners based at the Hale Clinic. Twenty of them are medical doctors, many are multi-disciplinary. Of the complementary medical therapies practised at the clinic, some are over 3,000 years old and others have developed in the last fifty years. Although they differ considerably in the way they treat illness, they all view the practice of complementary medicine as helping the individual organism achieve its natural harmony and balance, thereby making it much less susceptible to illness and disease. The clinic houses a natural medicines dispensary, complementary medical library and educational resources centre which provides a worldwide mail-order service.

The Hale Clinic logo was inspired by the ancient symbol of two interlocking circles called the Vescia Piscis, widely used in the Celtic and early Christian traditions. For the early Christians it represented the fish, and was also used in the sacred geometry of Glastonbury Abbey: it is seen as representing the blending of the masculine and feminine, yin and yang, the coming together of the conscious and unconscious worlds. The symbol's connection with healing inspired me to adapt it to reflect the philosophy of the Hale Clinic.

The outer circle represents a person's searching for wholeness. The two inner circles reflect the interconnection of body and mind. The eye in the middle represents our inner knowledge. The two snakes at the side have been taken from the Greek symbol of the god of healing, Asclepius. The lotus on both sides is an eastern symbol, reflecting the great contribution the oriental tradition has made to complementary medicine. The lotus also symbolizes the fact that although we have our roots in the mire, we can unfold over time to a reflection of serenity.

Autism

Imagine that the messages you are receiving from the world are so scrambled and distorted that ordinary things just don't make sense. Your world is a jigsaw puzzle of scattered pieces. This is what daily life can be like for people with autism. Not surprisingly, when you can't understand clearly what's going on and you can't communicate effectively with anyone, you retreat into your own world, turning away from speech and avoiding eye contact. You find it hard to understand other people's feelings, and other people find it hard to understand you.

Autistic children and adults try to cope in a number of ways. In an attempt to create order from the jumble of their senses, they may develop obsessive patterns of behaviour – insisting on going the same way, doing the same things. Or they may develop apparently irrational fears.

It is usually parents who first notice 'something strange' about their young child's behaviour. He or she may not play imaginatively with toys or other children, seems indifferent to what's going on, and/or talks 'at' people in an odd, repetitive way, paying little attention to their responses. Some autistic children also behave in a challenging way, screaming or biting and kicking other people, perhaps because they are anxious and frightened. One theory is that autistic children are supersensitive to certain sounds, which can make them irritable, frustrated and even hysterical. 'It's as though he's permanently at Heathrow Airport and hearing everything through the tannoy system,' said one mother of her autistic son.

For autism is far more than a problem of behaviour. It is a complex and variable form of disability affecting four times as many boys as girls. Three quarters of autistic children also have learning difficulties or other disabilities, while a tenth have a special skill such as music or art.

There are different theories about what causes autism. Research shows that a range of conditions – from maternal rubella and lack of oxygen at birth, to complications of childhood illnesses – can affect brain development before, during or after birth. Other experts believe that the MMR (measles, mumps and rubella) vaccination or food sensitivity may be to blame, although this is a highly controversial area. There is also a school of thought that over-compression of the skull during birth has caused head pain, which autistic children may try to relieve by head banging. From a bioenergetic or 'healing' perspective, autism is the manifestation of a great imbalance of energies at a cellular level. Healers describe these as 'very low-power energies over a wide range of frequencies which affect electrical, magnetic and chemical processes in the body'.

Whatever the cause, the result is a sensory processing disorder, so that the autistic person receives information in a distorted and disorganized fashion, in turn disrupting their ability to communicate. It's vital to spot autism early in a child's life if they are to be helped out of their isolation – and if their families are to receive the necessary support.

THE ORTHODOX APPROACH

Traditionally, autistic children have been put in residential schools and kept out of the community. 'Holding' or physically restraining children to modify their behaviour has also been tried, as have sedative drugs.

As yet there is no 'cure' for autism, but these days orthodox health professionals aim to help autistic people develop their social and communication skills so that they can become more independent and live fuller lives.

THE HALE APPROACH

The Hale Clinic approach to autism is unique and, provided the child is monitored by a child psychiatrist, the following approach to treatment is likely to be the most beneficial.

Autism is not like some illnesses, for which you take a pill and have an 80-90 per cent chance of success. It is a matter of selecting a range of treatments and educational tools which will help to improve the quality of a child's life. Each child's response to treatment will vary – from dramatic improvement to subtle change.

Many parents look at complementary medicine and see a whole range of possible treatments for their child. They are often very uncertain what action to take. At the Hale Clinic we have had considerable experience with autistic children, and this is our recommended approach.

Firstly, start treatment as soon as possible after autism is diagnosed. The younger the child is, the easier it is for any treatment to be effective.

Cranial osteopathy can be of great assistance and we advise seeing a cranial osteopath even if there has not been a difficult birth.

Secondly, see a nutritional/allergy specialist, in case food allergies are playing a part in aggravating the child's autism. Then try homeopathy with healing.

The child should now be in a position to gain the maximum benefit from Auditory Integration Training. The child's ears are first tested by an audiogram to see if he or she is oversensitive to certain sounds, in which case a course of treatment to normalize hearing would be recommended. Follow-up 'booster' treatments may also be needed. In addition, parent support groups are set up to help monitor progress.

Parents of autistic children are unsung heroes and heroines. They also need support, which may take the form of relaxation, healing or aromatherapy.

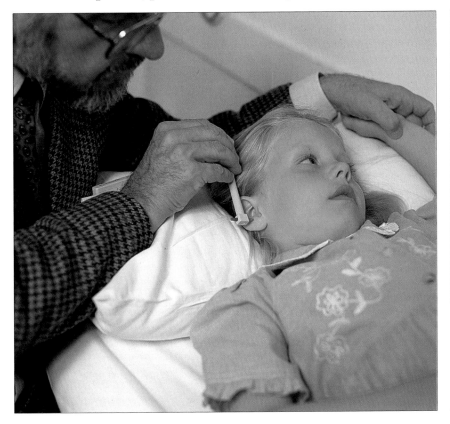

OSTEOPATHY

According to one osteopath, autism is not a syndrome but a wide spectrum mode of behaviour with multi-factorial aspects – behavioural, mechanical, emotional and biochemical. One possible treatment involves cranial osteopathy ('involuntary movement'). This subtle movement of the bones in the skull allows the body to find a fulcrum, enabling it to rebalance itself optimally.

Auricular diagnosis

AUDITORY INTEGRATION TRAINING

This therapy can be so pleasant – you mainly sit listening to some slightly strange music over headphones – that it hardly seems like a 'treatment' at all. Yet AIT can help autistic children to understand communication, to begin to speak, to interact with people and the environment, and to be more calm and less distressed by the world.

During AIT, sound frequencies are isolated and the music for the treatment session is electronically filtered and made louder or softer to emphasize frequencies in a random pattern. The effect is to make the brain pay attention – because it doesn't know what to expect. Through this treatment the way that auditory information is received may be improved, so that the autistic child is less likely to block out sounds and can begin to understand communication and auditory information. 'Afterwards, the children actually hear the world differently,' says an AIT therapist.

The effect of two half-hour sessions or one hour-long session a day over a ten-day period is to stimulate the auditory system, and sensory processing in general. 'The more we exercise our brain,' explains the therapist, 'the better it works for us.'

After AIT, children may be able to hear more accurately, with reduced sensitivity to sounds which previously caused them distress and fear. According to the same therapist, 'Children's self-esteem and mood improve. They don't all develop speech after AIT – it is not a "cure" – but they are more motivated to communicate. The first session can be difficult for a child who doesn't understand the concept of time or who doesn't like the sounds they can't block out.' However, once they are familiar with AIT, the children seem happy to co-operate: 'They do seem to enjoy listening – and they keep coming back for more.'

This is a therapy which takes commitment on the part of the parents, as it requires daily sessions for ten days, with subsequent follow-up sessions usually recommended at intervals of perhaps three to six months.

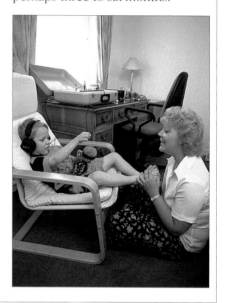

NUTRITION/AURICULAR ACUPUNCTURE

One homeopath, acupuncturist and nutritional therapist uses a two-pronged approach to help children with autism. 'I use auricular acupuncture (stimulating points on the ear),' he explains, 'working with both the nervous and the limbic (the part of the brain concerned with raw emotion) systems.' Autistic children generally won't put up with the insertion of needles into their bodies, so he uses a harmless device which looks like a pen torch, but is in fact an infra-red laser.

'I have to talk to the children about it, and sometimes rest my hand on their cheek, so if they move, the laser moves with them.' Each child requires stimulation to different points, according to individual sensitivities which are picked up through the pulse in the wrist.

The second aspect of this therapist's treatment of autism is to use nutritional therapy, assessing whether the child's system is

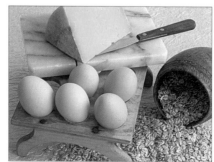

Avoiding certain foods can help autistic patients

burdened by allergy to particular foods. 'Tummy upsets may be a sign of sensitivity to milk products; scaliness of the skin suggests a problem with grains,' he explains. 'There is also a blood test we can perform to find sensitivities, but it is costly.' Eliminating certain foods – from eggs to cane sugar, from wheat to dairy products – can leave the child's body in a stronger state to deal with autism. Supplements such as magnesium and Vitamin B_6 may also help.

Together, the results of these therapies can be very gratifying. 'It's a matter of improvement rather than cure, but after about three or four treatments, the child may be less inwardly directed, responding when his parents speak to him and communicating better.'

PSYCHOTHERAPY/COUNSELLING

Autism is often confusing and distressing, not just for the autistic child but for his or her family. For this reason counselling often focuses on helping carers to manage their own feelings about and relationship with the child, as well as coping with the child's challenging behaviour. This kind of support needs to be long term and may involve counselling, medical input and periods of respite care.

'Psychotherapy or psychology can also help carers and families learn how to praise and reward appropriate behaviour,' says one psychotherapist, 'so as to foster positive development and to discourage negative or inappropriate behaviour. Most autistic children also need special schooling, and careful planning is needed to help the child make the transitions from home to school, between schools or from school to adult educational provision.'

BIOENERGETIC MEDICINE

Bioenergetics is a modern system of diagnosis using a computer to measure electromagnetic energy in the brain. Sensors attached to your body measure your physical reaction to over 3,000 conditions, treatments and compounds, including homeopathies, viruses, chemical toxins, fungi, amino acids and vitamins. Only a handful of therapists in the world use bioenergetic diagnosis, but they have found it effective for a wide range of disorders, including autism. 'It's like an electronic form of kinesiology,' explains one therapist. 'The body reacts to various substances it likes or dislikes, diagnosing for itself and indicating what is going on in the body.'

Autism, she believes, can be caused either by damage at birth or by a form of chemical damage – whether that involves a viral, a chemical or a fungal agent. 'Once we can pinpoint what caused autism, we can treat it. A colleague of mine has a severely autistic child, which could be because his wife was given pills for morning sickness while pregnant. This child was treated bioenergetically and with homeo-pathy, and now teaches other autistic children.'

Once diagnosis is complete using the bioenergetic computer, the causative factors are treated with homeopathic remedies. 'This is 21st-century healing,' says the therapist, 'using a computer to empower the earth's most intelligent system – you.'

HEALING

'Children with autism respond wonderfully to healing,' according to one healer. 'Their brains are working very, very fast so that all their senses are scrambled and I work to slow it all down.'

Some of the children she has treated have remarkable perceptual experiences, such as 'seeing' sound and 'hearing' colour. 'They are often very brilliant children, too,' she says, 'spiritual and very receptive.' Spiritual healing, she has found, can bring 'very good results' in the treatment of autism.

Another way of describing the healing process is to compare the healer to a 'low-power, multi-frequency laser machine, setting up a self-healing process centred on the pituitary and pineal gland area in the centre of the head.' The aim is to re-establish balance of cellular energies at a very subtle level. Some healers also call up colours – especially sky blue and indigo for problems such as autism – while listening intently to the responses of the patient. The result can be a kind of cellular reprogramming, which can help people with autism to adjust to their condition.

SELF-CARE

Flower Remedies: Bluebell and Sundew, both Australian Bush flowers, are said to be helpful in autism.

Aromatherapy: Soothing oils such as clary sage and jasmine may be useful in calming an overwrought child.

Another important aspect of self-care is to maintain good nutrition, avoiding foods that may burden the body through allergic reaction (see above under *Nutrition/Auricular Acupuncture*).

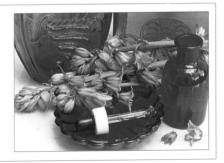

Multiple Sclerosis

A diagnosis of multiple sclerosis or MS is one which many people dread because we associate it with slow and progressive deterioration into disability. In fact, only a minority of those with MS will suffer its most crippling effects and there is much you can do to stay healthy and lead a normal life in spite of this disease.

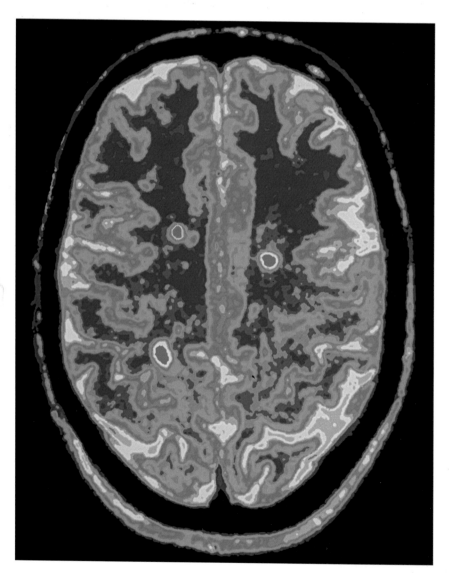

MS occurs as a result of damage to the nerve fibres of the central nervous system (the brain and spinal cord). This happens when the sheath of fatty tissue or myelin which insulates the nerves is attacked and becomes inflamed. Different people will have different symptoms, depending on which nerves have been damaged. The most common age of diagnosis is late 20s to mid-30s. It is rare to have MS after the age of 50.

MS symptoms are caused by patches of 'demyelination' (scarring) in the central nervous system and, depending on which nerves are scarred, movement, touch and sensation may be affected. MS is a very variable condition, but early symptoms often include tingling sensations or numbness which may affect a hand or a foot – sometimes described as 'walking on cotton wool'.

Other common symptoms are blurred or double vision, weakness or clumsiness of a limb, giddiness or lack of balance, disproportionate fatigue and the need to pass water frequently or urgently. Sometimes these symptoms simply disappear, never to be experienced again, but they may recur and worsen in a series of 'attacks' that may end in serious disability.

Researchers have been looking for the causes of MS for years, so far without success. It could be that a virus causes the inflammation of the myelin sheath, or inherited factors could be to blame. Complementary practitioners have linked MS to weakness of the nervous system which may be caused by stress, shock, infection or toxic metals. Another theory is that MS is linked to the effects of radiation from the sun.

THE ORTHODOX APPROACH

There is no conclusive test for MS and it often takes time – and a long period of anxiety – before it is suggested. Orthodox doctors treat symptoms as they arise, using a number of techniques. Steroid drugs may be given to treat the condition as a whole and these can stabilize symptoms by tackling inflammation. Other drugs are often prescribed to treat individual symptoms, such as muscle relaxants for spasms and analgesics if there is pain. Physiotherapy is also an important technique in the mainstream management of MS.

THE HALE APPROACH

Any symptoms that are obviously related to the nervous system, such as double vision, loss of co-ordination, etc., or any persistent problem that does not resolve, may have a neurological basis. Aches and pains, numbness or tingling should be taken to a doctor, who may well recommend consultation with a neurological specialist. Once a diagnosis of MS has been made, complementary medical opinion should be considered first line, since these therapies are aiming at a cure, whereas orthodox treatments are dealing with the symptoms and hoping for a remission. If your doctor has prescribed steroids, do not stop the treatment without medical supervision.

Advising on a treatment for MS is complicated because the condition can be aggravated by many factors, such as poor nutrition, stress, weak elimination, toxic metals or weakness in the nervous system. Also, assessing the improvement is not easy as spontaneous remissions are part of the pathology of MS.

The Hale Clinic approach would first address the nutrition/allergy aspect and recommend colonic irrigation to detoxify the system. This would be followed by homeopathy or Ayurveda combined with marma massage to build up the consititution generally. Marma treatment plays a very important role in the treatment of MS, by clearing obstructions from the nerve fibres and co-ordinating body and brain.

Healing can complement these therapies, helping the patient both physically and mentally, while Bach flowers, aromatherapy, yoga and T'ai Chi play their part as supportive treatments.

NUTRITION

Nutritional therapy can be used to modify and strengthen the immune system. This is helpful in treating MS, in which the body's immune system has turned upon itself. 'Treatment involves basic diet adjustment,' explains one therapist, 'minimizing intake of saturated fats from food like red meat. We also eliminate possible hidden food sensitivities and/or inhaled allergens, which could be important but unrecognized causes of MS.' With the use of vitamin and mineral drips and nutritional supplements, she also aims to combat harmful free radicals in the system. She advises the removal of amalgam dental fillings. 'Depending on the degree of disease,' she says, 'we can stabilize or improve the symptoms of MS.'

HOMEOPATHY

Homeopaths begin by treating MS constitutionally. This means looking at the individual, establishing the nature of their constitution and prescribing a remedy which matches how they are when well, to stimulate their normal state.

After that, a whole rang eof homeopathic remedies can help to support self-healing. For instance, if there is an exacerbation of symptoms or a loss of physical control, Aconite could be taken with the first six hours, followed by Phosphorus.

In the very early stages or when MS is first diagnosed, Lathyrus may help. Agaricus Musc can alleviate pain. The snake and spider poison remedies may also be beneficial.

However, for homeopathy to work properly, accurate prescription by a qualified homeopath is essential.

COLONIC HYDROTHERAPY

Colonic irrigation offers the benefits of detoxifying the body, says one therapist: 'In turn this helps the body's absorption of nutrients, allowing the body to feed and repair its tissues – which can halt the progress of MS.' And when MS has caused paralysis in the bowel, colonics can also help by bringing back some movement to the bowel.

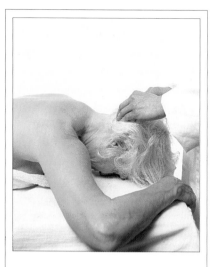

MARMA MASSAGE

A recent pilot study at a major London hospital has shown promising results in the treatment of chronic stroke patients for this ancient system of Indian health care, and similar techniques are employed in the treatment of MS. Ayurvedic doctors observed that there are 107 'junction boxes' or points in the body where the nerves and muscles meet. These marma points lie deep within the body and, as they are directly connected to the nervous system, they link the body and brain.

'Marma is a neuro-muscular therapy,' explains one of the few Western practitioners to use marma therapy. 'It clears obstructions from the nerve fibres and co-ordinates the brain and nerves.'

After the first 45-minute session, a further 6-20 half-hour treatments are recommended. 'Marma can stop MS attacks,' claims the therapist, 'so that symptoms disappear – depending on the level of damage.' He also teaches self-care: 'Diet and exercise are very important parts of the treatment, enabling you to lead a normal life.'

AYURVEDA

While he stresses that the symptoms of MS vary from person to person, and that it is easier to treat someone in the earlier stages of this disorder than someone who is already in a wheelchair, one practitioner maintains that Ayurveda is highly effective in treating neurological weakness. 'Ayurvedic oral and external preparations are made to stimulate motor nerve functions. *Panchakarma* (revitalizing) therapy is most useful. Some other detoxification treatments may be prescribed according to the individual case. Certain types of yoga are also helpful.'

A course of Ayurvedic treatment could last from six months to two years or longer, involving at least one consultation a month.

The practitioner tells of how he treated a nurse colleague who was suffering from numbness in her lower limbs and mild symptoms of weakness. 'After one year during which I treated her with Ayurveda and acupuncture, all of her symptoms and weakness disappeared. She is still working in our practice. She has needed no treatment during the past two years and is completely free of symptoms of this disease.'

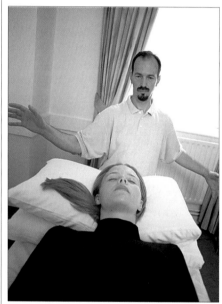

ENERGY HEALING

In MS, one healer believes, the messages of the nervous system have become 'misrouted': 'I work on the spinal cord and the muscles and nerves in the back to try to repair damage in the early stages of MS. Healing also helps to improve the circulation of the blood in the legs and spinal area.'

Healing can help in the early stages of MS, working directly on the nervous system, and patients can expect alleviation of symptoms, stabilization of the condition or remission.

SELF-CARE

Nutrition: Diet adjustment including supplements are an important part of keeping well with MS, according to one nutritionist, while alcohol and tobacco (potent free radical generators) should be avoided.

Aromatherapy: At home, aromatherapy oils may be massaged on to affected limbs or used in the bath to uplift. Vaporizers may also be used to affect mood. Oils such as geranium and rose are particularly beneficial.

SUPPORTIVE TREATMENTS

Light Therapy/Reflexology
'We work on the central nervous system using reflexology in conjunction with light therapy,' explains one therapist. 'Both of these treatments are effective in improving the nerves and the blood supply. Light dilates the blood vessels, and if we catch MS early we can keep the nerves healthy, stabilizing the symptoms.'

Flower Remedies
Snowdrop (a Pacific remedy) is said to dissolve energy blocks and personal holding patterns that prevent the free flow of energy. It also strengthens the will to dissolve paralysing fear, making it excellent for problems of paralysis such as MS.

Aromatherapy
Aromatherapy massage helps to calm the nervous sytem. The properties of the essential oils chosen for the treatment will reflect the patient's needs, offering emotional and physical support. Oils may be uplifting, antispasmodic and stimulating to the circulation.

Remedial Yoga
Yoga has a range of benefits for people with MS, both physical and mental, strengthening muscles, stimulating nervous-system response and stretching out constricted muscles. It also increases blood and lymph circulation, which can become sluggish if MS has reduced muscle tone. Mentally, yoga teaches us how to utilize the strength derived from the breath, re-establishes our sense of control over our bodies, and centres and calms the mind.

Acupuncture
There is no 'cure' as such for MS, but acupuncture can help relieve the pain that often accompanies this illness, improving general wellbeing and making life more bearable. This is a slow and long drawn-out process, however, and may involve weekly treatments over the course of perhaps a year, with regular follow-up treatments after that.

Chi Kung/T'ai Chi
These gentle exercises, which can be practised at home as a self-help therapy, may also be used to relieve pain. More fundamentally, though, Chi Kung and T'ai Chi are about restoring balance to the whole body. For MS, the 'first Chi Kung' exercises are particularly beneficial.

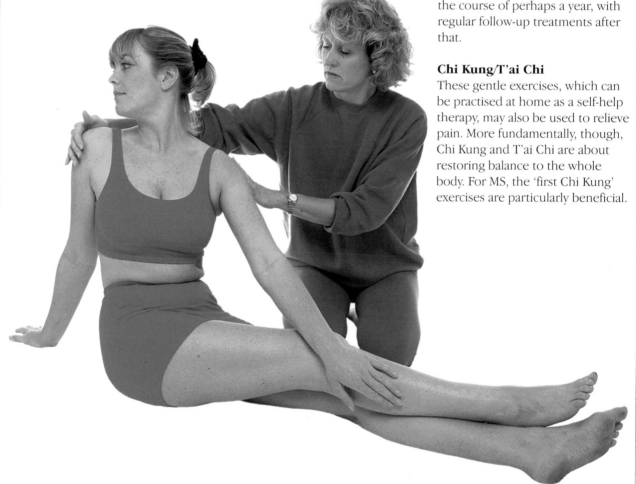

Parkinson's Disease

Once known as the 'shaking palsy' and widely seen as a disorder of elderly people, Parkinson's disease is increasingly common in the Western world where we are living longer and longer. Most people are diagnosed over the age of 60, but younger people are not immune: in fact one in twenty people with Parkinson's is under the age of 40 when diagnosed.

The symptoms vary greatly between individuals and may appear very gradually. Shaking, or tremor, is a common sign, usually beginning in one hand or arm only to diminish when the affected limb is being used. This can be an embarrassing symptom, but it is often very slight and usually has little impact on daily life.

Stiffness or rigidity of the muscles is another common symptom. It means that people with Parkinson's may have trouble getting up from chairs, or in doing up buttons or generally getting around. This can be compounded by the third major symptom, slowness of movement (bradykinesia). This makes it difficult to 'get going', so that walking is an effort; the sufferer may also come to a halt and have difficulty in starting again.

Other symptoms are caused by the interaction of these three sets of problems, with the result that people with Parkinson's may have altered posture, difficulties in balance, speech and writing, as well as an absence of facial expression. Parkinson's can also be very tiring and sometimes swallowing is a problem too.

In practice what all this means is that Parkinson's can dramatically upset your quality of life, affecting everything you do from getting dressed in the morning to being able to smile at your nearest and dearest.

So what causes this progressive neurological disorder – and what can be done to remedy it? In over 170 years since it was first pinpointed, scientists have not been able to come up with a cause for Parkinson's, although we do know that it is neither inherited nor contagious. It begins when – over the course of many years – there has been a loss of cells from the part of the brain which controls movement. These cells normally produce a chemical messenger known as dopamine, which works with another chemical messenger called acetylcholine to enable us to perform smooth, controlled movements. Once 80 per cent of the dopamine-producing cells in our brains have been destroyed, the symptoms of Parkinson's become noticeable.

THE ORTHODOX APPROACH

Conventional treatment involves prescription drugs as part of a package of treatments which also includes exercise, diet, physiotherapy, speech and occupational therapy. Drug treatments aim to restore the balance between dopamine and acetylcholine. This is done by taking medication either to increase our levels of dopamine, or by blocking the action of acetyl-choline, or both.

For most people who are diagnosed as having Parkinson's, drugs can initially be very effective. However, long-term treatments can cause severe side effects, including confusion, hallucinations and fluctuations in the ability to perform movements. So far, no ideal drug has been found, and the search goes on.

THE HALE APPROACH

Any neurological condition such as numbness, tingling, lack of co-ordination, visual problems, etc., should be examined immediately by a doctor, who may choose to refer you to a neurological specialist. Once a firm diagnosis ruling out any emergency situation has been established, then complementary treatments are far more likely to be beneficial than orthodox drugs. Advances are being made rapidly in both drug and surgical treatment for Parkinson's and keeping in touch with your specialist and managing any drug regime accurately is important. Anti-Parkinson's drugs may not be effective after a few years, and therefore complementary therapies that help to delay the onset of the use of orthodox drugs are most beneficial.

The combination of acupuncture and Marma massage can be very effective in the treatment of Parkinson's. Alternatively, homeopathy can be used in the early stages in order to delay the onset of symptoms. Reflexology can play a similar role in delaying the onset of the disease.

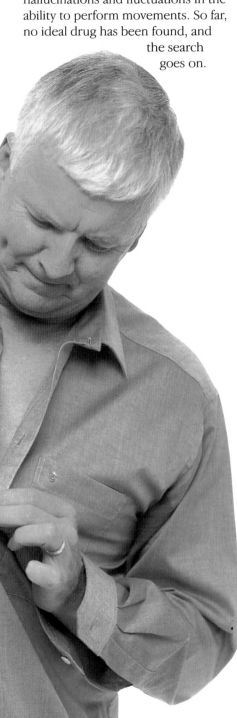

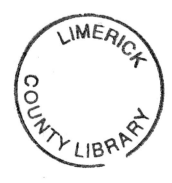

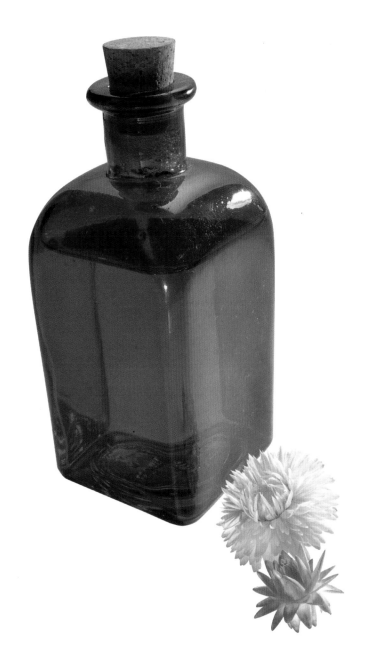

MARMA MASSAGE

The ancient techniques of marma massage combined with special exercises can be helpful in relieving the symptoms of Parkinson's disease. There are many marma points in the neck, an important articulation area of the body, which the therapist massages in order to stimulate blood flow. The marma points in the legs are also massaged. The effect is to improve blood flow to the brain, bringing much-needed oxygen to the brain cells.

A further benefit of this treatment is that it stimulates the nerves, sending messages to the brain to 'wake up' or adapt further brain cells.

Depending on the severity of your symptoms, between six and twenty sessions of marma massage can reduce shaking and trembling.

FLOWER REMEDIES

A helpful flower remedy for Parkinson's, according to one therapist, is Poison Hemlock (Pacific): 'This can dissolve emotional, mental and physical paralysis, especially of the physical structure of the nervous system.'

HOMEOPATHY

Parkinson's is a 'disease of deficiency' according to one homeopath, 'and therefore homeopathy can help by stimulating the body to manufacture the deficient substance, dopamine.'

He sees homeopathy as particularly beneficial in the early stages of Parkinson's, when it can help in delaying the onset of symptoms. The type of remedy prescribed depends on the type of symptoms, and 'by using a homeopathic remedy which matches the normal constitution of the individual we can enhance the patient's receptivity to drug treatments'.

ACUPUNCTURE

According to acupuncturists, Parkinson's disease arises when the blood supply to the liver is insufficient. Long-standing blood deficiency leads to lack of energy and stagnation of both energy and blood. The tendons and muscles rely on nourishment by the blood and liver yin in order to move and ensure proper motor control. If they do not receive this nourishment, the symptoms of Parkinson's will occur.

The branches and roots of the disease have to be treated simultaneously: new blood should be created to clear wind; energy and blood circulation must be regulated; and kidney yin should be treated to nourish liver blood and calm the mind. Regular nourishing and a blood-forming diet with some form of exercise are important.

SUPPORTIVE TREATMENT

Reflexology
Parkinson's disease may be helped by reflexology, but it must be a long-term, regular course of treatment. A member of the patient's family could be taught to give basic home treatment in between clinic visits. Reflexology may slow the progression of the disease and ease daily life.

SELF-CARE

Daily exercises which also promote blood flow to the brain support the massage treatment. These are simple neck exercises in which you move your head to one side and hold for the count of five before moving it to the other side for a further count of five. Repeat ten times.

Once you are familiar with your own marma points, you can continue with gentle self-help massage at home, as well as practising the neck exercises every day.

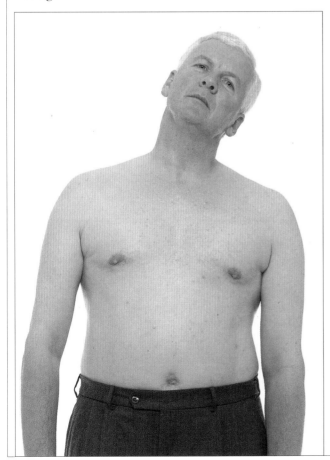
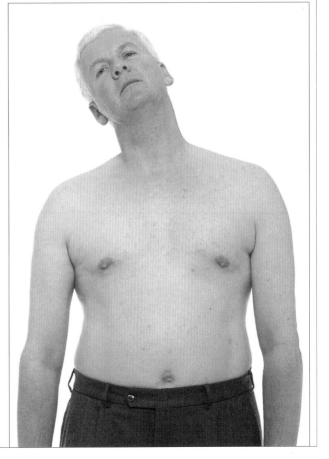

Epilepsy

Time was when the word 'epilepsy' was spoken in hushed tones: ignorant of its causes and helpless to prevent it, people reacted to this condition with fear and hostility. Today epilepsy has emerged from the shadows. We now know that it is no more than a tendency to have recurrent seizures, and people with epilepsy are the same as anyone else in every other respect. And these days medication to control seizures is widely available, so that most people with epilepsy are able to live full and active lives.

In simple terms, epileptic seizures happen when changes in brain chemistry cause the complex electrical messages travelling between our billions of nerve cells to become scrambled. Some people lose consciousness; others show hardly any symptoms. But after a matter of minutes or even seconds, the brain cells are back to normal and the seizure is over.

There are over forty different types of seizure, affecting different individuals in very different ways. They fall into two categories; 'generalized' (involving the whole brain) or 'partial' (originating in one part of the brain).

'Tonic-clonic' seizures (once known as 'grand mal') are the most common of the generalized types. In this kind of epileptic 'fit', you may fall down unconscious, your body stiffening (the tonic phase) and then jerking uncontrollably (the clonic phase). During the seizure you may make strange sounds, dribble, bite your tongue or be incontinent. It all lasts for no more than a few minutes but, while the person having the seizure can't remember what has happened, it can be distressing to witness.

Another kind of generalized attack is the 'absence seizure'. Once known as 'petit mal', this is a lapse in awareness in which you may stop

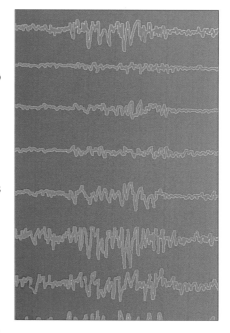

what you are doing, stare or look as if you are daydreaming for a few seconds – before carrying on as usual. It is more common in children (especially girls) and in teenagers than in adults. Although some people may have many 'absences' a day, they can be hard to spot and diagnose. Generalized seizures also include 'atonic' seizures or 'drop attacks', in which the person suddenly falls down; and 'myoclonic' seizures, in which the muscles jerk briefly.

'Partial' seizures may be 'simple', with a range of symptoms including jerking, pins and needles, dizziness and strange distortions of sensation – such as *déjà vu*, or things seeming abnormally large or small. These symptoms are sometimes known as an 'aura' and may be early warning of a more generalized seizure to come.

Alternatively, 'partial' seizures may be 'complex', causing people to act oddly – for instance swallowing repeatedly or appearing drunk. These behaviours are called 'automatisms' and the person having the seizure is unaware of what is going on.

One in every 130 people in the UK has epilepsy, making it the most common serious neurological (i.e. to do with the brain and nervous system) disorder in the country. It can affect anyone, and at any age. For most people with epilepsy there is no clear cause, but for the minority some kind of damage to the brain following a stroke, a blow to the head, an infection (such as meningitis) or a difficult birth may be to blame. Sometimes a tendency to seizures can be inherited. There are also common 'trigger factors' which can make seizures more likely – alcohol, stress, fever, lack of sleep and (in women) changing hormones, for example. And although it remains a controversial point, some people believe that certain foods can trigger seizures.

THE ORTHODOX APPROACH

Conventional medical treatments consist of anti-epilepsy drugs which act by calming the nerve cells in the brain, or by raising the seizure threshold. Drugs can control seizures for 80 per cent of people with epilepsy, but there may be unpleasant side effects, ranging from drowsiness and rashes in the short term to poor concentration, irritability, acne and weight gain in the long term.

THE HALE APPROACH

Epilepsy is not cured by orthodox treatment. Complementary therapies can be far more efficacious and should be used as early as possible.

The risk of falling downstairs or of fitting when driving a car or using potentially dangerous tools requires that epilepsy be controlled and therefore orthodox treatment is essential. Any fit should be reviewed by a doctor, referred to a neurological specialist if required, and the condition should then be monitored by the medical profession and anti-epileptic drugs used until the doctor recommends withdrawal.

It is particularly important for people suffering from epilepsy to strengthen their constitution and reduce stress levels. Epileptic attacks may be triggered by many different factors, so treatment should not focus on a single aspect – such as diet – but aim to make the whole system function at the optimum level.

We would recommend epileptics to check that they are following a good nutritional programme and that no allergies are aggravating the problem. Acupuncture, homeopathy and Ayurveda can also be used to strengthen a patient's general constitution. The electro-magnetic energy fields of many epileptics is disturbed, so healing can play an important role here.

Learning the Buteyko breathing technique gives patients a tool to reduce the incidence of epileptic seizures. Self-hypnosis and stress management can help limit the ability stress has to trigger an attack, and yoga, Chi Kung and T'ai Chi will help harmonize the patient's mental and physical state, further reducing the risk of an attack.

AYURVEDA

According to this traditional Indian system of medicine, epilepsy is a *vata*-oriented problem affecting the head. *Vata* is the force in the body that controls the central nervous system and it is associated with air and the ether. Treatment takes a number of forms, starting with oral herbal preparations in liquid and/or tablet form.

Panchakarma detoxifying treatments are also considered appropriate for people with epilepsy. 'Because the bowel is responsible for *vata*,' says one Ayurvedic practitioner, 'laxatives and enemas may be used to reduce abdominal pressure and cleanse the gastro-intestinal system.'

Thirdly, a special herbal treatment called *shiro dhara* may be prescribed. This involves lying still for about an hour while warm herbal oils are slowly dripped on to your forehead and then massaged into your scalp. This may be followed by a general herbal oil massage to the rest of your body.

Relaxation, meditation and specific yoga postures are also part of Ayurvedic treatment for epilepsy, while inhalation may be suggested when needed to reduce pressure on the sinuses.

ENERGY HEALING

Science has not as yet come up with an explanation for the mechanism of healing, but some healers describe their technique in terms of working with the electromagnetic field, or aura, which surrounds us all. 'I slow down the nerve function in the brain, making it more co-ordinated,' says one. 'This helps avoid the electrical storms which cause epilepsy. I would suggest perhaps six sessions of around thirty minutes each – and see how they go.'

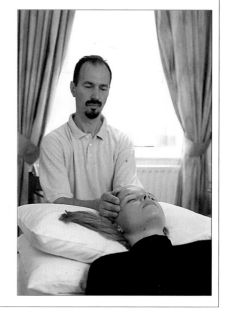

ACUPUNCTURE

Contributing factors to this disease include diet, heredity, negative emotions and other diseases. Anger and fear lead to stagnation of the liver energy, which impairs the function of the spleen, resulting in the formation and accumulation of phlegm. Fear may impair kidney and liver yin (cooling energy), leading to excess heat in the body, which condenses body fluids into phlegm. Depression and stress may lead the phlegm upwards to disturb the heart and mind, producing an epileptic attack.

Treatment programmes depend on the individual case, but may include clearing phlegm, strengthening the spleen and stomach to produce blood (in cases of sallow complexion, nausea, loose stools and emaciation), nourishing the heart, liver and kidney yin (in cases marked by insomnia, dizziness, soreness of the lumbar region and constipation) and normalizing hyperactivity of the liver (in cases of irritability and mental restlessness).

In an emergency when no needles are available, pressure applied by the thumb between the upper lip and the nose should help the patient to regain consciousness.

Epilepsy is a condition whose root causes and symptoms are often treated together. Patients should initially continue to take their orthodox medication, decreasing it gradually as the condition improves.

HOMEOPATHY

Homeopathy stimulates the body's own natural healing reaction and can make epileptic seizures less frequent. Remedies prescribed would depend very much on the individual case. Homeopaths would suggest three or four consultations, with follow-up visits at six-monthly intervals. Dietary changes may complement homeopathic treatment, which can bring significant improvement to the health of people with epilepsy.

NUTRITION/ALLERGY TREATMENT

'There is considerable evidence that food allergy, intolerance or even chemical sensitivity may be one of the causes of epilepsy,' believes one registered naturopath, homeopath and osteopath at the Hale Clinic. He points to evidence that certain gases, aerosols, pesticide sprays, smoke and exhaust fumes, solvents, drugs and food additives can very occasionally precipitate allergic epileptic seizures.

A trial, held at the Great Ormond Street Hospital for Sick Children in London in 1982 and 1983, showed a dramatic improvement in the health of children suffering from migraine – of whom a proportion also had epileptic seizures. After these children stopped eating foods to which they were allergic, not only did their migraines stop, their epileptic seizures also disappeared.

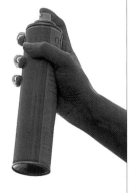

BUTEYKO

How can a method which teaches a healthy breathing technique have an impact on epilepsy? The answer, according to one Buteyko teacher, is that correct breathing influences practically every major system of the body – including the nervous system, cardiovascular system, immune system, hormonal system, pH balance and the body's take-up of oxygen. Through these complex systems, he argues, breathing influences the pathology of electrical impulses, enabling us to reverse the process which causes seizures.

'These are enormous factors, and when we normalize our breathing, epilepsy reduces. No person who breathes normally has epilepsy: all people with epilepsy hyperventilate, breathing between three and five times as much as they should.'

In this practitioner's experience as a Buteyko teacher, he has seen people with epilepsy learn the correct breathing method – only to find that they don't notice much of a change at first: 'Then they have a seizure and find they can diminish its effects while it is happening by practising a breath-retention technique. They get better at the technique and find that eventually they can stop a seizure. This enables them to cut down on symptomatic medication, until they find they don't require it.'

FLOWER REMEDIES

Ranunculus – buttercup (Petite Fleur and FES) – is said to be helpful when there are imbalances in the brain, especially epilepsy. It is particularly good for the treatment of children.

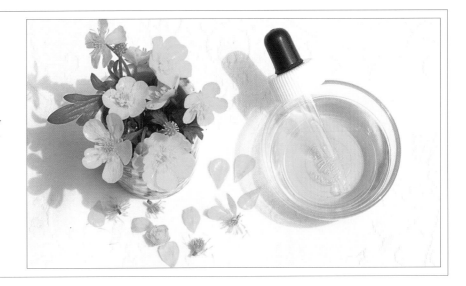

SUPPORTIVE TREATMENTS/ SELF-CARE

Self-Hypnosis/Stress Management

As stress is one of the triggers which can spark off epileptic seizures, it makes sense to learn techniques to manage the stresses of daily life. One practitioner teaches self-hypnosis and relaxation as part of a range of techniques aimed at managing stress.

'Relaxation helps prevent the build-up of stress,' he explains, 'and if you reduce your stress levels then epilepsy may be less frequent and easier to manage.'

Coupled with a healthy diet and exercise regime, this therapist helps you reassess your lifestyle to gain a clearer understanding of – and control over – the problems that give rise to stress in the first place.

Remedial Yoga

Once the symptoms of epilepsy have been stabilized, yoga as taught by a therapist can help to revitalize the body and mind, encouraging blood flow to the brain, rejuvenating and stimulating the brain function.

Yoga also balances the endocrine system and soothes the nervous system, helping you to focus within yourslf and bringing a sense of bodily

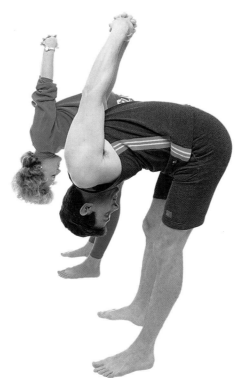

strength and feelings of balance.

The forward bend illustrated here should not be attempted by anyone whose epileptic symptoms have not been stabilized.

Chi Kung

'Heartbeat listening' is a very good exercise for the epileptic patient, restoring a sense of harmony and calm to the disrupted system. Chi Kung exercises allow the client to reclaim a sense of control both before and after a fit. Committed and long-term practice of the Chi Kung exercises (especially in combination with the 'third fundamental' T'ai chi exercise) will significantly ameliorate symptoms and may even get rid of epilepsy altogether.

In addition to the effect of food and chemicals, emotional upsets can set off seizures. Therapies which can help control the effects of such upsets include autogenic training, mental imagery, meditation and bio-feedback, all of which have been shown to reduce the number and severity of epileptic seizures.

Shingles

Anybody who has ever had the childhood disease of chicken pox can develop the painful, blistered rash of shingles, technically known as herpes zoster. The chicken pox virus lies dormant in a nerve root for years, only to be reactivated later in life when the characteristic rash appears on the area of skin supplied by the affected nerve. The reactivation is sometimes a result of contact with someone – usually a child – carrying chicken pox, but it can also arise from stress or when the body is particularly run down.

The first symptom of shingles is severe pain, for no apparent reason, on one side of the body, usually on the chest, back or neck. A few days later, the blistering rash appears and covers the painful area. It normally disappears in two or three weeks but it can leave scars where the crusts have formed. Although the rash clears up quite quickly, the pain (known as post-herpetic neuralgia) can persist for months, if not years, afterwards.

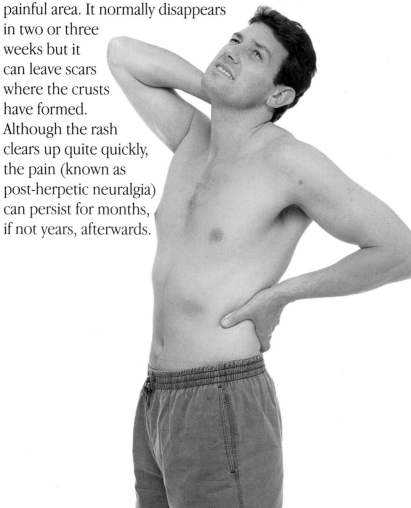

THE ORTHODOX APPROACH

If the complaint is caught early enough and treatment starts within say 24 hours of the rash appearing, antiviral drugs will reduce the duration of the illness and lessen the risk of post-herpetic neuralgia. Strong pain-killers may also be prescribed. If shingles affects the forehead, the doctor will examine your eyes to make sure that the cornea has not been harmed (sight can be damaged if treatment comes too late), and special eyedrops will be prescribed to protect the eyesight. It is wise to wear loose-fitting clothing so that the blisters are not rubbed and irritated. Cool baths may help relieve the pain.

THE HALE APPROACH

A diagnosis of shingles is best made by a doctor, since other conditions can mimic shingles. Once a diagnosis has been made, complementary medical treatment should be considered first line. The use of antiviral drugs is slowly but surely creating the development of resistant strains of the herpes virus that causes shingles, so socially and ecologically naturopathic treatments should be used first. Any herpetic lesion that is internal or associated with the eyes should be monitored by a doctor.

Shingles is a most unpleasant illness and many people are unaware how quickly and effectively it can be treated by certain complementary therapies. The Hale Clinic would recommend acupuncture, homeopathy or

Ayurveda, combined with an appropriate nutritional programme. There are also some natural topical ointments which will considerably reduce the pain.

Patients recovering from shingles often feel very depressed and debilitated: hypnotherapy will help reduce the lingering pain and encourage them to feel more positive about their lives again. Healing, Chi Kung and Moor treatment will also act as supportive therapies, helping patients on the road to recovery.

ACUPUNCTURE

According to the theory of ancient Chinese medicine, shingles is caused by overheating along with viruses and toxins in the body. As one acupuncturist explains, 'The principle of treatment is to tackle the overheating, to get through the blockages and to balance the body.'

He estimates that it normally takes between about two weeks to clear up shingles. 'Acupuncture alone is excellent for shingles, and for the accompanying pain,' he says.

HYPNOTHERAPY

Post-shingles pain can linger for a long time, often causing depression, and hypnotherapy can be most effective in dealing with this attendant aspect of the disease. When the patient is in a hypnotic state, visualization techniques can be used so that he or she sees the virus being expelled from the body and sees him/herself being well again.

HOMEOPATHY

One homeopath reports that 'most cases of shingles show good improvement' using homeopathic remedies. He estimates that three to four consultations are usually adequate to produce results. The best known homeopathic remedies for shingles are Bellis per. and Hedera helix (ivy). Other commonly used remedies include Rhus tox. for the blistered, itchy skin, Apis mel if the skin burns or stings, and Mezereum for extreme pain and itching.

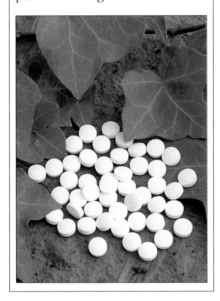

SUPPORTIVE TREATMENTS

When combined with other remedies, the following therapies can be highly beneficial: the therapeutic properties of a Moor therapy drink or body treatment; the ancient Chinese exercise of Chi Kung, which balances the body's energies and brings a sense of wellbeing; and the powerful effects of healing energy.

NATUROPATHY

There are dietary factors that are known to help or hinder the development of this painful disease. Specifically, there are two amino acids, lysine and arginine, which have an antagonistic effect on each other - arginine promotes herpes and lysine suppresses it. Therefore, foods rich in arginine and low in lysine are to be avoided. These include peanuts and other nuts, chocolate, various seeds (sunflower, poppy, sesame), cereal grains (bread, breakfast cereals), raisins, gelatine and carob. Instead, choose foods which have a higher ratio of lysine to arginine, such as eggs, beans, fish, chicken, potatoes, milk, meat and brewers' yeast. One naturopath also recommends that you drink red bush (Rooibosch) tea, which contains a bioflavonoid called quercetin that is useful in combating the herpes virus. In addition, aloe vera and liquorice can be taken internally and/or applied topically to help the rash.

Finally, for local, topical application, he recommends two treatments. Firstly, propolis, which has a 'tremendous anti-viral effect'; and secondly lithium, an element found to inhibit herpes. It can be used in the form of an ointment containing lithium succinate with Vitamin E and zinc. 'When applied to the blistered area four times daily, it can reduce the duration of the pain and discomfort considerably, easily by half,' he says.

Rooibosch tea

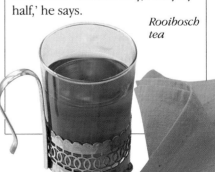

Stress

Stress is notoriously a double-edged sword. We need a certain amount of stress to keep us on our toes, healthy and motivated. But too much of it and we can crash into nervous breakdown; too little and we feel bored and apathetic. Stress is so much a buzz word of the '90s that you might think we knew all about how to manage our lives to avoid its extremes. Yet on the contrary, stress thrives untram-melled in the lives of many of us, whether it is caused by pressures of work, tension in relationships, the difficulties of raising a family, all of these combined or a range of other factors.

The consequences for our health can be overwhelming. An estimated three quarters of all medical complaints are stress-related, which means that 75 per cent of the people in doctors' waiting rooms could benefit from some sort of advice on how to reduce stress in their lives. The effects of stress can be both obvious and subtle. Some people show up with noticeable symptoms such as rashes or headaches. Often, however, the physical effects are less evident and so more potentially dangerous in the long term; they could include high blood pressure, ulcers and stomach disorders, panic attacks or rapid or irregular heartbeat.

Stress may be at the root of a host of disorders, from migraine to strokes, from constipation, colds and eczema to impotence and insomnia. Indeed, many complementary practitioners argue that stress – by undermining our immune systems – is a factor in almost all cases of ill health. Harder still to measure are the effects of stress on the quality of our lives and the lives of those around us. Stress may be at the root of phobias, compulsions, anxieties and nervous habits which can make the

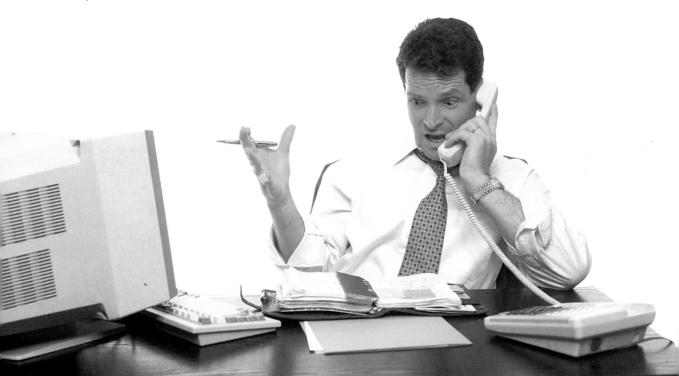

simplest of our daily routines intolerable. Stress can steadily wear away at confidence – until we wake up one morning wondering what happened to the person we once were.

Stress can also lead us into unhealthy habits of smoking and/or drinking, because it seems at first that a few glasses of wine or a cigarette will calm us down and help us cope. The reality is the opposite: alcohol is a depressant, tobacco a toxin, both can be addictive – and by depleting our energies they make it harder to manage stressful situations in the long run.

THE ORTHODOX APPROACH

Conventional medicine will often treat the physical symptoms of a stress-related disorder – such as ulcers – with drugs. Emotional and psychological symptoms – such as anxiety – may be treated by a combination of drugs and counselling. While these techniques can bring rapid relief of symptoms, unless the root causes of stress are tackled, the symptoms are likely to recur.

THE HALE APPROACH

Drug treatment for stress should be used only as a last resort; the complementary therapies listed here are the first step. If physical symptoms are showing, your doctor should be kept informed and allowed to monitor your progress.

Although stress, in certain conditions, can stimulate us to great achievement, we cannot remain in a permanent state of stress without doing long-term damage to our physical and mental wellbeing, as well as hurting our relationships with people in our close proximity – our family, friends and colleagues. We cannot avoid all stress and be forever floating through life on a 'cosmic cloud', but we need to find special times to experience tranquillity.

Nearly every complementary treatment practised at the Hale Clinic will help you towards some sort of peacefulness, and it is impossible to give a description of every treatment in this section. However, the following descriptions should enable you to select either a single therapy or a combination from the various categories.

Many of these treatments will help bring calmness in the short term; however, stress is a permanent feature of many people's lives today and choosing a permanent stress-reducing programme is often a necessary survival mechanism in the frantic world in which we live.

Acupuncture, homeopathy and Ayurveda are very good at strengthening a patient's constitution, mentally and physically, so that they are in a stronger position to withstand stress. These treatments are also effective in treating severe cases, when a patient needs to be calmed down very quickly.

You should avoid eating foods which aggravate stress, such as sugar, coffee, tea and chocolate. Stress often weakens the digestion, so it is particularly important to eat foods that are easy to digest.

Improved digestion will have a positive effect on our ability to handle physical and mental stress and prevent illness associated with a poor diet and weak digestion.

Likewise, the combination of poor diet and stress can seriously effect our elimination system, which again compounds stress levels. Colonic irrigation, lymphatic drainage and the Hale Clinic Liver Detox Diet (see page 160) will help the elimination system to work better, making you feel healthier and better able to cope with stress; it will also prevent the development of such stress-related illnesses as irritable bowel syndrome.

When we become stressed, our musculo-skeletal system may be affected. Osteopathy and chiropractic are not generally associated with the relief of stress, but manipulation of the vertebrae, soft tissue work and cranial osteopathy can make us feel much calmer. Likewise, special massage treatment such as marma, *tuina* (Chinese massage), Indonesian and Thai massage and tangent therapy can gently relieve the build-up of stress in the muscles, as well as calming the mind.

The essential oils of aromatherapy induce a feeling of calmness. Reflexology, by massaging special points in the foot, can also have a great calming effect. I often advise a massage once a week, possibly on a Friday if you are work a conventional five-day week, so that you can enjoy the weekend fully. Many people go out for a meal or to the cinema to relax, but often the rebalancing effect of the correct massage can be more beneficial (although laughter and having fun are among the best antidotes for stress).

By training you to breathe correctly, the Buteyko Technique gives you a tool which you can use at any time to calm you down. Light therapy, which you can have as a treatment or practise at home by installing a full-spectrum light box, will also help

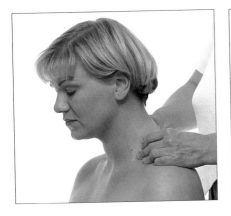

will also help create a peaceful environment.

The fact that many illnesses are related to stress shows the power the mind has over our physical wellbeing. But the mind can also be trained to redirect our thoughts and behaviour into a more positive *modus operandi*. Research into hypnosis has shown how it can remove the physical and mental symptoms of stress. Moreover, patients can be taught self-hypnosis techniques which they can use to reduce stress levels.

Many people are apprehensive about seeing a psychologist or counsellor, but so often these therapies can help us to understand the way in which our emotions are creating a stressful environment, holding us back from positive experiences and preventing us enjoying life to the full. Just as we look after our physical bodies, with good nutrition and exercise, so we need to understand our mental and emotional states in order to express and realize our true individuality.

The exercise systems of yoga, T'ai Chi and Chi Kung help to calm the body, mind and emotions.

It is interesting that working on the body (e.g. with massage) can calm the mind, while working on the mind (e.g. with hypnosis) can calm the body. Equally, healing by cleansing the aura fields around the body can bring a state of peace and tranquillity to both body and mind.

BodyHarmonics

This is an integrated approach to therapy, drawing on 3,000-year-old traditional Chinese, Indonesian and Thai medical techniques (left). Its originator calls it BodyHarmonics because she likens the body to a musical instrument. When we are 'well tuned' and our energies are in harmony, we can experience a wonderful feeling of wellbeing.

'Your body demands individual tuning,' she explains, 'but unlike a musical instrument it contains your life history. The "harmonics" of your body are unique, having developed through your interaction with the world from the moment of your conception.'

Treatment for any kind of emotional problem – which can cause high levels of stress – usually begins with a session of acupuncture, which can be highly effective in relieving the various components of emotional pain. Stress often takes a heavy toll on the neck, shoulder and back and, after acupuncture, massage is essential to disperse the tension that has built up in the soft tissues.

For this *tuina* – Chinese massage, a vigorous form of manual pressure combining soft-tissue massage and joint manipulation – is used. 'Its unique rolling action eases pain and liberates powerful healing forces,' the therapist believes.

Clinical Aromatherapy

'Clinical aromatherapy is a holistic treatment promoting relaxation and self-healing within a safe, nurturing environment,' says one practitioner. And when you feel relaxed, safe and cared for, you may also feel free to discuss the reasons why you are feeling stressed – so relieving the pressures you are under and working towards possible solutions.

At the first consultation the practitioner takes a detailed case history and carries out an examination, then blends organic or wild cultured essential oils to suit your particular symptoms, emotions and mood. She uses these in massage – tailored to your individual needs – to calm the nervous system, as well as giving advice on diet, exercise, meditation and relaxation techniques.

'Treatments take up to an hour and a half,' she explains. 'Massage to relax the muscles, including acupressure to help balance the body's energies and induce deep relaxation, gives the patient a much-needed rest from life's merry-go-round.'

Aromatherapy oils can also be used for inhalation or in baths as part of your self-care strategy at home. Cedarwood, petitgrain, Roman chamomile, lavender, sweet marjoram and sandalwood are all soothing oils which may be useful for stress-related problems.

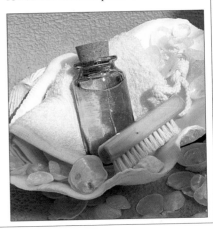

STRESS MANAGEMENT/ SELF-HYPNOSIS

'I can't cope!' 'I've had enough!'
'I never have time for myself!'
'I can't seem to stop worrying!'

These are all cries which stress managers recognize as signs of stress getting out of control and taking over our lives. Through stress-management techniques which are often coupled with learning hypnosis, stress managers work to identify sources of stress and to reduce and eliminate them.

'I aim to teach people how to become positive, effective and relaxed while finding a new balance,' explains one. 'Self-hypnosis uses the power of your mind to relieve symptoms and alter unwanted behaviour patterns.'

The list of stress-related conditions which he believes stress management may help is long, but it includes anxiety, agoraphobia, asthma, bed-wetting, eating problems, executive stress, grief, hay fever, impotence, irritable bowel syndrome, migraine, obsessive compulsions, pain reduction, panic, phobias, fear of public speaking, problems with relationships, feelings of rejection, lack of self-confidence, skin disorders, sleep problems, travel fright and weight control.

Most courses in stress management take from five to ten sessions and, according to the same therapist, 'In most cases when people are willing to make changes in their lives, there is permanent release from symptoms.' By the end of the treatment, patients will also have learned techniques for self-hypnosis, which will help them manage stress better in the future.

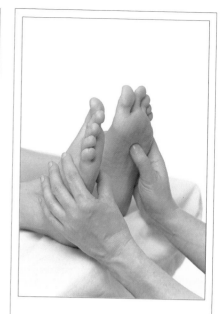

REFLEXOLOGY

A reflexology session would begin with a comprehensive case history, helping to identify the causes of stress in your life. A full treatment, unblocking energies throughout the body, follows, after which the reflexologist concentrates on those areas which have specific problems.

By its very nature as a massage of the feet, reflexology is a relaxing treatment which reduces nervous tension and stimulates the body's own self-healing properties. It is also an essentially natural treatment, involving no medication or interference with the body. And once you are aware of the points on your feet – or hands – which can be pressed to alleviate your individual symptoms of stress, you can administer 'self-help' at home by massaging these points.

If you are severely stressed, a course of six reflexology sessions over three weeks may be recommended, followed by 'top-up' treatments as and when you feel the need.

COLONIC HYDROTHERAPY

The colonics therapist tackles stress on two fronts. Firstly, you will be advised on how to change your diet in order to eliminate nutritional stressors. When you take away stimulants like tea and coffee, which increase the body's toxic load, you are likely to find that – quite suddenly – your body is able to relax.

Secondly, colonic irrigation reduces your body's toxic burden, clearing quantities of toxic material. Therapists explain that the rest of your body will respond, so that you feel less overloaded – and less stressed.

HELLERWORK

'Stress is always embodied,' says one Hellerwork practitioner. 'Imagine someone with perfect posture – could they be stressed?'

Your relationship with yourself and the Earth is determined by the effortlessness with which you deal with gravity. Stress is like carrying a heavy suitcase. Putting the suitcase down makes everything feel lighter and easier, but most people cannot imagine *how* to put the suitcase down. Hellerwork gives you the experience of feeling lighter, both physically and psychologically. Stress builds up over time and is stuck in the body, accumulating with each stressful event. Hellerwork reduces the chronic stress build-up and teaches you how to manage stress in the future.

COUNSELLING/ PSYCHOTHERAPY

Many counsellors regard stress as a state in which the demands being made of us exceed our abilities to cope with them – and because we all respond differently to stress, counselling and psychotherapy treat stress in a range of different ways.

For instance, if we can identify those aspects of our own behaviour which contribute to stress – and those which diminish it – we can learn to improve things in our lives. On the emotional front, too, we need to develop an understanding of those feelings which cause us stress if we are to find positive and effective ways of dealing with them. The nature and quality of our relationships with work colleagues, friends and family are a vital part of this larger picture.

Sometimes we have negative thoughts and mental images of ourselves as unable to cope, which add to stress. Counselling can help to challenge these and substitute more positive patterns of thinking, so that we can feel better about ourselves and cope more easily with the ups and downs of life.

Counselling can also help us to identify the physical signals of stress so that we can nip the problem in the bud. Maintaining healthy diet, sleep and exercise patterns will support the range of effective coping skills which counselling can help to develop.

FLOWER REMEDIES

Just as stress makes itself felt in many different ways depending on who we are, there is an enormously wide range of flower remedies which could help you cope with its symptoms.

Goat's Beard (Pacific), a calming and relaxing remedy, is believed to activate the thymus gland to deal with long-term problems of stress. Black-eyed Susan (Australian Bush) is for speedy people, always on the go, who find they suddenly have too much on their plate. Hau (Hawaiian) is a calming, healing and balancing influence for those overcome by nervous stress to the point of breakdown.

Chamomile (FES) is said to calm the nervous system in people who find that stress affects their stomachs, and can also be useful if you suffer from panic attacks. For stress caused by your environment – such as living in the city – Indian Pink (FES) is recommended, while Crowea helps if you feel 'frazzled' and off balance.

Fairy Duster (Desert Alchemy) is a flower remedy for those of us – especially children – who overreact to situations, veering from the hyper to the despairing. Macrocarpa may suit you if you have been chasing your own tail and feeling 'burned out', while Hop's Bush (Australian Living) can ease symptoms in those who can't sleep or relax as a result of stress.

SELF-CARE

Relaxation or meditation is a powerful way to combat the effects of stress, even if you can only find a few minutes of peace each day. Assertiveness training that helps you politely but firmly to say 'no' to too many burdens can soon lighten your load, while common-sense health measures like maintaining a good diet, eating well and trying to get a good night's sleep will stand you in good stead. Vitamin B complex can also provide a useful boost at times of stress.

Taking an aromatherapy bath at home, using essentials oils for inhalation – from your pillow at night or from a handkerchief – can alleviate symptoms.

SUPPORTIVE TREATMENTS

Nutrition
Nutritional consultants aim to remove toxins (which are chemical stressors) and stimulants (certain foods, drinks and allergens) from your body. Extra nutrients are also recommended in order to counteract stress.

You may need between three and six treatment sessions, which would involve detoxification, identifying food allergens and other underlying causes of stress, as well as establishing an individual diet and exercise regimen designed to suit your individual needs.

Marma Massage/Exercises

If stress has the effect of overloading the brain, marma massage works by 'creating a space' in the brain cells, according to one practitioner. This space acts as an extra shock absorber, giving your brain the capacity to do the job of dealing with stress.

Once that space is available, yoga breathing of two counts for the in-breath and three counts for the out-breath will re-establish the balance and rhythm of your system. The yoga 'tree pose', which involves concentrated balancing, helps you to forget stress by 'balancing' your mind.

Classical music – which should be listened to between 6 and 7p.m. – is also excellent for relaxation.

Light Therapy

There is a direct correlation between rising stress levels and lack of light. A combination of light therapy and reflexology is particularly beneficial for those suffering from stress. Light therapy reduces stress by increasing serotonin levels in the brain, thereby making the world seem an easier place. After a series of sessions the patient feels both relaxed and energized at the same time.

Moor Therapy

The Moor contains over 300 medicinal herbs, including some with a calming effect on the body. Taken internally and as a body wrap, it is both relaxing and uplifting.

Remedial Yoga

Yoga is a therapy which relieves stress by calming both mind and body, giving us focus and stability while improving the quality of sleep. Physically, yoga stimulates blood and lymph circulation and helps balance the endocrine system, allowing your

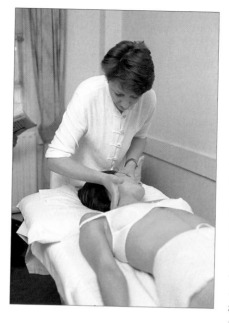

body to relax. Its breathing techniques can also help with relaxation and give you control over the rate and rhythm of your breathing.

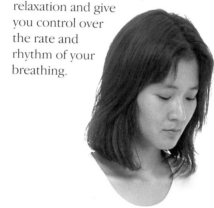

Tangent Therapy

Stress usually builds up over a period of time, eventually affecting the weakest part of the body and person. The tangent therapist (left) assesses the weakness and shows the patient how to move forward. Following a detailed consultation, treatment is chosen and may consist of aromatherapy massage using acupressure points, and exercise. The essential oils used in aromatherapy reach the brain and circulate around the body, making the patient feel peaceful and calm (for suggested oils see under *Clinical Aromatherapy*, above). To reduce stress levels, lifestyle changes and detoxification using food herbs may be advised.

Chi Kung/T'ai Chi

These exercises are all about restoring the balance of yin and yang throughout the body, warding off disease which – according to traditional Chinese medicine – can follow from an imbalance of energy. For stress and stress-related symptoms the exercises known as 'Second Chi Kung' and 'Triple Heater' are especially helpful as a supportive treatment.

Shiatsu

All sorts of stress-related illnesses respond to this gentle form of Japanese massage. The therapist will aim to locate the source of the trouble and work on the relevant meridians to improve the flow of energy through the body.

Insomnia

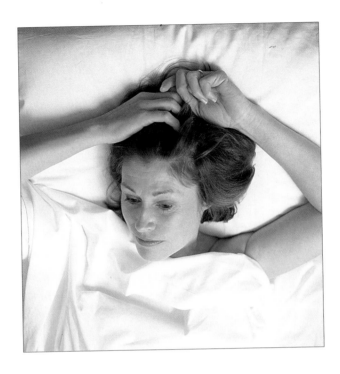

There are very few people lucky enough to be able to say that they have never lost a night's sleep for one reason or another. Even if you are one of the fortunate few and fall into a deep slumber the moment your head hits the pillow, worry, unfamiliar surroundings, noise and pain are just some of the reasons why almost everyone experiences insomnia (sleeplessness) on occasions.

Sleep gives our bodies the opportunity to repair themselves and our minds a chance to rest. Without enough sleep, we feel irritable and inefficient, and we are less able to concentrate on our daily tasks. Each individual needs a different amount of sleep, ranging from a brisk five hours to an indolent twelve, although seven hours is about the average. The amount of sleep we need to revitalize and function efficiently during the day also changes as we grow older. Young babies sleep for up to 18 hours each day, but by the time we are elderly, this total has been cut to somewhere in the region of five or six hours. We also tend to wake more during the night as we age and take longer to get to sleep in the first place.

These are normal sleep patterns that alter as we progress through life. Insomniacs, on the other hand, have regular difficulty in falling asleep, wake frequently and are restless throughout the night, and often wake early only to feel tired during the day. The effects of a few broken nights are not serious but, for insomniacs, sleeplessness can last years. They frequently find themselves in the relentless, vicious circle of overtiredness and worrying so much about the need for sleep that they cannot relax enough to drop off.

THE ORTHODOX APPROACH

If the cause of sleeplessness is readily recognizable and treatable, then the appropriate treatment will be given – sufferers from some forms of depression will be given antidepressant drugs to relieve insomnia, painful diseases which interfere with sleep can be treated with painkillers, and so on. In cases where the patient finds him/herself in the vicious circle of sleeplessness and overtiredness, sleeping pills or tranquillizers may be prescribed to break the pattern. However, these can very quickly become addictive, perhaps after as little as a month of regular use, so caution should be exercised. Sleeping pills may also aggravate the insomnia in the long term.

THE HALE APPROACH

Sleeplessness, unless very prolonged or total (no sleep at all), can safely be assessed by complementary practitioners initially. Orthodox doctors will generally have recourse to drugs, which do little to illuminate the cause of the problem and may in themselves worsen it.

The Hale Clinic's approach to insomnia looks at the reasons behind a patient's inability to sleep properly; we will advise an appropriate treatment that addresses the root causes of this problem, so that long-term improvement can be brought about.

As with many illnesses, a good place to start is with nutrition. Certain foods such as coffee can act as stimulants which keep us awake, while adequate intake of vitamins and minerals can be important in helping us get a good night's sleep. Allergic reactions can affect sleep – a certain food eaten at 7.30 p.m. can activate adrenaline which will wake you up at two in the morning.

Acupuncture is very effective at stopping insomnia very quickly. Like homeopathy and Ayurveda, the treatment will address the physiological, the nutritional and the emotional issues which might have initiated the problem. The volume of research on psychosomatic medicine testifies to the strong link between our minds and our physiological state.

Hypnosis is another very effective treatment. It looks to see if there are any underlying psychological causes, calms the mind and body and teaches the patient self-hypnosis techniques to use at home.

For those who wish to go into greater depth with the psycho-logical issues behind the insomnia, we would advise a period of treatment with a psychologist.

There are a range of supportive treatments and self-care advice detailed in this section which will further enhance the quality of your sleep.

ACUPUNCTURE

In traditional Chinese medicine, it is believed that the organs are governed by the five elements and that insomnia is caused by a deficiency of the heart (symbolized by fire) and the kidneys (symbolized by water) and the way they interact. In order to treat the condition, it is the acupuncturist's job to make sure that the heart and kidneys communicate well with each other. By inserting needles at points along specific meridians in the body, they can restore the balance between the yang (positive, aggressive) energy of the fire and the yin (passive, gentle) energy of the water – and so the insomnia is cured. Depending on the severity of the condition, improvement may be experienced after as few as two sessions, though follow-up treatments may be necessary to prevent a recurrence.

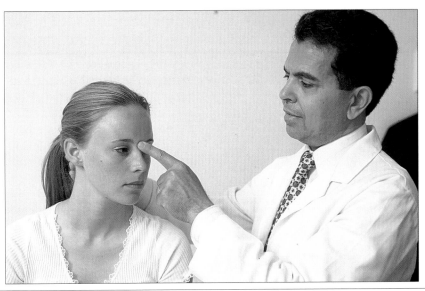

PSYCHOLOGY

When the cause of insomnia is mental or emotional rather than physical, psychology can be a helpful support therapy to other treatments. Gathering information about any underlying causes for insomnia helps to identify specific anxieties, and then, through discussion and therapy, clients are helped to recognize these problems so that the insomnia can be handled.

HOMEOPATHY

When the cause of insomnia is linked to depression or to physical or psychological factors such as tension, pain, emotional arousal, discomfort, disruption in your surroundings or a change in environment, then Passiflora Lehning Drops (containing Avena sativa, Passiflora, Belladonna, Secale and Valerian in low homeopathic dosages) are very effective. Other specific remedies may include:

• If the mind is very active at bedtime, sleep troubled by dreams, person wakes up about 4 a.m. – Lycopodium.

• Troubled by a fear of not being able to sleep, and by nightmares when sleep comes – Ignatia.

• Waking between midnight and 2 a.m., restless and worried – Arsenicum.

AYURVEDA

According to the principles of Ayurveda, the causes of insomnia may be physical, mental or environmental. If the cause is physical, treatments to reduce *Vata* (the driving force which controls the nervous system and all energies in the body) are indicated. Ayurvedic oral preparations to maintain good bowel movements and special herbal preparations which have a hypnotic effect or are calming to the nerves are given. *Shiro dhara* (herbal oil treatment to the scalp) is recommended, together with a special oil massage. *Vireka* (oral laxatives) are also given to detoxify.

Relaxation and yoga are prescribed for mental and emotional causes.

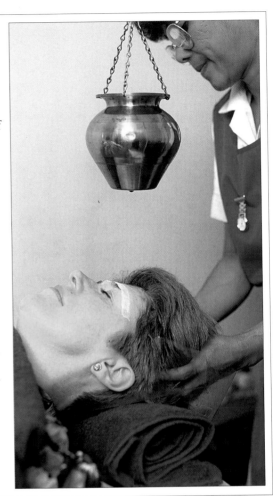

NUTRITION/ALLERGY TREATMENT

'When patients come to me with insomnia, my first line of attack is to look for something they're taking or eating, such as unidentified food allergies or hypersensitivities,' says one naturopath. He explains that there is often a six-hour delay between consumption of the offending food and a feeling of wakefulness, so eating at eight o'clock may cause insomnia at two. If you are prone to sleeplessness, then you should steer well clear of known stimulants such as tea, coffee, chocolate or cocoa, but this therapist also adds alcohol to the list, saying that it can significantly interfere with the quality of sleep. When examining what we consume as a cause of insomnia, it is worth bearing in mind that certain herbal tonics also contain botanical stimulants, and numerous over-the-counter and prescription medicines contain caffeine.

Nicotinamide, a form of Vitamin B_3, appears to produce similar effects to those of the benzodiazepine (tranquillizing) drugs. As an insomniac, it may be wise to have a blood test for your Vitamin B_3 status so you can take the appropriate dosage of a B_3 supplement before bedtime. Magnesium and yeast-free vitamin B_6 should be taken at the same time.

HYPNOTHERAPY

Practitioners can teach relaxation techniques that are known to be very effective in inducing sleep. Discussion while under hypnosis may also be used to reveal the causes of poor sleep when there are underlying emotional or psychological causes.

SELF-CARE

Aromatherapy

Essential oils may be used in vaporizers in the bedroom, in relaxing warm baths or in tissues in the pillow. Relaxing oils include lavender vera, Roman chamomile and ylang ylang.

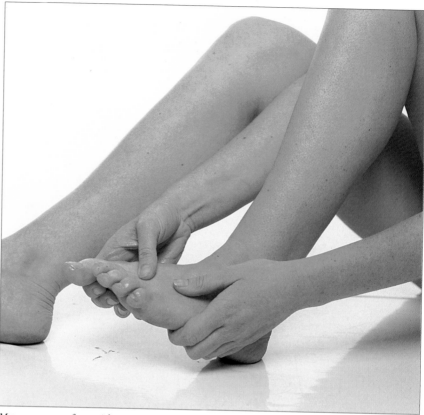

Massage your feet with sesame oil before going to bed

SUPPORTIVE TREATMENTS

Reflexology

This massage and stimulation of reflex points on the foot can be very successful, particularly in association with other therapies, in relaxing a person who has difficulty in sleeping or for dealing with underlying problems. For example, if tension is an underlying cause, the solar plexus reflex (in between the first and second metatarsal) is massaged along with the adrenal reflexes (in the middle of the feet) and the pituitary reflexes (centre of the pads of the big toes).

Aromatherapy

Massage with essential oils can induce deep relaxation and calm the mind, encouraging sleep. The massage works over tense muscles, releasing them, improving blood supply and calming the nervous system. When under extreme stress people run on adrenaline and often use stimulants to keep themselves going. Aromatherapy breaks this cycle, allowing the patient a caring, relaxing environment.

Flower Essences

Verbena (Petite Fleur) is one of the most potent essences for insomnia, although there are many from which to choose. One expert also suggests Hops Bush from Australia (Living range) as being very good for the restlessness and inner turmoil that often accompany insomnia.

TIPS

The following advice from the traditions of Indian medicine should ensure a good night's sleep:

• Drink hot water one hour before bedtime.

• Wash your feet before going to bed and massage them with sesame oil.

• Put a bucket of cold water or an ionizer by your bed.

• Retire around 11 o'clock.

• Sleep only on your left side.

• Never sleep with your feet pointing south.

Depression

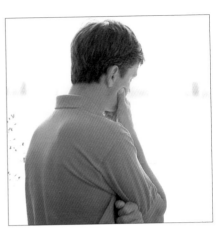

If there is one thing we can say for sure about depression, it is that it is very complex. This rather bland word covers the whole range of negative human experience from 'feeling blue' to terrifying anxiety and suicidal despair, as well as physical symptoms ranging from flu-like aches and pains to a sense of profound tiredness. Depressed people – and one in five of us will come into this category at some point during our lives – tend to feel very cut off from the rest of humanity. The stigma which traditionally surrounds 'mental illness' makes the sense of misery even worse and stops many people from seeking help. But depression is not anyone's 'fault'; it is a recognized illness which can be effectively treated in a whole range of ways.

And as befits a complex condition, depression has a range of causes as wide as life itself. Stressful events which cause a deep sense of loss – such as bereavement, divorce, physical illness or the loss of a job – can trigger depression. Some people believe that bottled-up anger and frustration also turn into depression.

There is evidence that depression runs in families, although no one has ever found a gene for depression. Perhaps growing up with depressed parents is enough to make us depressed; it's certainly true that our childhood experiences are crucial to our long-term mental and emotional health.

Chemistry also has a part to play in depression: when you feel very low, chances are that your brain is lacking in vital nerve messengers called neurotransmitters, although whether this is cause or effect is not clear. Similarly, hormonal changes (as women with PMS know all too well) can make us feel depressed. People who suffer from depression linked to Seasonal Affective Disorder (SAD) may have an imbalance of the hormone melatonin, which is produced in the brain during the hours of darkness.

THE ORTHODOX APPROACH

Orthodox doctors look for the following symptoms in identifying depression: feelings of worthlessness and guilt; impaired concentration; loss of energy; thoughts of suicide; loss or increase of appetite and weight; insomnia or oversleeping; agitation or a sense of being slowed down. If you have had four of these for two weeks or more, without another illness which could be causing them, you are likely to be diagnosed as depressed.

Until recently, orthodox medicine relied chiefly on drug treatments to lift the symptoms of depression. Modern anti-depressants work to increase the quantities of neurotransmitters in your brain, although getting a drug to suit your symptoms without unpleasant side effects is often a matter of trial and error.

Yet while anti-depressants can give us the lift we need to tackle the causes of depression, most of us don't like taking pills for what we perceive as a problem of mind, body and spirit. Increasingly, modern doctors are taking a two-pronged approach: prescribing drugs, but also referring depressed patients to counsellors who can help identify the roots of the problem.

THE HALE APPROACH

Depression is principally endogenous (caused by a lack of chemicals in the brain) or exogenous (caused by external events). This differentiation is important, since drug treatment is often required for the former, whereas good counselling can put an end to the latter without recourse to drugs. A counsellor or psychotherapist is a good starting point, and referral through them to a doctor or psychiatrist would be beneficial. Complementary therapies will speed up most treatments.

Many different events in a person's life, both physical and mental, may trigger depression. It is important for the individual patient to be properly advised at the outset which treatments are likely to be most effective for them. For example, some depression may be aggravated by physiological problems such as hormone imbalance, blood sugar problems, allergy or lack of vital nutrients for brain chemistry. In these cases nutritional advice or light therapy may be necessary. Other patients may benefit from acupuncture and homeopathy, which address both the physical and the mental aspects of depression. With others, psychotherapy, hypnotherapy or counselling will be necessary. For many patients a combination of treatments will be necessary.

The Hale Clinic would therefore advise seeing our complementary medical consultant or a psychologist, who can advise patients suffering from depression on the best course of treatment for their particular case. If it was felt appropriate, we might refer a patient for another medical opinion regardng medication.

LIGHT THERAPY

Light therapy uses a broad spectrum of visible and invisible wavelengths to counteract the effects of not enough daylight in our lives. As one light therapist explains, 'Modern living has cut down drastically on our bodies' exposure to natural daylight, yet we need broad-spectrum light in order to stay healthy.' For instance, UVA light stimulates the skin's production of Vitamin D – and without Vitamin D we are unable to absorb vital minerals such as calcium, magnesium and phosphorus from the food that we eat.

Light can also lift our spirits – because it increases the production of seratonin (the 'feel good' hormone) in the pineal gland. Most of us feel better when the sun comes out, and by mimicking this effect through a specially designed light box, light therapy can combat depression, leaving you with a feeling of exhilarated wellbeing.

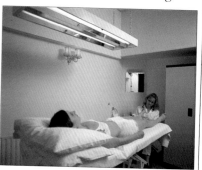

HYPNOTHERAPY

Hypnotherapy, perhaps more than any other complementary therapy, shows how much power your mind really has when it comes to influencing health. At the very least, hypnotherapy helps you to relax without drugs, reversing the stress effects which so often contribute to depression. It is especially useful in relieving depression in people who are terminally ill or undergoing acute medical treatments.

For one practitioner hypnotherapy is a form of psychotherapy. 'I begin with a guided relaxation and then I use hypnotherapy to reassure, comfort and uplift,' he says. 'It helps people to express their feelings because when you are sufficiently relaxed your unconscious has the ability to rise close to the surface. Hypnotherapy makes it possible to listen to – and talk to – the unconscious. For instance, it can help to imagine and visualize feeling better. At the same time I employ a range of counselling techniques.'

He stresses the importance of his role as a careful listener: 'In the way depressed people describe themselves you can often find the way out. One of my patients came to me after a year of worsening depression. She was intelligent, well-to-do and had a great deal to live for, but she had thoughts of suicide, low spirits, insomnia and loss of appetite and libido. There was clearly a spiritual component to her depression and she told me that she had lost the ability to pray; I encouraged her to try to pray – and that was the catalyst which began the process of her recovery.'

A person's qualities, successes and achievements are often submerged by depression. It is important, by slowly but surely developing strategies for change, to re-empower a sufferer so that they learn to recognize their qualities and inner strengths.

HOMEOPATHY

Both chronic and acute depression can be helped by homeopathy, although you should contact a doctor immediately if you or' someone close to you is having thoughts of suicide.

Not only is depression tremendously variable, but homeopathic remedies are very individual. 'There are some 200 to 300 homeopathic remedies for depression,' explains one practitioner, 'but in simple terms, low-potency remedies of 30x or below work on mental symptoms, while high-potency remedies of 200x or above treat mental symptoms of depression.'

Homeopathy is 'excellent' for the depression which follows distressing life events (often called reactive depression): 'It also works well for depression caused by lack of chemicals (often called endogenous) when prescribed in conjunction with nutritional supplements such as zinc and Vitamin B_6.' In addition to homeopathy, some form of counselling or psychotherapy is essential to understanding why you have become depressed.

While you are advised to consult a qualified practitioner, this homeopath suggests that if, for example, you feel depressed after deep grief or heartbreak you may benefit from Ignatia 200x or Natrum mur. 200x, to be taken in three doses, one each night. If this is the right remedy for you, depression should begin to lift within a week.

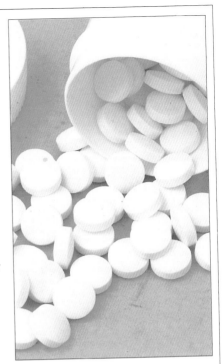

PSYCHOTHERAPY

Psychotherapy, which gives you precious time and space to talk about how you are feeling – and why – with a qualified practitioner, can be enormously beneficial in coming to terms with complex and deep-seated depressions. One psychotherapist works with individuals as well as groups to address the events in your life which may have contributed to depression.

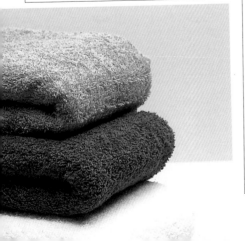

NUTRITION

If it's true that you are what you eat – and 98 per cent of your body's cells replace themselves each year – food is essential to your mental and physical health. One nutrition consultant uses a combination of psychological and physiological methods to combat depression: 'I ascertain whether depression is blood-sugar related, or (in women) cyclical and hormone-related. The therapy is very individual,and varies according to the symptoms. I may use nutritional supplements because brain biochemistry – and hence mood – can be altered with nutrients.'

She aims for 'total cure' when depression is hormonal or sugar-related, although she finds that improvements may be more gradual in depression which is fundamentally psychological.

HEALING

In healing, the body, mind and soul are seen as one entity in which good health depends on harmony. It can be a powerful form of therapy for depression, which so many of us experience as a kind of profound discord. One healer perceives depression as a tangible weight which she works to remove from the patient's spirit. 'I find that I can literally reach in and pull out all those negative emotional states which people store up from childhood onwards,' she says. Sometimes, when people have severe psychological difficulties, she suggests they have psychotherapy first and come for healing later. But with depression and/or anxiety states which follow illnesses or the usual painful losses in life, she finds that 'when people are ready to let go of depression, healing can be instant'.

SUPPORTIVE TREATMENTS

Acupuncture

Depression is traditionally associated with the liver, so an acupuncturist would concentrate on the liver meridian to regulate the flow of *chi* (vital energy) in the body. 'Improvement or cure' might be expected within six sessions.

Aromatherapy

Massage with essential oils working on specific acupressure points helps lift patients out of depression, enabling them to help themselves and be positive about change. Advice would be given on diet, exercise and counselling or psycho-therapy may be recommended.

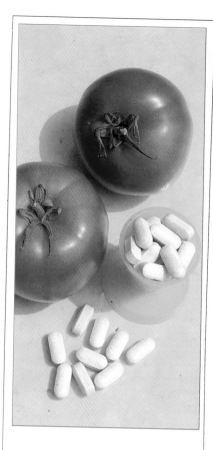

SELF-CARE

Aromatherapy

It is important to look for the root cause of the depression in order to choose the most appropriate oils, whether for massage, to put in the bath or to inhale. Mandarin is particularly good for calming nervous tension, anxiety and feelings of isolation; ylang-ylang also relieves tension and boosts low self-esteem; bergamot or rose help counteract the lethargy that often goes with depression.

Flower Remedies

All flower remedies deal with the emotions, so you will need to look carefully and honestly at your particular symptoms to find the appropriate treatment. Sweet Chestnut (Bach) is one remedy that may be used when you really feel you can't cope any more; Wild Rose (Bach) stimulates those who have lost interest in trying to make life any better.

Yoga/T'ai Chi/Chi Kung

By balancing the body's energies, these exercises can help reduce stress and remove toxins from the system. They enable you to slow down, find your own centre and restore mental balance.

TIPS

If you are feeling under pressure, try to cut down on your work load and to take some time off – perhaps going out with your partner or a close friend. Avoid tea and coffee and increase your intake of B vitamins (found in many foods, including cereals, wheatgerm, milk and green, leafy vegetables) and Vitamin C (found in fresh vegetables and fruits, including tomatoes). You can also apply your own DIY light therapy, making the most of natural light by going outside whenever possible, especially at midday, or get a full-spectrum light box to use at home. Try to leave off contact lenses and glasses in order to expose your eyes to daylight – and perhaps take a midwinter break in a sunny resort.

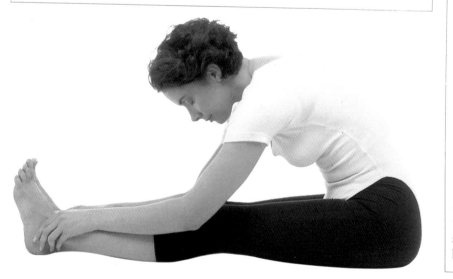

Eating Disorders

They are high-profile problems, often in the news, linked to celebrities. Yet most of us have little real understanding of anorexia and bulimia, which remain notoriously difficult to treat. Perhaps this is because eating disorders are on one level about food – refusing food, bingeing on food, 'purging' food – yet they can also involve complex emotional and psychological problems.

In anorexia nervosa, people (mostly young women) starve themselves, sometimes to the point of death. Anorexics often become skeletally thin, yet they don't see themselves that way. Emotionally they may become irritable, isolated, depressed – even suicidal. Excessive exercising is sometimes a part of the picture, coupled with loss of sleep.

With extreme weight loss also come the unpleasant symptoms of malnutrition and dehydration. As body fat is lost and muscle protein broken down to provide energy, women's periods will stop, teeth will decay or be lost, the blood will lose important minerals, there will be increased risk of osteoporosis in later life – and there may also be inflammation and even rupture of the stomach and oesophagus. Sometimes anorexics experience the growth of downy hair all over the body. And although anorexia can be successfully treated, it has one of the highest death rates of all psychiatric illnesses.

In bulimia nervosa (which is more common than anorexia and often follows it), binge eating is followed by self-induced vomiting, periods of starvation and/or purging with laxatives. People with bulimia – mostly women, and generally of an older age group than anorexics – also go through emotional extremes, often feeling out of control, helpless and lonely.

Because self-induced vomiting is a source of shame, people with bulimia are often devious and deceptive about their problem, going to the bathroom after meals to 'get rid' secretly of what they've eaten. Habitual vomiting can also erode tooth enamel and cause sore throats, while menstrual disorders may follow and again the risk of osteoporosis is increased.

So what leads (mostly) women to such desperate measures? The Eating Disorders Association believes that anorexia and bulimia may be ways of avoiding other, more painful emotional problems, or of coping with long-buried stresses. Their figures show that a third of anorexics and bulimics who seek therapy have been sexually abused.

Alternatively, it may be a way of exerting control, especially tempting to women who may feel that their bodies are about the only thing in life they *can* control. People with eating disorders commonly see 'control' over eating as the answer to other problems – until anorexia or bulimia begins to make them so ill that the condition becomes the number one concern.

These problems are not helped by the fashion industry's promotion of unnaturally thin models. The pressure an already stressed person feels to strive for this public image of beauty may be the trigger that starts the illness.

Another theory (held by a naturopath at the Hale Clinic) is that some eating disorders have a straightforward physiological origin, beginning with food allergy which results in food 'addiction'.

And so, even after a decade of publicity for eating disorders, the picture remains confused. Only in the last 20 years have anorexia and bulimia been recognized by the medical profession as 'diseases'. Meanwhile there are up to 200,000 people in the UK with eating disorders – yet only 1,500 places are available at specialist treatment centres. However, people with anorexia and bulimia can and do get better – especially when the disorder is recognized early and treated.

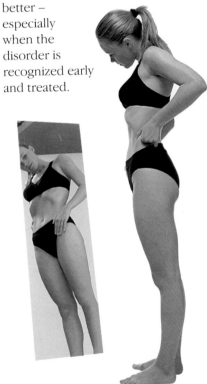

THE ORTHODOX APPROACH

Orthodox treatments try to address the emotional and psychological issues as well as the question of body weight. They usually include some form of counselling (such as psychotherapy, or group or family therapy) together with weight monitoring and advice on diet. There may also be treatment with drugs. Cognitive behaviour therapy has been found to be especially effective for people with bulimia.

THE HALE APPROACH

Once a counsellor trained in eating disorders has been found, through either your doctor or the Hale Clinic, orthodox treatment should be necessary only on the advice of the counsellor.

Anorexia and bulimia can benefit both from treatments which are orientated towards the physical body and from therapies such as hypnosis and psychology which are focused on the mental state. Each case is individual to that particular person, but in general terms the Hale Clinic approach would be to focus on strengthening the physical body. This could be achieved by seeing an allergy/nutrition specialist and an acupuncturist or homeopath to build up the constitution in general.

At the same time we would advise a course of psychology or hypnosis to deal with the emotional background which allowed the illness to take hold in the first place.

NATUROPATHY

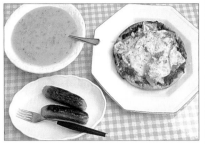

The naturopath mentioned above believes that in certain cases there are clear physical causes – and so relatively simple remedies – for many eating disorders. He regards them as a sort of food addiction, comparable in effect to being hooked on nicotine or alcohol: 'If you have a sensitivity to food, you will develop an inordinate desire to have it. Why does this craving develop? Because when your body has a food allergy, you develop antibodies to that substance. As soon as those antibodies are released into your system, they call for the same substance again because they (the anitboides) are there in excess – paradoxically fuelling the addiction.'

So how do eating disorders, with all their emotional complexities, develop from here?

'Perhaps you are a teenager who is a bit sensitive to grains such as wheat, rye and barley. You find you have a craving for bread and biscuits. But you don't want to get fat (you've been told fat girls have problems getting boyfriends) and so bread becomes an enemy in your mind. If you go without food and therefore do not trigger the craving-producing antibodies, you find it's easier than having a little bit, which does trigger them.

'But if you have a sausage (often containing 30-40 per cent wheat), or some tinned soup (which probably contains flour), your craving is triggered again because if you eat food to which you are allergic you will never be fully satisfied. So you raid the fridge, demolish the bread and then the pizza from the freezer – anything. Still your craving is not satisfied. You don't know it's just the wheat (in this example only). You feel "possessed". So you stop eating altogether – and then you feel a lot better. You feel lighter, cleaner, triumphant! It is a glorious feeling, better than eating.'

This, believes the naturopath, is how anorexia can develop, while bulimia is the other side of the coin: 'In bulimia, people go the other way, trying to satisfy their craving by bingeing.'

He treats eating disorders by firstly explaining this scenario, and then by looking for the foods that trigger the cycle of craving and cutting them out of the diet. This can be done by a process of simple blood tests.

BIOENERGETICS

Toxicity is a causative factor in food cravings. High consumption of refined sugar and exposure to chemicals, petrochemicals and pollution stresses the intricate function of the endocrine system. The resulting subtle imbalances and malabsorption of vitamins, minerals and amino acids cause food cravings and cellulite. By supporting and detoxifying the system, we can restore a healthy balance. Bio-energetic testing combined with homeopathic treatment creates a dynamic and supportive solution to this increasing problem.

COUNSELLING/ PSYCHOTHERAPY

Psychological therapy for eating disorders starts by assuming that low self-esteem generates excessive concern about weight and shape – which in turn leads to the excessive dieting and/or purging behaviour of anorexia and bulimia. Yet when we set impossible goals for how we should look, failure inevitably follows, setting up a vicious circle of even lower self-esteem and worsening eating disorders.

Treatment focuses on identifying the origins of the problem and how this has led to anorexia or bulimia. Counselling pinpoints negative thinking patterns about weight and shape, which may be keeping the whole process going. Attention is also paid to basic eating patterns.

A crucial element of treatment is the development of problem-solving skills, because the eating disorder is often a smoke screen for other problems which seem insurmountable. Losing and then regaining control of an eating pattern becomes an important way for people to hold on to the illusion of being in control of their lives. But repeated 'failures' simply reinforce the desire to try even harder to achieve unrealistic goals in order to boost ourselves up again.

Because these problems are so closely associated with our self-image, treatment can take from four months to two years, and follow-up appointments may be needed to prevent relapses.

COLONIC HYDROTHERAPY

Eating disorders can – amongst other things – put your entire digestive system in turmoil and colonic irrigation can help to return it to health. 'Colonics can encourage healthy bacteria,' says one practitioner, 'soothing bowel inflammation, detoxifying the system and helping with rehydration.' However, given the link between eating disorders and 'purging' behaviours, it is important to approach this therapy with care: 'It is suitable for people who are in recovery from eating disorders which may have lasted many years.'

ACUPUNCTURE/CHINESE MEDICINE

In Chinese medicine, practically everything about the way we live – and the way we have lived since babyhood – is seen as having an influence on our health. So when it comes to treating eating disorders, practitioners look at the broader picture of our day-to-day existence.

'The important thing is the diagnosis,' says one, 'and I ask a lot of questions about your everyday life – including food, social life, stress and relationships. For instance, English people drink cold drinks from the fridge, they sit on the floor or the grass, and they open the window while sleeping. Over many years this causes damp and cold in the body which – because the blood doesn't travel well if you are not warm enough – can disturb your health. Cold blood causes cold organs and weakens the body.'

The organs of the body co-operate in complex ways, with implications for our emotions: 'The different organs help each other like a company: the kidney should help the liver, the liver should help the heart and so on. Strong, lasting emotions (especially anger) can disturb the liver, but when the body is strong it can control the emotions properly. If the body is weak, however – perhaps because it has had too much cold for many years – it cannot do this.

'If you have too much stress in your life (maybe from work or a relationship) this affects your liver, which then produces too much "fire" in your system. This in turn affects stomach function so that food is burned too quickly – and therefore you feel hungry all the time. The spleen works to transport this food in the body, but if by overeating you put too much stress on the spleen (which has many functions) your stomach will feel bloated and you will feel tired and heavy. You think "I ate too much" – and you want to get rid of the food, maybe by vomiting.'

Through acupuncture, this therapist works to re-establish healthy energy in the organs of the body, restoring the correct relationship between them. 'I have used acupuncture to help patients with eating disorders,' she says, 'and it has been very successful. It is not that serious: after a period of time patients feel better and happier.'

HYPNOTHERAPY

One hypnotherapist at the Hale Clinic also sees eating disorders as comparable to addiction. 'There is often the same pattern of behaviour – particularly denial and deviousness – as in alcoholism,' he says, 'and it isn't until eating disorders are honestly recognized that I can help.'

But at the point where an anorexic or bulimic has reached an understanding of what is wrong, the techniques of psychotherapy and hypnotherapy may be combined to tackle the roots of this disorder.

'I may use hypnotherapy to discover why a person should want to harm (usually) herself.' Often the therapist finds that an accumulation of sadness over the years, or sometimes a traumatic incident that the patient has chosen to forget, can lead her to seek an outlet through food. 'If the emotional reasons for the psychological problems can be expressed and acknowledged, then there can be change.'

This therapist finds that hypnosis, which creates a state of profound relaxation, helps both in discovering the roots of a problem and in allowing him to make positive suggestions to the unconscious 'as to how it might like to behave in terms of more healthy, balanced eating, and feeling more in control around food'. He has treated people with eating disorders who have 'responded very well', although he stresses that it can be a slow process, especially when people need to shed weight. Treatment could involve up to five sessions across a six-week period initially, and depending on progress he assesses how to take it from there.

Both bulimia and obesity are closely linked to the binge/purge mentality. It is therefore important to develop strategies to intervene and disrupt the existing behavioural patterns, to enable the patient to realize that he or she has the ability to change. Hypnosis is a powerful tool which can facilitate these strategies for change.

Anorexia is distinct from bulimia or obesity and can often be traced to family dysfunction. Using family therapy to get members to change their behaviour can bring swift benefits for the patient.

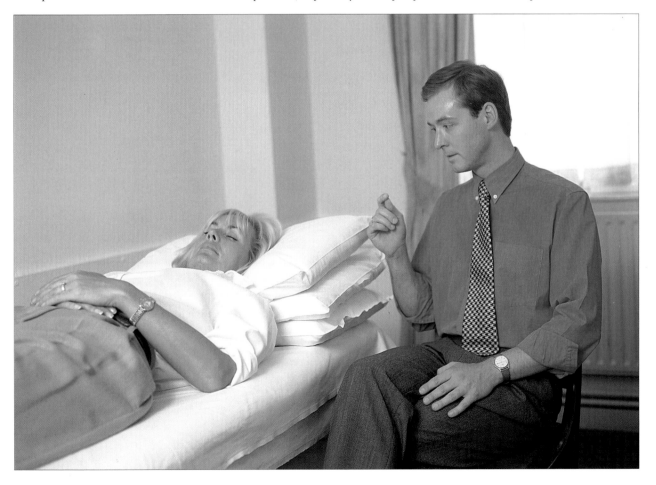

SUPPORTIVE TREATMENTS

Chi Kung/T'ai Chi

These traditional Chinese health exercises are especially beneficial for those of us who feel stressed and depressed by the rollercoaster of eating disorders. The exercises can help us to centre ourselves, calming the mind and emotions. And as *chi* (intrinsic) energy circulates, it energizes the internal organs, leaving us revitalized and refreshed. The 'Open and Closed' Chi Kung exercises (which can be learned in two or three lessons and then practised at home) are particularly recommended: they are to do with digestion and can help to restore balance within mind and body. Physical balance and breathing in harmony with the exercises are very important parts of this self-help practice.

Yoga

Yoga as therapy can help people with eating disorders by focusing their awareness on their own bodies, making them aware of their physical needs and relaxing the anxiety which can upset eating patterns. Yoga also aids digestion, redirects the energies and strengthens and calms both mind and body. Above all, it gives us back a sense of control over ourselves, empowering us to make changes.

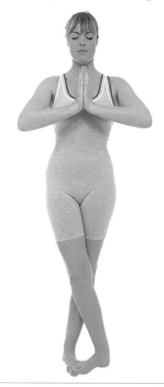

Energy Healing

Healers are sometimes able to relieve conditions which conventional medicine has difficulty in treating. By channelling a higher source of energy to realign and correct a patient's electro-magnetic field (aura), healing can help to eliminate the kind of negative emotions which are often at the root of eating disorders, empowering the patient to regain control of her health.

Homeopathy

Homeopathy would aim to treat the underlying problem causing eating disorders, possibly working in conjunction with a psychotherapist. Constitutional treatment based on the individual case is most appropriate with anorexia, but specific remedies to counteract the 'bingeing' aspect of bulimia may be recommended:
• If the patient puts on weight on the buttocks and thighs, and responds badly to expressions of concern – Natrum mur.
• If the patient is overweight, shy and anxious – Calcarea.
 Zinc supplements may also be suggested.

SELF-CARE

Moor Therapy

This treatment would begin with an in-depth health and lifestyle questionnaire. Further sessions would focus on specific problems, aiming to detoxify, heal and strengthen the whole person. Moor therapy may take the form of a drink or a detoxifying body wrap.

Flower Remedies

Pawpaw (to help absorption of nutrients, Five Corners (a remedy suitable for lack of self-esteem) and Sea Palm (which works on the stomach, satisfying cravings for emotional and physical nourishment) may all be recommended to help combat eating disorders. These remedies can be taken separately or in combination.

 In addition, for anorexia nervosa one therapist recommends Pretty Face (FES) and Peppermint (Petite Fleur). For bulimia she suggests Manzanita (FES), Sea Palm (Pacific) and Orange Honeysuckle (Pacific).

Nutrition

You can be your own food detective by looking for the signs of food allergy in your daily diet. 'If you drink orange juice or milk and then get thirstier, be suspicious,' says the naturopath quoted above. 'You can be addicted to almost anything, but to find out the truth, you have to be honest with yourself.'

Relaxation

The hypnotherapist quoted above suggests using relaxation tapes at home: 'It's useful to practise sitting and being quiet at home if you feel in difficulties. Words, images and/or affirmations used in the therapy can also be helpful at home.'

Obesity

There are few words in our culture more loaded with negative meanings than 'fat'. To be fat – especially for women – is often to feel like a social outcast. In contrast to being overly thin ('You can never be too thin,' as the saying goes), to be overly large is commonly regarded as a sign of greed and laziness – not to mention 'unhealthiness'.

Yet the truth is far more complex and some researchers have concluded that the health risks of moderate obesity (about 11kg/28lb over the conventional height/weight chart limit) have been greatly exaggerated. Indeed, there is evidence that it is healthier than excessive thinness. It is perfectly possible to be fat and fit, while trying to get thin can seriously damage your health. Excessive dieting can actually lead to long-term weight gain because your body is programmed to get back to a physiological 'set point' as soon as possible – and while you have been dieting your metabolism has slowed down, making it more difficult to lose the weight next time round. However, true obesity (defined as a 20 per cent excess of body weight) is a different matter and does cause physical problems. If your weight is enough to restrict movement it may be difficult to take exercise. Arthritis may also be exacerbated by weight, and obesity may be a cause of late-onset diabetes as well as of cancer of the colon and rectum in men. It has also been associated with heart disease and high blood pressure.

But why do people become obese in the first place? The answer lies in a complex interaction between eating styles, genetic inheritance, exercise and your physiological set point. Moreover, people may become or remain obese for various psychological reasons such as fear of a relationship – being fat may be seen as a form of protection.

Other factors involved in the complex process of weight gain include food allergies, nutritional deficiencies, chemical toxicity, a sluggish metabolism, lack of exercise, a diet high in refined and processed foods, insulin imbalance or impaired thermogenesis (the mechanism by which fat is burned to produce heat).

There may also be further psychological complications of guilt, self-loathing and fear of 'forbidden' food, driving the vicious circle of dieting and bingeing – as well as causing one of the most serious health problems of being fat, namely stress.

THE ORTHODOX APPROACH

Despite (or even because of) all our efforts to get thin, 98 per cent of people fail to maintain weight loss. However, conventional doctors still seem to have little other than diet sheets to offer. But they believe that lack of exercise is a major contributing factor – young girls in particular often starve themselves unnecessarily and unsuccessfully when more exercise would go a long way towards solving their problem. A new drug called sibutramine, said to make the brain believe the stomach is full, is likely to become available on prescription soon.

THE HALE APPROACH

Doctors will be the first to admit that dietetics and nutrition are not taught well in medical school. Provided the reason for your obesity is not a glandular condition or other disease process, complementary therapies are the best starting point. Initially, ask your doctor for an assessment to rule out these factors. In most circumstances, you should avoid orthodox 'slimming pills' wherever possible.

The right weight for any individual is the subject of much debate between the fashion industry, feminists and health-care practitioners. However, the subject of this section is obesity, which I define as being not just plump, or rather fat, but seriously overweight to the extent that your health is put at serious risk.

The causes of obesity are complex – they could be genetic, physiological or psychological. The Hale Clinic cannot treat the first of these, but we have developed a programme which addresses the physiological and psychological causes of obesity.

We begin with hypnosis, to put the patient in the right frame of mind to lose weight and to make them aware of the weight-reducing programme they will be following. The hypnotherapist/psychologist also looks at any psychological issues that may be an impediment to losing weight (though this will not be relevant in every case).

Then the programme proceeds as follows:

• Developing a good nutritional programme and making sure there are no deficiencies in vitamins, minerals, etc.

• Checking for any allergic reactions to food which could be causing bloating and weight gain.

• Assessing hormonal, digestive and elimination functions to ensure that they are functioning correctly; if necessary, advice is given on how to improve these functions. Consulting an Ayurvedic practitioner will identify your particular body type; the practitioner will then be able to advise you on which foods to eat.

• Assessing the musculo-skeletal system to see if there have been any back injuries – which could affect a person's weight. Ideally at the same time, while taking account of any back problems, a specially tailored exercise programme should be started. This might begin with yoga or T'ai Chi and walking and build up to running and/or working out in a gym.

• After a few weeks of following this programme, the patient does a Buteyko breathing course for a week. This will considerably reduce appetite, detoxify the body, help reduce allergic reactions, improve digestive elimination and boost hormonal functions.

In certain cases a quick drop in weight can bring psychological issues to the fore, so continual contact with the hypnotherapist/ psychologist is important. A lifetime commitment to changing the pattern of breathing is necessary if weight is to be kept in check.

PSYCHOTHERAPY/ NUTRITION

One therapist uses a combination of psychological and physiological approaches to address problems of obesity. These include NLP (neurolinguistic programming), a form of hypnotherapy. 'We look at the pattern of eating: why you eat, when you eat and so on,' she says. 'Are you eating out of habit, do old patterns and beliefs need to be changed? Is you mind stopping you from eating healthily?

'I would look into whether certain foods are causing weight to stay on because of sensitivities – and may recommend a blood test for food intolerance.'

She also checks for thyroid imbalance and discusses the possibility of blood-sugar imbalance. 'Then, exercise and food elimination diets – for people with food sensitivities – can help.'

Treatments and how long they take are variable and tailored to the individual. Results are variable, too. The therapist says she sometimes sees a very gradual improvement, but at other times treatment 'can produce amazing results'.

HYPNOTHERAPY

'Nine times out of ten,' says one hypnotherapist, 'clients come to me having tried many, many diets. But those diets haven't worked. People are often in great distress; they want something done now, but reductions in weight must be achieved gradually. Treatment can take months and involves a permanent change in eating habits, as opposed to dieting.'

Hypnotherapy opens up a two-way process in which the therapist both listens to and helps supply suggestions to the subconscious. He attempts to discover the cause of the problem. 'Some people describe an addiction to food. There may be a compulsion to eat, the roots of which lie in the past. Some people may have a secondary gain in making themselves unattractive. Through hypnotherapy I can work out a sensible eating programme, coupled with positive suggestions to the subconscious to promote maintenance of that programme.'

ACUPUNCTURE

One specialist in Chinese medicine uses a combination of acupuncture and Chinese herbs to balance the body's metabolism, eliminating blockages in the flow of energy along the meridians.

'By regulating energy balance in this way,' he says, 'and by also addressing diet and exercise, it is possible to help people lose around 6kg (14lb) in weight over a two-month period.'

COLONIC HYDROTHERAPY

While colonic irrigation is not used as part of a weight-loss programme in the sense of 'purging' the body, it can be helpful if weight gain has been caused by excess toxicity in the body. 'If the body is holding on to toxins which are stored in the fat cells,' explains a colonic therapist, 'colonic irrigation can help by detoxifying the system. This enables the body to break down the fat cells.'

She finds that this form of treatment can also help reduce cravings for food because, by improving the metabolism and the absorption of nutrients, it is aiding the body to get what it needs from food more efficiently.

AYURVEDA

By introducing an eating regimen that is appropriate for the individual constitution – moving away from heavy, oily, cold foods to light, dry and healing foods – the practitioner helps the client to build digestive capacity and shed excess weight.

BUTEYKO

'There is no person who is obese who breathes correctly,' according to the Hale Clinic's Buteyko teacher, 'and there is no person who breathes correctly who is obese.'

The Buteyko Method aims to normalize breathing by retraining the complex involuntary mechanisms which govern our breathing. The thinking behind this is that if we breathe too much we absorb not more but less oxygen. This is because we need to maintain a specific level of carbon dioxide in our blood in order to make use of oxygen.

So how can changing our breathing help with obesity?

'When your breathing is normalized,' explains the teacher, 'your metabolism increases, burning up more energy.' He sees obesity as a symptom of 'over-breathing'.

'If your breathing is dysfunctional, your metabolism becomes alkaline and your body cannot produce a range of hormones such as insulin, which regulates the level of sugar in the blood. When your pH (acid/alkaline) balance is correct, however, your body can absorb the right amount of protein from the food you eat, and therefore you will not feel so hungry.'

The Buteyko exercises are taught either in groups or on a one-to-one basis. You need to follow them up with about 20 minutes of daily exercise. Bona fide Buteyko practitioners offer a money-back guarantee of substantial improvement to any patient they have agreed to treat for obesity. 'People with obesity can get remarkable results,' says the teacher.

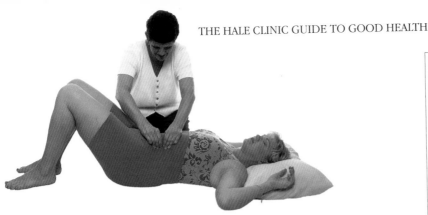

BODYHARMONICS

This integrated and holistic therapy is based on a fusion of Chinese, Thai and Indonesian techniques. The treatment of obesity involves deep abdominal massage which minimizes the appetite and adjusts the functioning of the internal organs so that the body gets rid of fatty tissues by itself. BodyHarmonics also raises energy levels so that you feel lively and energetic.

Weight losses on this programme are typically up to 3.5kg (8lb) in a series of 15 daily sessions and up to 7kg (16lb) in a month.

SELF-CARE

Flower Remedies
Those suitable for obesity include Old Man Banksia (Australian Bush), Hound's Tongue, Nicotiana, Pink Monkey-Flower, Tansy (all FES), Poison Hemlock (Pacific) and Pink Rose (Petite Fleur).

SUPPORTIVE TREATMENTS

Remedial Yoga
The practice of yoga increases the circulation of blood through the body, relieving feelings of sluggishness and stimulating digestion. It also stimulates the endocrine system, which controls the workings of the major organs. Yoga can relieve compression around those organs, helping to release toxins from the body.

On the emotional level, yoga can help you feel more positive about yourself and in control of your body, encouraging a sense of strength and vigour.

Chi Kung
In Chinese medicine, fat is viewed as unspent energy. Chi Kung exercises and breathing restore the flow of energy, allowing the body to return to its natural shape. 'First Chi Kung' exercises are especially recommended. Once mastered, they can easily be practised at home.

Moor Therapy
Moor therapy, based on a natural herbal drink containing 300 medicinal herbs, plus vitamins, minerals, trace elements and enzymes, treats the whole body – with the by-product of reducing appetite. Treatment begins with six initial sessions with a therapist who employs counselling and massage techniques according to need. You also take a teaspoonful of Moor drink three times a day. Treatment may last from six months to two years.

Healing
While there is no 'quick fix' for obesity through healing, it can be a process which enables people to take responsibility for their own health. The healer is in some ways a vehicle for the transfer of energy, which can give you the strength and awareness to make radical changes in your lifestyle. In this way healing for obesity can bring a shift in consciousness which allows you to find your own solutions.

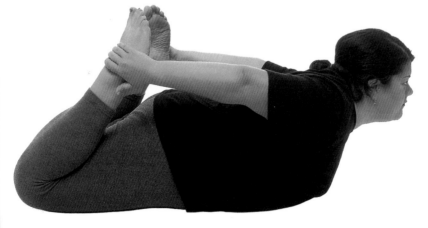

Bereavement, Loss & Separation

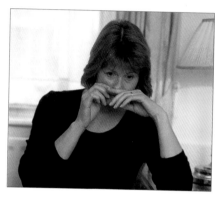

There's only one thing surer than taxes, as the saying goes, and that is that none of us lives forever. Inevitably, and increasingly as we get older, we lose loved ones – and come closer each time to our own mortality.

How do we deal with this most fundamental truth about being human in a society which prefers not to think about it? Death is the great modern taboo: talking about such things can cause shock and offence, while anyone who has been bereaved will know the embarrassment and reticence which surrounds the subject. Widows often say they are shunned by former friends; some people seem to find it easier to cross the road to avoid you than to offer their condolences.

These days, caring for the terminally ill happens increasingly outside the home in specialist units and hospitals. Not only does this remove loved ones from us in their last days, but it removes death and dying from our normal experience. And as we have become estranged from this powerful and potentially devastating process, our ability to cope with it has diminished accordingly.

Yet bereavement, together with other kinds of loss or separation from loved ones, can have serious consequences for our health, with the potential to undermine sleep patterns, appetite, mental health and physical energy and wellbeing. In the early months of a bereavement, you may experience distressing physical symptoms, including headache, dizziness, tiredness, diarrhoea, nausea, tightness in the throat, difficulty with breathing, palpitations and chest pain. There is evidence too that serious illnesses like cancer are more common in people who have suffered a recent bereavement.

Loss is also a well-known trigger for insomnia. Research shows that many people suffer from disturbed sleep patterns for several years after a bereavement. In a recent survey, 13 per cent of people who could identify a cause for their insomnia attributed it to a bereavement. On average, their insomnia lasted four years.

Bereavement, loss and separation are also major precipitating causes of depression. Clearly, the death of a loved one is a considerable loss, but the break-up of a marriage, the loss of a job or home, separation from your child or partner can also have devastating effects. Many women suffer a deep sense of loss in midlife when their children leave home. This 'empty nest syndrome' may be compounded by other simultaneous losses – a sense of lost youth and perceived attractiveness, the loss of elderly parents, the loss of fertility, even the loss of hopes and dreams for the future.

Many factors influence how well we deal with the bereavement, loss or separation, ranging from our previous experience of loss, to the strength (or otherwise) of our social support systems. The conventional view of grieving is that it is a process which has several stages, beginning with numbness or a sense of unreality, then moving on to a mixture of complex emotions including guilt, fear, longing and anger. Depression and despair may follow; it is only after a year or two, perhaps more, that life returns to some semblance of normality.

THE ORTHODOX APPROACH

Orthodox treatments for the symptoms of loss or bereavement include antidepressants and/or bereavement counselling.

THE HALE APPROACH

All treatments for loss or bereavement should be in association with and with the support of a professional counsellor, whether he or she is found privately or through recommendations of friends, your doctor's surgery or the Hale Clinic.

Everyone is faced with a great loss at some time in their life – be it the loss of a job or an important relationship or a bereavement – and those times will always weaken us physically and emotionally. It is particularly important to seek help in order to reduce your risk of developing an illness while you are in this weakened state.

Homeopathy and acupuncture are particularly helpful in strengthening you physiologically and emotionally, as well as dealing with suppressed grief and grief in general. Mental and emotional help can be given by counselling, psychotherapy, hypnotherapy, aromatherapy and healing, which in turn will help the physical condition of your body.

In times of great stress, we often forget to look after ourselves, so try to keep to a healthy diet and use flower remedies and aromatherapy. All these treatments can help you through the difficult time – and always remember that with the passage of time your grief will diminish.

NUTRITION

There is an old saying that 'man is what he eats and what he drinks, how he breathes and what he thinks.' This fits with what we all know from experience – that the food we eat can affect our mood and vice versa.

If you have recently been bereaved, for instance, your appetite may well be changed, along with your breathing and your thinking. And there are certain foods which are best avoided when you are suffering from grief. Heavy meals can have a depressing effect, slowing you down and making you feel sluggish. This is because they tend to release hormones into your system which have an adverse effect on your emotions, making you feel low and irritable.

'And one should keep wel away from alcohol,' according to one nutritionist, 'because alcohol is the great magnifier and can make a sad situation feel even worse.'

HYPNOTHERAPY

To enable an individual to come to terms with loss is to re-emphasize the qualities that someone who has passed away has contributed to the life of the bereaved person and to those of other people. Death is not a finality; people's qualities and influences live on through those with whom they have interacted. It is important to reassert a positive, happy vision of the deceased person and reduce the negative vision of illness and suffering.

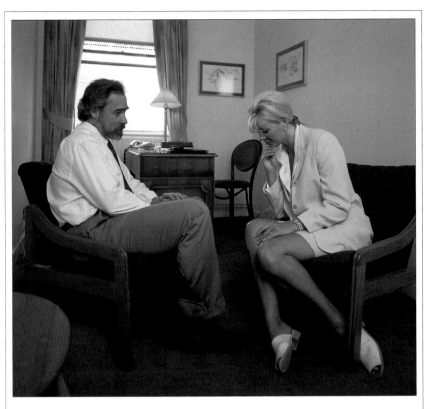

COUNSELLING/ PSYCHOTHERAPY

The essence of supportive counselling and therapy for loss and bereavement has several strands, according to one psychotherapist: 'I aim to help a person recognize their loss and the changes associated with it, including a whole range of feelings, positive and negative. These powerful emotions are normal and not to be feared.' He works to support positive coping, adjustment and change, ultimately fostering the development of emotional attachments to others.

A recently bereaved patient wrote to this counsellor using a sailing analogy. The therapist's job, she wrote, is 'to go around the bay teaching people how to sail, how to build their boats, service and maintain them, how to manage the rudder, how to choose the right equipment, how to sail with other people and how to learn to enjoy spending time on your own boat, with or without other people. He also helps you to enjoy going on other people's boats and how to forecast, avoid and deal with adverse weather and sea conditions.'

She went on to describe how the therapist 'first used a tow rope so I would feel safe when the business of sailing alone was too much for me' – but added that ultimately she would be able to sail alone, steering her own course and maintaining her own ship.

Through this kind of supportive counselling, the therapist forms a good working alliance with the person who has suffered a loss, believes the therapist. Through therapy, we can express our fears, gradually moving on to greater self-sufficiency with the confidence to pursue new relationships and with a new sense of purpose.

HEALING

One healer who deals with those who have undergone a loss or bereavement uses healing – in combination with a careful review of diet – to ease the suffering.

'The therapy works in two ways,' he explains. 'On one level there is energy replacement through bio-electromagnetic transfer. This can give a "kick-start" or "jump-lead" energy lift to replace the energy field of the loved one.' At the same time he aims to effect a shift of consciousness at the spiritual level.

Results, he claims, can be quite dramatic: 'In one case, the person had experienced a total loss of energy, including the loss of her sense of smell, together with digestive complications. All this was resolved through healing.'

This therapist recommends around three to five sessions involving a laying on of hands, enabling a transfer of energy to the patient's aura. He also looks at common-sense dietary issues and may recommend supplements of amino acids and B complex vitamins, together with exercises aimed at improving blood circulation.

HOMEOPATHY

Homeopathy can be very helpful both immediately after a bereavement and for long-term grief when a person has difficulty coming to terms with the loss. The two remedies most often used are Ignatia in the acute stage – when the person either cannot cry or cannot stop sobbing – and Natrum mur., often used for long-standing grief.

COLONIC HYDROTHERAPY

According to traditional Chinese medicine, the emotions of grief and fear reside in the bowel. Modern Western therapists who treat bereaved people say that they often find a link between an occasion of loss or bereavement and the time at which a person's bowels stopped working properly. In one sense it could be said that people are 'holding on to' fears and griefs in their bowels, explains one colonics therapist, and as colonic irrigation helps them to 'release' their toxic material, these mental and emotional states are also released.

Before colonic irrigation the therapist takes a full case history, sometimes using iridology to help diagnose the source of the problem. Nutrition is also discussed before the irrigation procedure is started. Often the client expresses long-hidden feelings during treatment, and these emotional explorations may persist after the session is over.

ACUPUNCTURE/BODY HARMONICS

Acupuncture can be very effective for people suffering emotional pain, explains one practitioner, especially if they find themselves stuck in a rut and unable to find a way forward. They may be feeling broken-hearted, perhaps after a failed relationship, and suffer pain as if the heart itself were physically broken. The feelings of hurt, sadness, anger, resentment, loneliness and restlessness remain with them 24 hours a day, often causing serious problems of sleeplessness and bodily malfunction. The acupuncture point on the inside of the wrist is particularly effective for 'mending a broken heart', while pressure on the point on the brow helps to relieve stress.

If the stress that accompanies this kind of emotional upset has caused pain in the shoulder, back or neck, soft-tissue massage – based on traditional Chinese, Thai and Indonesian techniques – can be effective in easing the accumulated tension. Many people find this kind of treatment brings a drastic change to their view of life, almost as if they had discovered a 'miracle drug'. Others respond more slowly and may need up to ten sessions.

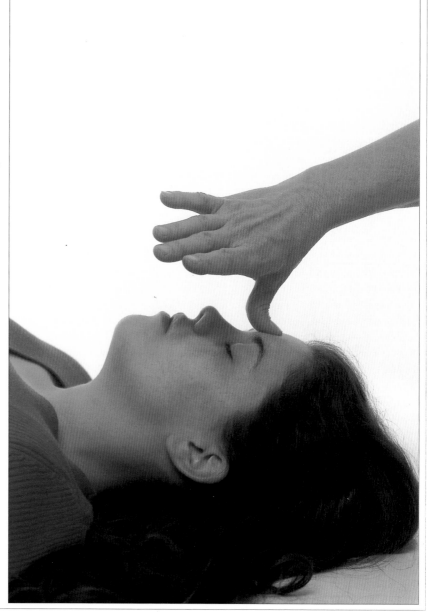

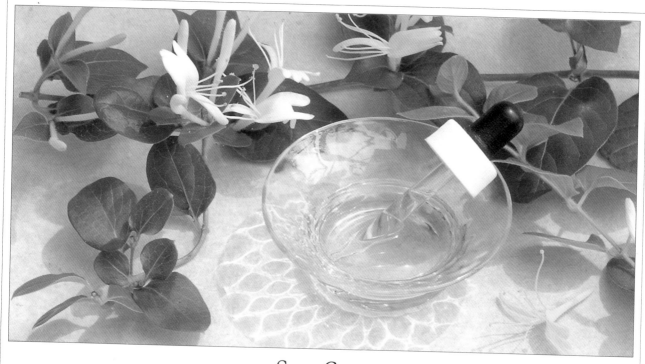

Self-Care

Flower Remedies

There are many different flower remedies to aid letting go through the grieving process, according to one therapist: 'Pear Blossom (Mosters) helps for any kind of grief or loss in the short term; Ashoka Tree (Aditi Himalayan) is for deep, long-term grief. Honeysuckle (Bach) is for people who look back to the past with feelings of "if only".'

Supportive Treatment

Aromatherapy

The loss of a close friend or relative is inevitable, but people who have suffered such a loss often begin searching for a therapy to help them relax and forget everything, and aromatherapeutic massage may soothe.

If a few months have passed since the loss, grief may have manifested itself physically, appearing to the patient as a new and sudden symptom. One practitioner of aromatherapy, massage and Chinese medicine says she often sees grief manifested in the lungs. The patient's *chi* (intrinsic) energy becomes deficient and breathing less full. The voice may be low, even inaudible, and the chest sunken, causing the shoulders to round as if protecting the lungs. Essential oils are able to excite an emotional response that frees the grief in a breakthrough for the patient. Breathing returns to normal, and calmness and acceptance replaces sorrow.

Physiologically the aroma of certain oils helps patients come to terms with loss and uplifts them in daily life. Frankincense and sandalwood are particularly good for calming the mind and relaxing the body.

Tips

A vital part of self-help when you are suffering loss is to talk about your feelings – and to ask for help. The British stiff upper lip has probably led to a great deal of chronic depression and long-term illness. Far better to seek out a counsellor or close friend, or to contact one of the organizations which offer support and a listening ear.

Exercise – whether that means long walks in the country or yoga or lengths of your local pool – can help to take the edge off your negative feelings, restoring normal appetite and patterns of sleep.

Phobias

It is estimated that about one person in every ten has a particular phobia which causes them attacks of extreme panic that can occur at any time and in any place. Anyone who has experienced the symptoms of a mild panic attack - whether because you nearly missed a flight or train, or because a spider scuttled out from behind the shower curtain - may begin to imagine how a phobia sufferer might feel, but it is hard to conceive just how widely a phobia can affect a person's life.

According to one psychologist, phobias are characterized by four factors:

- A persistent, irrational fear of an object or situation.
- A powerful desire to avoid the object or situation.
- Significant distress associated with the problem.
- Recognition that the fear is unreasonable or irrational.

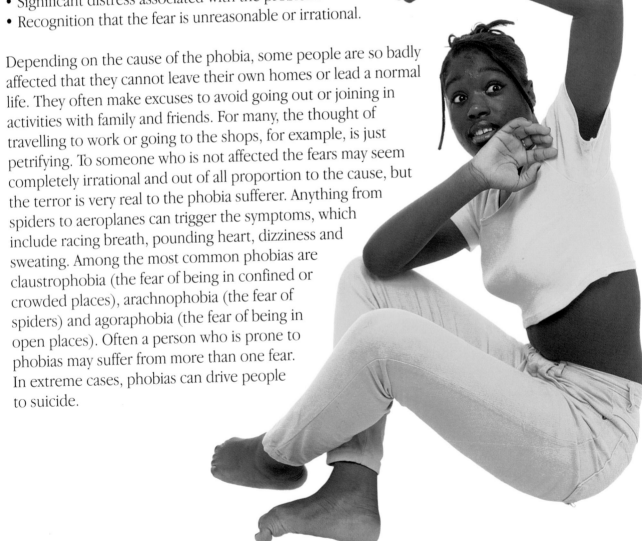

Depending on the cause of the phobia, some people are so badly affected that they cannot leave their own homes or lead a normal life. They often make excuses to avoid going out or joining in activities with family and friends. For many, the thought of travelling to work or going to the shops, for example, is just petrifying. To someone who is not affected the fears may seem completely irrational and out of all proportion to the cause, but the terror is very real to the phobia sufferer. Anything from spiders to aeroplanes can trigger the symptoms, which include racing breath, pounding heart, dizziness and sweating. Among the most common phobias are claustrophobia (the fear of being in confined or crowded places), arachnophobia (the fear of spiders) and agoraphobia (the fear of being in open places). Often a person who is prone to phobias may suffer from more than one fear. In extreme cases, phobias can drive people to suicide.

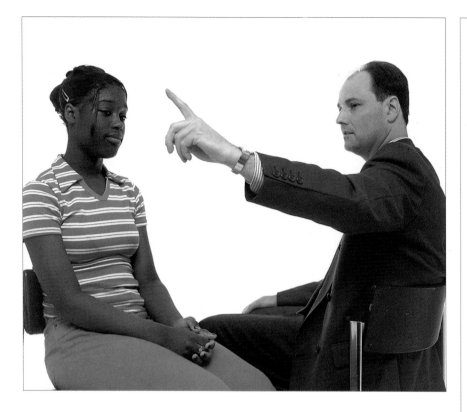

THE ORTHODOX APPROACH

In some cases, a doctor will prescribe tranquillizers. However, it is now widely accepted that these can give only short-term relief and they are known to be highly addictive, so many doctors are starting to recommend forms of psychotherapy instead.

THE HALE APPROACH

Phobias, like other obsessive, compulsive or neurotic disorders, are best dealt with through psychotherapy, although psychiatric drugs may benefit in an acute phase. An initial assessment by a psychiatrist with referral on to psychological care is best supported by complementary treatments to speed up the process.

Something can almost always be done to help phobias and often considerable improvements can be gained in as little as eight to ten weeks. Patients do not have to suffer indefinitely from phobias.

EMDR, hypnosis and psychotherapy can be very effective in treating this disorder and all have their own specific techniques, usually combined with a discussion with the patient which looks at the original cause of the problem and the development of positive strategies to help cope with it in the future.

For patients who do not wish to go this route, there are some very effective homeopathic remedies for phobias. Sometimes the benefits can be felt very quickly, although other patients may find that the phobias take some time to disappear.

Art therapy and healing are very helpful supportive treatments.

EMDR

In the late 1980s, Francine Shapiro did some research concentrating on rapid eye movement, using Vietnam War veterans. She obtained impressive results in alleviating and resolving traumas associated with war. Eye movement desensitization and reprocessing (EMDR) therapy developed from these findings. A patient tracks the therapist's finger backwards and forwards with their eyes to produce rapid eye movements. These stimulate the brain, allowing it to process information that may hitherto have been 'frozen' if it were of a traumatic nature, and to reprocess it and draw a logical conclusion. In this way, a client can see a phobia for what it is and thereafter is able to encounter it again and again without re-stimulating the old fears.

One EMDR practitioner says, 'One of the benefits of this process is the speed at which positive results can be achieved. On average, 8-10 sessions are required. The first few sessions involve confidence building and relaxation strategies. Successive sessions consist of gaining an understanding of the problem through EMDR and developing a new approach to it. Self-hypnosis techniques can be taught alongside EMDR to provide additional support'

Some people notice nothing more than an improvement in the control of their phobia, but most achieve a total resolution of the problem.

HYPNOTHERAPY

Therapeutic hypnosis works on three levels when dealing with phobias. Firstly, on a conscious level by helping the patient to gain insight and perspective into the problem and realize that he or she has choices. Secondly, using regression under hypnosis to the time of the first incident, allowing the subconscious to treat the phobia as something that belongs in the past with no bearing on the future and, finally, positive suggestions made under hypnosis offer coping strategies and solutions.

One hypnotherapist reports, 'Hypnosis is used to defuse phobias and their symptoms. In 8-10 sessions involving counselling, problem solving and regression hypnosis most clients achieve a total resolution. Some simply obtain an improvement and a very small percentage gain no overall benefit but, in this case, I would realize it after the first few sessions and would not continue.'

Another hypnotherapist tells of a case where a 48-year-old woman suffered from ophidophobia, a morbid fear of snakes. Her phobia was so bad that she actually hallucinated, seeing snakes coming out of the taps when she ran a bath. Obviously, this limited and tormented her life. The first few sessions were spent getting used to the 'feel' of hypnosis, using relaxation exercises and discussing her fear and how it had arisen and grown. A step-by-step approach was used – starting with calming suggestions, looking at a book with drawings of snakes, and asking the patient to draw how she felt about the fear. The treatment culminated in a trip to London Zoo to come face to face with a live snake. In this case, progress was steady because the patient put in a lot of effort between sessions. The therapist says, 'As with any recovery, a patient will flourish in one part of the treatment and go more slowly in others.'

HOMEOPATHY

The homeopathic remedy varies depending on the cause of the phobia and the form it takes. For example, Argentum nitricum is commonly used for claustrophobics who fear being trapped. However, if your claustrophobia takes the form of fearing crowded, closed places such as lifts or underground trains, then Pulsatilla may be recommended. When the phobia is accompanied by severe shock that leaves you feeling weak and faint after an attack, Arnica may be suitable. Aconite is good for agoraphobia.

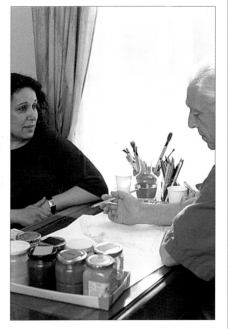
Art therapy

SUPPORTIVE TREATMENTS

Healing
Spiritual healing uses its energy to cure or relieve the symptoms of sufferers. In the case of someone who is phobic, the first thing one healer would do would be to realign the patient's own energies and work through their aura (the energy field that surrounds each of us). She would 'look into' the patient to discover the root cause of the phobia and then deal with this.

Some healers work solely through the patient's aura, others may also touch the patient during treatment to encourage the flow of energy.

Art Therapy
It is commonly held that phobias often result from childhood traumas. Art therapy plays a vital role in the holistic approach to dispelling these fears by recalling the traumatic experience through image-making (drawing, painting, modelling, etc.). Patients are encouraged to express what is in their unconscious directly and spontaneously in a symbolic/ pictorial form. The visual image produced in art therapy reveals aspects of the patient's self and the nature of the inner conflict, providing the possibility of release and resolution.

The art therapist accompanies patients in their search, helping them to reflect on and make sense of inner feelings and experiences, and allowing them to regain their capacity to relax and lead a normal, creative life.

SELF-CARE

Yoga/Relaxation

'Obsessional behaviour and emotional fears are often a feature of anxiety states,' says one yoga therapist. 'A state of persistent anxiety can result in hyperventilation. This pattern can become a habit which creates a cycle of anxiety that is very difficult to break. The symptoms of anxiety make us feel more anxious. Yoga helps us to relax the body and regularize our breathing patterns. We can have an effect on the autonomic function of breathing and this knowledge gives us confidence. Because we can have an effect on the body, it can also conquer that feeling of being out of control.'

The principles of yoga promote a holistic approach to healing and so, used in conjunction with other therapies, yoga can help you to deal with the psychological, emotional and physical aspects of phobias.

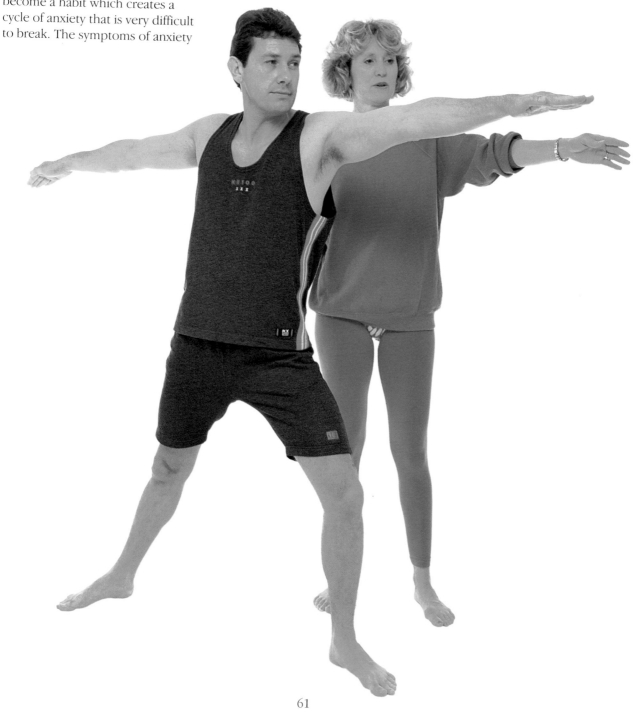

ME

It has disparagingly been called 'yuppie flu', reflecting the fact that this is an illness which people neither understand nor accept. Yet the World Health Organization has classified myalgic encephalomyelitis (ME) as a disease of the nervous system, while in Britain the Department of Health recognizes it as a 'debilitating and distressing condition'.

ME can be a severely disabling and chronic condition which has a devastating impact on your daily life, work and personal independence – an impact often made worse by the prejudice and disbelief which surrounds this complex disorder. People with ME have often enjoyed good health before coming down with a range of symptoms affecting their muscles, such as fatigue and pain, together with various symptoms which suggest a change in brain function. ME can cause loss of concentration and short-term memory, dyslexia, nausea, clumsiness and disturbed balance.

There may also be problems with vision and sensitivity to light, as well as sensitivity to noise and misjudgement of distance. People with ME are often depressed and may suffer from mood swings. They may also have problems with bladder control and changes in their bowel function.

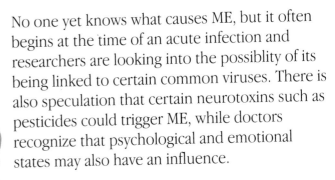

No one yet knows what causes ME, but it often begins at the time of an acute infection and researchers are looking into the possiblity of its being linked to certain common viruses. There is also speculation that certain neurotoxins such as pesticides could trigger ME, while doctors recognize that psychological and emotional states may also have an influence.

Getting over ME can be a long, slow process taking several years and involving relapses, but it is possible to recover in time. However, some people merely show some improvement while a minority never get over their symptoms and become invalids.

ME can hit at any time, whatever your age or background, and although it most commonly starts between the ages of 20 and 40, children as young as seven can be affected.

THE ORTHODOX APPROACH

Conventional medicine has no 'cure' as such, although there are therapies aimed at individual symptoms, ranging from antibiotics for infection and sedative drugs for sleep disturbances, to exercises and special diets. There is also broad agreement that it is important to be diagnosed as early as possible and to rest properly during acute states and relapses. Doctors believe that people with ME should pace their activities, gradually increasing their levels of activity while accepting that progress may be slow and erratic.

THE HALE APPROACH

Many doctors still do not accept ME as a condition. If yours falls into this category, have no hesitation in approaching another member of the practice. There is a blood test called Viral Protein One which is positive in around 60 per cent of people with ME symptoms and this should be checked, since ME is really a diagnosis of exclusion (i.e. one that can only be made when all other causes have been ruled out). Because of this you need to find a doctor who can monitor you while you go through complementary treatments.

Choosing a complementary treatment can be particularly confusing for patients suffering from this debilitating condition. The factors that can aggravate the illness are so very diverse (stress, poor nutrition, problems with digestion or elimination, poor posture) that it is often difficult to decide which single therapy or combination of therapies is the best approach.

Improving the nutrition of ME sufferers usually alleviates the condition. In a significant number of cases patients are able to resume normal life after dietary changes. Special emphasis is placed on correct digestion and elimination, two systems in which malfunction can lead to the onset of ME. Removing 'allergic' foods from the diet can also bring about a great improvement.

Treatments that strengthen the constitution are an important part of a campaign against ME: a patient can choose from homeopathy, acupuncture or Ayurveda.

Many ME patients have great tension round the neck and shoulder area, often caused by stress or many years spent hunched over a computer or desk. This restricts blood flow to the brain, causing severe fatigue and short-term memory loss. The blood flow to the brain is greatly enhanced by bio-energetic healing. This treatment is particularly effective with ME, especially long-term cases. It has even had success with patients who have been wheelchair-bound for a number of years. Alternatively, Marma massage is very effective in increasing the blood supply to the brain.

Support treatments are particularly important with ME because anything a patient can do to strengthen their system will alleviate the condition.

The Buteyko breathing method will help strengthen bodily functions like digestion, elimination, hormonal activity and respiration. The patient can also practise its techniques as a self-care tool. Likewise light therapy will help improve bodily functions and increase energy levels. Aromatherapy and Moor treatment have a generally beneficial effect.

It is often difficult for ME patients to do strenuous exercise, so the gentle-but-powerful exercises of yoga and T'ai Chi can be of great assistance.

BIO-ENERGY HEALING

One therapist's diagnosis is done by passing her hands over the patient's body, a few inches away from it. Although she can then tell which organs are healthy and which are not, she prefers to work with the patient's medical doctor, so X-rays and blood tests also form part of the diagnosis. Treatment involves 'feeding' positive energy into the patient with one hand while drawing negative energy out with the other. This balances the body and helps restore it to health.

She sees herself as a 'transmitter of life energy. In the case of ME this is absolutely vital, for ME is a condition of great energy depletion. An ME patient is simply unable to draw from the cosmos the life energy he needs to support himself, so I help make that link for him. ME patients tend to use too much mental energy and to be unable to draw on good supplies of physical energy to support what they are using.'

A single treatment session takes 20-30 minutes, and the therapist likes to see a patient three times on consecutive days, then three times the following week. The number of treatments needed varies with the individual and the severity of the condition, but many begin to respond almost immediately.

Although she does not talk about 'curing' ME, this therapist has had great success in enabling people who have been seriously ill for a number of years to lead healthy, active lives.

NUTRITION/ALLERGY TREATMENT

A new form of treatment enables certain people with ME to recover within five days, claims a naturopath at the Hale Clinic. If extreme fatigue is a predominant symptom, it could be that you are effectively being 'poisoned' by various toxic alcohols, which are the result of increased bacterial fermentation in the intestines. Even small quantities of these alcohols can cause muscle tenderness, reduced reflexes, depressed respiration, other nervous-system symptoms and profound tiredness. A simple blood test will tell whether toxic alcohols are present.

Extremes of bacterial fermentation may also be linked with a so-called 'malabsorption syndrome', meaning that important nutrients are not being absorbed from the intestine – making ME symptoms worse. Supplements to reverse this situation can have a dramatic effect within days, once the malabsorption has been improved.

Another aspect to this treatment involves tackling what naturopaths call 'allergic tension-fatigue syndrome', in which 'delayed food allergy' contributes to the symptoms of ME. When this syndrome is suspected, the nutritionist recommends excluding the offending food item from your diet.

This combined nutritional and allergy treatment is relatively quick and straightforward, involving three consultations, a blood test and several food supplements and medications.

ACUPUNCTURE

Acupuncture, with its capacity for strengthening the immune system by regulating the energy balance in your body, can bring improvements in the symptoms of ME. A course of acupuncture and Chinese herbs may involve from six to twenty sessions with a therapist, during which you will also be offered advice about diet and exercise.

LIGHT THERAPY

Light therapy can have the effect of boosting the immune system as well as the blood circulation. And your blood, according to one light therapist, is a 'living battery', providing your organs, glands and tissues with nutrients and oxygen.

People with ME may be confined to bed or housebound because of fatigue, which means they are getting very little natural light. Light therapy can remedy this lack, and those ME sufferers who avoid daylight because they are sensitive to it often react well to the full-spectrum provided by this therapy. For people who can't go out, an added advantage is that a light box can be brought to your home. It also improves muscle tone and heart function, thus increasing strength – so vital for the ME sufferer.

Treatment sessions generally last for an hour, and some ME sufferers quickly respond to light therapy, which helps them return to normal functioning.

AYURVEDA

Ayurvedic treatment for ME begins with detoxification using *panchakarma* techniques, which include 'purification', detox-ification, massage and 'rehabil-itation'. The aim is to restore balance or 'homeostasis' to the body. Oral medicines are prescribed to balance the *doshas* or forces which control the workings of the body. Harmful *doshas* are eliminated. *Rasayana* treatment may also be given while *agni* helps improve the appetite.

One Ayurvedic physician tells of a teacher he has treated, aged 38, who had been off work for six months with ME. Within three months of starting Ayurvedic treatment she was back at work.

HOMEOPATHY

ME has a wide variety of symp-toms – and so a wide variety of possible homeopathic treatments. If, however, your overriding sympton is fatigue, there are four main remedies which may help.

Aconite, if used swiftly at the first signs of relapse, can help keep fatigue at bay. Vertrum Alb. may be preferable if you are fatigued to the point of collapse. Carbo animalis is for general but less severe collapse. Carbo veg may be prescribed if the fatigue is accompanied by respiratory and abdominal problems.

'With ME,' says one homeopath, 'homeopathy can be an effective support therapy to speed healing, but psychological and other deeper factors will have to be tackled by delving into the psyche as well as nutritional issues.'

MARMA MASSAGE

According to Ayurvedic Marma medicine, ME sets in after a serious infection or prolonged period of stress, which creates a negative environment and a lack of energy and life force. In addition to the debilitating symptoms of ME, patients become prone to further infection because of a weak immune system.

Marma massage therapy helps increase the supply of blood and oxygen to the brain, oxygen being a major source of energy. If the brain receives the maximum oxygen and blood, the mind and body are able to produce enough strength to heal the whole system. In increasing the supply of these substances to the brain, the goal of Marma massage therapy is therefore to re-establish co-ordination of mind and body, to reduce overall toxicity, to increase energy and to help the patient fight his or her way back to normal life.

Although each case is unique, improvement is likely to occur after 3-6 months of regular (weekly) Marma massage sessions.

SUPPORTIVE TREATMENTS

Aromatherapy
Aromatherapy and light massage help to reduce the muscle pain which so often accompanies ME. It can also improve circulation, stimulate the immune system, uplift the mood, improve breathing and relaxation, counter depression and heighten self-esteem.

Treatment generally consists of one-hour sessions, involving massage with individually chosen essential oils. It is often supported by acupressure, healing, reflexology and breathing/relaxation/meditation techniques to help strengthen and heal.

Buteyko
Many people with ME become breathless very easily after even slight physical effort. The Buteyko Method, which is aimed at normalizing your breathing, counters this lack of oxygenation to improve symptoms of chronic fatigue.

How you breathe can also have a dramatic impact on many of the body's other important functions, including the absorption of nutrients, the immune system and your hormonal activity. As such, Buteyko can effectively support other treatments for ME.

Length of treatment varies with the needs of the individual. Bona fide Buteyko practitioners offer a money-back guarantee of substantial improvement to any ME patient they have agreed to treat.

SELF-CARE

Remedial Yoga
Yoga encourages improvement of health on many levels, stimulating the musculature as well as circulation of the blood and lymph. Their effect is to increase energy levels, counteracting symptoms of lethargy and sluggishness. Yoga also teaches you to improve your breathing patterns.

Flower Remedies
Flower remedies which may help people with ME include those which address the immune system, such as Pansy (which has anti-viral properties, from the Pegasus range), Koenign Van Daenmark (also Pegasus), Combine Shrimp, Old Brush and Thyme (all Petite Fleur).

Moor Therapy
Daily doses of the Moor herbal drink (a combination of 300 medicinal herbs, minerals, vitamins, enzymes and trace elements) aim to lift your energy levels, especially when the treatment is supported by massage and counselling.

Light Therapy
You can administer your own light therapy by sitting near a specialized light box for an hour or more each day.

Chi Kung
Chi Kung, which in Chinese means 'the study of the vital force through exercises and meditation', is a technique of fluid movements which enable us to be aware of *chi* (intrinsic) energy in our bodies, and to balance it. As a form of self-help it can bring an immediate sense of rejuvenation and vitality. The exercises can be learned in two or three lessons and subsequently practised at home. For ME the exercises known as 'Second Chi Kung' can be most helpful, while 'Triple Heater' Chi Kung exercises are also recommended.

In addition Chi Kung supports other complementary therapies which encourage the body to heal itself.

Acne

THE ORTHODOX APPROACH

Spots are the bane of many a teenager's life, but true acne, which almost always begins at the painfully self-conscious period of puberty, is unsightly and can cause acute embarrassment at best, and very real distress and depression at worst. The good news for acne sufferers is that with today's methods of treatment, bad scarring can almost always be avoided.

Most adolescent boys and many girls suffer from acne vulgaris to some degree. This is caused by a plug of skin cells obstructing the flow of sebum (an oily substance secreted by the sebaceous glands) at the neck of the hair follicles. When sebum becomes trapped in a follicle, bacteria multiply and the follicle becomes inflamed, taking on the appearance of a spot.

It seems that acne blights teenage boys in particular because changes in levels of sebum secretions are linked to the increased levels of androgen (male sex hormones) produced at puberty. Acne can also run in families. The condition can be aggravated by some drugs, including steroids, barbiturates, and drugs used in the treatment of tuberculosis and epilepsy.

Acne occurs mainly on the face, in the centre of the chest, on the upper back, on the shoulders and around the neck. The most common acne spots are open comedones (blackheads), closed comedones (whiteheads), papules, pustules, nodules (firm swellings below the skin) and cysts (larger, fluid-filled swellings in the skin). Frustratingly, as spots heal, others tend to appear and the scars they leave often appear as small, depressed pits.

The increase in natural oils that are produced from the scalp often leads to acne around the hairline. This condition is compounded by putting hot oils or pomades on the hair. In the same way, using cosmetics with oily bases leads to an increased tendency to acne. If you do suffer from acne, regular contact with mineral or cooking oils such as in a restaurant kitchen can make the condition worse, so pick your Saturday job with care.

Over-the-counter or prescribed topical treatments (applied to the skin) such as benzoyl peroxide, retinoic acid, antibiotic lotions and creams containing sulphur act by unblocking pores and removing sebum, and promote healing. Ultra-violet light is also known to be beneficial, so get out in the sunshine or take an occasional sun-bed. If topical treatment fails, long-term therapy (lasting at least three months) using oral antibiotics often helps.

In the case of severe acne, the use of retinoid drugs can improve the condition, but these will not usually be prescribed until other forms of treatment have failed, and must be used cautiously because they can lead to liver damage. They can also cause foetal malformation, so must not be given to a woman who might become pregnant.

Acne cysts can be treated by intralesional therapy (injection of drugs into the acne spot) which can help prevent scarring. For those who already carry severe acne scars, dermabrasion (removal of the top layer of affected skin under general anaesthetic) is occasionally used to improve the appearance. However, you will still be left with a rough complexion and it is an extremely painful treatment that would only be considered as a last option in extreme cases.

Some beauty salons offer a cosmetic treatment for mild acne scarring whereby collagen is injected into small acne pits to plump them out. It is reported to give perceptible results but the effects are not permanent and the treatment has to be performed repeatedly.

THE HALE APPROACH

Acne, whilst socially debilitating and personally disfiguring, is rarely a life-threatening condition and treatment can therefore be sought from complementary practitioners as a first line. Orthodox treatments are rarely prescribed on the basis of looking for an underlying cause of the condition, and therefore tend to be effective when they are being used, but not always in the long term. Complementary treatments will examine your entire lifestyle and are far more likely to help find a cure.

Oxypeel is exceedingly effective in the treatment of both acne and the scarring it causes. After the treatment, the acne rarely returns.

However, if patients wish to address the hormonal imbalance which originally aggravated the condition, then homeopathy, acupuncture, Ayurveda and Irish herbs or nutritional therapy can be of great benefit. If the acne seems to be strong related to a person's mental state, hypnosis may be helpful.

NUTRITION

In the treatment of acne the aim of nutritional therapy is to balance the hormones that cause the sebaceous glands to produce too much sebum. To achieve this the nutritionist would employ detoxification, identification and treatment of any food allergies, and treatment of any underlying diseases that might be causing the acne. A total cure can be achieved after three to six sessions.

AYURVEDA

According to the principles of Ayurvedic medicine, acne is caused by stagnation of *doshas* (humours or channels) in the body. The main *doshas* involved are *Vata* (air – the driving force, controlling the nervous system and all the energies in the body) and *Pitta* (fire – all digestive and metabolic processes, bile, enzymes, etc). In certain cases the third *dosha*, *Kapha* (phlegm, fat, water, lymphatics, mucous membranes) may also need attention. 'A complete cleansing is the way to improvement,' says one Ayurvedic practitioner. 'Mainly *panchakarma* (revitalizing) therapy would be given for detoxification. A suitable diet would consist of mainly low-acidic foods, with no meat or dairy products.'

ACUPUNCTURE

According to Chinese medicine, if the spleen is weak it produces phlegm and blocks proper liver function. A stressed liver produces excess heat. Heat and phlegm combine to cause congestion along the meridian that flows from the abdomen to the face, and this leads to skin trouble. Acupuncture tones the spleen and relaxes the liver, removing the phlegm and preventing a recurrence of the complaint. Once blood can travel freely, skin problems disappear.

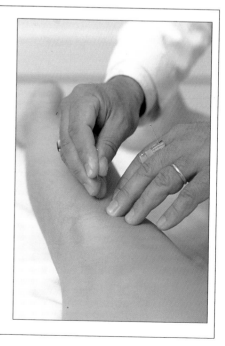

HOMEOPATHY

Because a homeopathic remedy is a highly diluted form of a natural substance that, in a full-strength dose, would produce the symptoms of the illness in a healthy person, symptoms sometimes get worse before they improve. This means that an acne sufferer may see more spots emerge before a homeopathic remedy produces a cure. Be patient.

Homeopaths treat each patient individually but, as a gross generalization, Kali bichromicum is recommended for chronic acne, and Sulphur for infected pustules that get worse after washing. When Sulphur aggravates, Hepar. sulph., Rhus tox and Ignatia often give good results. If the cause of the problem is an imbalance or a sensitivity to the male hormone testosterone, remedies may be given to rebalance this. Psorinum is a good general remedy.

HYPNOTHERAPY

Hypnotherapy relies on the therapeutic use of hypnosis to diagnose, treat and cure a condition. According to one hypnotherapist our skins can be viewed as a projection screen on to which our emotions are thrown. When we are embarrassed, for example, we blush. The natural progression of this theory is to accept that skin conditions can sometimes be an expression of an underlying emotional problem or repressed emotions. 'I take a thorough case history and listen carefully to the person,' says the hypnotherapist. 'With any talking therapy, the co-operation between the practitioner and patient must be there or else you will not advance. My work is only the offering of guidance – it is the client who leads me and not the other way round. My words are dictated by what they say to me. But I do encounter people with very bad acne and they can be helped.'

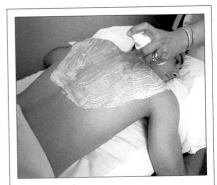

OXYPEEL

Oxypeel treatments work on the principle of biological exfoliation gradually removing the blemished layers and/or disintegrating the cells, which are then replaced naturally by healthy skin. The treatments are based on well-researched and balanced formulations using therapeutic chemicals, enzymes and natural plant extracts. 'Oxypeel treatments are progressive in nature,' their inventor explains. 'An improvement is apparent after two to three treatments, but the number required would depend upon the severity of symptoms. Oxypeel treatments were introduced in 1983. The formulations are constantly being reviewed and sometimes they are adjusted to meet the specific needs of a patient.'

SUPPORTIVE TREATMENTS

Healing/Chi Kung
Used in conjunction with other complementary therapies and a healthy diet, both these treatments – which are based on rebalancing the body's energies – can be beneficial for acne. A healer channels energy from an outside force into the patient to rebalance the body. Chi Kung (a traditional Chinese therapy which uses seven basic exercises, often in conjunction with the eight fundamental T'ai Chi exercises) is especially useful for dealing with the causes and results of acne such as adolescent emotional problems, embarrassment over appearance, resentment, etc. Skin 'chi breathing' helps alleviate superficial symptoms.

SELF-CARE

Flower Remedies
Although there are several flower essences from which to choose for skin conditions, Luffa (Pegasus) and Spinifex (Australian Bush) are particularly recommended for acne.

Nutrition
Obviously, you can continue to follow a diet prescribed by a nutritional therapist after your regular treatment has ended, and any improvement should be maintained. In general terms you should avoid refined carbohydrates, red meat, tannin, caffeine, inorganic iron (i.e. iron supplements, because they are constipating and antagonistic to Vitamin E), female hormones found in milk, and extra iodine (found in some table salt). Eat a low-fat diet and use corn (maize) oil for cooking. The group of fatty acids known as Omega 6 have been shown to be beneficial in combating acne.

TIP

Wash affected skin twice daily to prevent spreading spots - washing any more frequently will simply dry out the skin. Tempting though it may be, spots should not under any circumstances be picked or squeezed. This only worsens the condition and can lead to scarring.

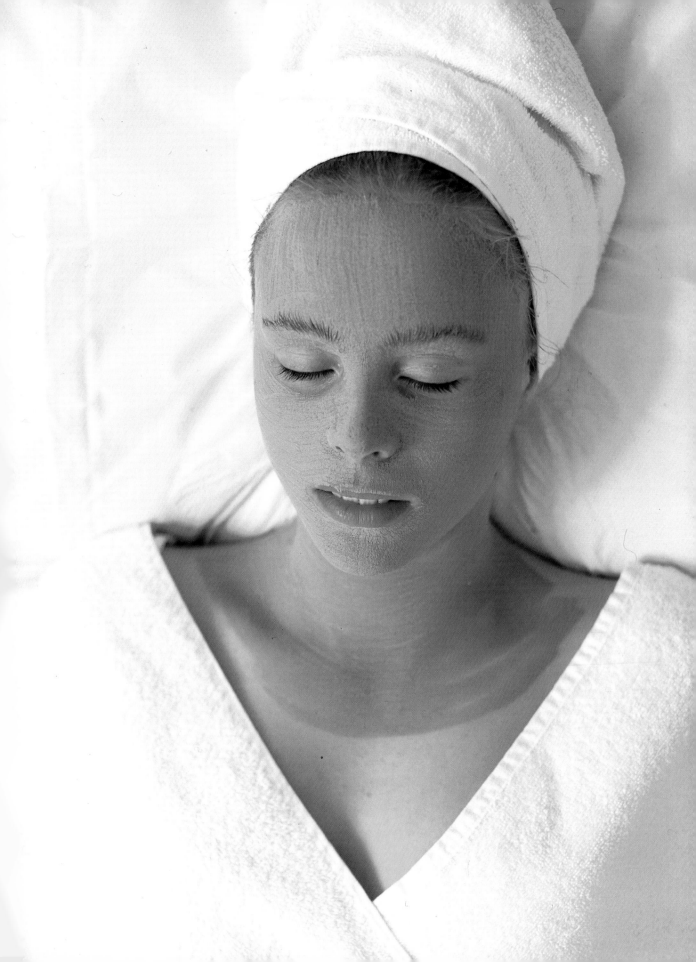

Allergies

You get an allergy when you develop a super-sensitivity to something that normally doesn't cause any problems. For example, peanuts are normally a tasty snack but for an unlucky few they can be a death sentence. Your mouth and throat swell up, you can't breathe and if you don't get a shot of adrenaline quickly you may die. Most allergies aren't deadly, but they can make life miserable.

Often allergies appear at the point where the allergen comes into contact with the body. The red, flaking, scaly skin of eczema (see page 74) may be a response to washing powder; the nose and eyes of a hay-fever sufferer run when they pick up pollen; a few people get swollen lips from eating eggs, others sneeze uncontrollably anywhere near a cat.

Although almost every part of the body can be affected with different symptoms by an allergy, the underlying mechanism is the same – a mistake by the immune system. We all have blood cells called lymphocytes which are the body's home guard, constantly on the look-out for invaders such as bacteria and viruses. When they come across something that they recognize as not part of the body's own proteins they produce antigens, which in turn produce antibodies (known as IgE) to neutralize it. When someone has an allergy, for reasons that are not yet clear, normally harmless substances like dust mites, cat hair or shellfish trigger off those antibodies. The swelling and redness are caused because the IgE antigens cause cells in body tissue, called mast cells, to produce histamine and other chemicals, which can quickly produce all sorts of effects from a runny nose or wheezy chest to a skin rash or upset stomach.

The IgE reaction provides the medical profession with a convenient marker of an allergy response. You can find it, for example, in people who have been poisoned by shellfish once and ever after react with immediate nausea and vomiting to the merest morsel of it. Some doctors do allow that a food may be associated with some chronic condition and in such cases they will advise either a skin test – putting tiny samples of possible culprits on the skin for 24 hours to see if any produce a reaction – or an elimination diet – removing certain foods from the diet to see if the condition clears up.

The most obvious approach is to find out what is causing the allergic reaction and avoid it. When something is hard to avoid, like pollen, then the most direct way of reducing the effect of histamine is with another body chemical called adrenaline. There is now a range of anti-histamine drugs based on adrenaline which are useful for conditions like hay fever or nettle rash.

Another approach is the vaccination. Minute amounts of whatever it is the patient is sensitive to – pollen, bee stings, etc. – are injected so that the real thing stops having such a dramatic effect. Corticosteroids are also prescribed in severe cases.

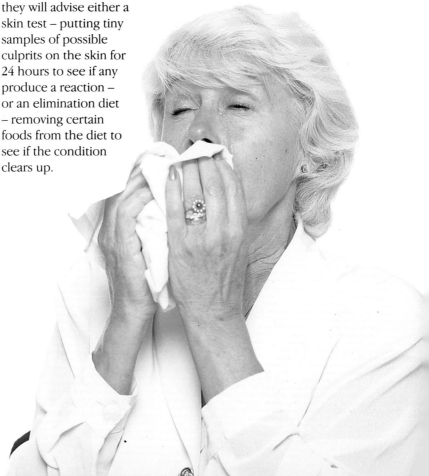

THE HALE APPROACH

Complementary treatments for allergy are safe and more effective at isolating a cause and therefore finding a more permanent cure; orthodox treatment is only symptomatic. You can therefore consult a complementary practitioner without the necessity of involving your doctor.

When looking at the subject of allergy, there are three key issues to keep in mind:

1. The identification of the allergy
2. The fact that some people will be allergic to certain substances, e.g. shampoos, no matter how healthy they are otherwise
3. The need to bring the body back to a state where it is not allergic.

The Hale Clinic would recommend a variety of tests to identify the cause of the allergy. The practitioner's input can be invaluable here, especially if the 'agent' causing an allergic reaction is an unusual one. The patient can then either remove the substance permanently from their diet or lifestyle, or have a vaccination which will build up a tolerance to the offending substance (see below under *Nutrition/Allergy Treatment* for further details).

If a patient wishes to pursue the treatment of allergies further, the question needs to be asked – why are some people 'allergic' and some people apparently not? Most allergies are caused by a weakness in the immune system, which is where treatments such as homeopathy, acupuncture, Ayurveda, the Buteyko Method and colonic irrigation can be of great assistance, strengthening the whole system so that the body is less likely to exhibit allergic symptoms. Supportive treatments such as healing, light therapy, Chi Kung, Shiatsu, remedial yoga and aromatherapy also offer that sort of help – strengthening the body in order to eradicate the allergic response.

If a patient suffers from a multitude of allergies, it is particularly advisable to follow this second approach as well as avoiding the *main* causes of allergic response. The Hale Clinic would not encourage a course of treatment whereby the patient ended up able to eat only two or three foods. If a patient is that badly affected, it is essential for their immune system to be strengthened, not for foods to be continually removed from their diet.

NUTRITION/ALLERGY TREATMENT

The digestive system is the key to our health, which is why many of the chronic illnesses and low-grade symptoms – aches and pains, swellings, frequent minor infections, insomnia, regular stomach upsets – are due to hidden food allergies. Conditions associated with food allergies include migraine, eczema, thrombosis, arthritis, colitis, ear infection and childhood hyperactivity. When the digestive system is working properly, allergies are not a problem, but stress, a modern diet of refined foods and high fats, antibiotics and a range of other factors can reduce its efficiency. When this happens, partially digested food particles can leak from the gut into the bloodstream, where they trigger off an immune response, which resembles an allergic response.

Yet it is not only the conventional IgE response but also an IgG response, produced by the B lymphocytes system, which shows the existence of food allergies and can be easily tested for. The IgG antibodies tag on to the food particles, signalling to the clean-up cells in the blood that they should be removed. When the removal system is overwhelmed, these tagged particles are dumped all over the body, where they cause chemical reactions that in turn produce those runny noses, stiff joints and constricted blood vessels of the typical allergic response.

Once the allergic foods have been identified with a blood test they are eliminated from the diet and the patient is encouraged to vary his food intake, not having the same foods within four days while the digestive system repairs itself. Selenium, zinc, Vitamin B complex and thymus extract can help supply necessary nutrients during this period. The bioflavonoid (an extract of plant material) quercetin can reduce the amount of histamine produced by the mast cells, as can Vitamin C and bromelain.

Checks will also be made for an imbalance in the bacteria in the gut, liver problems or a candida infection which can make the bowel more leaky.

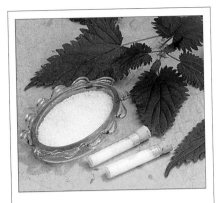

HOMEOPATHY

Although homeopathy normally takes a holistic, constitutional approach, it is possible to treat the specific symptoms of certain allergies. So in the case of urticaria or hives, for instance, there is one treatment – Apis – for burning and swelling of lips and eyelids, made worse by warmth, and another – Urtica – for a rash caused by stinging nettles made worse by touching, scratching or bathing with water. There are others for hay fever, middle-ear infections, hyperactivity and so on.

Desensitization – giving progressively stronger doses of what causes the problem – can work in some cases, but the condition may return more strongly after a few months. If you suspect a food allergy there are a number of remedies given for specific effects. For instance:
• When cold foods make the symptoms worse – Arsenicum, Culcamara or Nux. When raw foods make the symptoms worse – Pulsatilla, Ruta or Veratrum.
• When milk makes the symptoms worse – Aethusa, Calcarea or China.

There are also specific remedies for candidiasis, the fungal infection which can cause a leaky gut.

BIOENERGETICS

A combination of bioenergetic testing and homeopathy can pinpoint and treat not only the allergic reaction but also the underlying cause which originally aggravated it. Unless the endocrine system is rebalanced, the symptoms of one desensitized allergy will quickly be replaced by another. By treating the causative factor, bioenergetics aims to ensure an overall return to health.

BIOLOGICAL MEDICINE

Food allergies can take many different forms – from stomach aches and rashes to fatigue, aching joints and depression. First tests are done to pinpoint the foods involved. There are three ways of detecting them: an elimination diet, cytotoxic testing (which checks for anything that may be toxic to the cells) and a blood test for IgG4 antigens. You can then either simply cut the offending foods out of your diet or, if you want to be able to carry on eating them, you can have regular shots of a vaccine – known as Enzyme Potentiated Desensitization (EPD) – which gradually restores the body's tolerance of those foods. Anything between three and twelve vaccinations over one to two years are needed to remove most or all allergic responses.

A similar procedure is followed for inhalant allergies, such as hay fever. In these cases the test is for IgE antibodies and far fewer vaccine shots are required. One or two may clear up hay fever completely.

BUTEYKO

Teaching people to breathe correctly ensures that the level of carbon dioxide in the lungs is the correct one. Everyone who has an allergy breathes too much, diluting their supply of carbon dioxide. When the CO_2 levels are down this has a direct effect on the immune system, because CO_2 is one of the key regulatory chemicals in the body: a lack of CO_2 means that the antigens in the body do not bind to foreign material as fast as they should.

In some allergies the problem is that the body has become super-sensitive to a given substance. Correcting the CO_2 levels can bring the threshold of sensitivity back to normal.

Bona fide Buteyko practitioners offer a money-back guarantee of substantial improvement for any allergy patient they agree to treat.

COLONIC HYDROTHERAPY

This involves a gentle flushing out of the colon with warm, purified water (with the possible addition of herbal or other implants) to remove accumulated matter. The effect of the treatment is the detoxification of the system as a whole and, more specfically, of the colon or large intestine. This allows the colon to function much more efficiently in terms of absorption, mobility, bacterial balance and elimination of waste. Colonic hydrotherapists also look at the patient's nutrition and often recommend avoiding certain foods, such as dairy products.

SUPPORTIVE TREATMENTS

Healing
'We can work on the adrenal cortex to produce more cortisone – the body hormone that is anti-inflammatory,' explains one healer. 'If the patient comes with swellings or rashes we can get rid of them. Healing also speeds up the circulation to clear out allergens through the kidneys as quickly as possible.'

Light Therapy
This is generally relaxing and improves circulation which has an overall beneficial effect on allergies. It can be particularly helpful in the case of inflammations on the skin such as eczema and psoriasis.

Trichology
Topical preparations are used to soothe the skin and reduce irritation. In some cases a low-powered laser is used to reduce the level of inflammation. Patients are advised to avoid substances to which they are sensitive. They are also recommended to make lifestyle changes such as cutting out alcohol and spicy food and reducing their intake of refined carbohydrate. Most patients experience results within two months.

Chi Kung
There are exercises – which vary for each individual – that will concentrate energy and transfer it to the part of the body that is causing problems. Once mastered, the Chi Kung exercises are ideal for self-care at home.

Shiatsu
Eczema, hay fever and asthma are the most common expressions of allergies and all are exacerbated by stress. Shiatsu massage balances and relaxes the whole of the body and, coupled with specific dietary advice and exercise, can dramatically alleviate the symptoms of allergy.

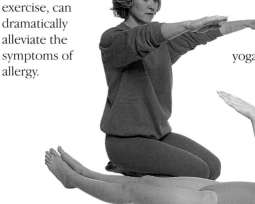

Aromatherapy
Peppermint is often used to relieve hay fever symptoms, as it helps to clear the head. Chamomile and lemon balm are useful both for hay fever and for allergic skin reactions.

Remedial Yoga
Allergies occur as a result of a hypersensitivity in tissues of the body, and yoga is one way to bring the body back to a more centred and balanced response to our environment. Yoga is also valuable because allergies often involve the adrenal system, which becomes overworked by stress, and yoga helps reduce the effects of stress. Allergies create a feeling that the body is under attack and yoga returns an element of control.

Jala Neti – 'nasal washing', taught at the Hale Clinic by a remedial yoga teacher – can also help with hay fever. You can learn the technique in one 30-minute session and will then be able to practise it at home.

SELF-CARE

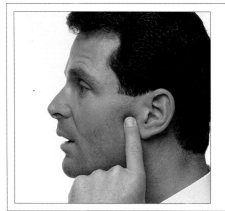

Indian Medicine
Pressure points: find the point where the upper and lower jaw meet on the left side and press it for 30 seconds once a day.

Diet: Drink a minimum of eight glasses of water throughout the day. Have no fried foods but eat papaya.

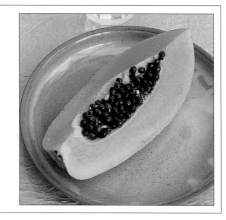

Dermatitis & Eczema

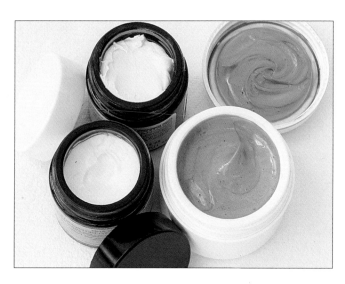

THE ORTHODOX APPROACH

Applying corticosteroids and/or other drugs to kill the micro-organisms is often helpful. Difficult though it may be, it is important to avoid scratching and, as far as possible, exposure to irritants such as detergents.

In the case of contact dermatitis, the rash is a reaction to some substance that comes into contact with the skin. It may be a direct toxic effect or an allergic response. People who cannot wear cheap pierced earrings without getting sore ears are experiencing a form of contact dermatitis. The most common causes of irritant and allergic contact dermatitis are detergents, nickel (e.g. in bracelets, watch straps, necklaces, fasteners on underwear), chemicals (e.g. in rubber gloves and condoms), certain plants (e.g. ragweed), certain cosmetics and some medication in the form of creams, lotions or drops. The rash may be treated with corticosteroid medication and, obviously, further contact with the cause of the rash should be avoided. If the cause is not known, it may be possible to identify the offending substance using a patch test.

Photodermatitis occurs in those whose skin is abnormally sensitive to sunlight. The numerous people who complain of heat rash (itchy spots or blisters that appear in the sun or very hot weather) during their holidays are simply experiencing photodermatitis in its most basic form.

The price we pay for living in a modern, civilized, sanitized convenience world is that we are in contact with more pollutants, additives, chemicals and detergents than ever before. As a direct result, the incidence of allergies has exploded in recent years. Allergies can take many forms (see page 70 for further details), but when manifested as an inflammation of the skin, an allergic reaction is often diagnosed as dermatitis – better known as eczema. That said, there are cases where dermatitis appears without any known cause but, in its commonest form, atopic dermatitis usually affects people with a family history of asthma (see page 132) and hay fever (see under *Allergies,* page 70), the other common allergies. The other most prevalent forms are seborrhoeic dermatitis and contact dermatitis (eczema).

Seborrhoeic dermatitis is a red, scaly, itchy rash that develops on the face (particularly the nose and eyebrows), scalp, chest and back. On the scalp, it is the most common form of dandruff. The rash often develops at times of stress but its exact cause is not known. It is believed to be an overreaction to the natural yeasts in the skin and it seems that keeping the yeast levels low helps to keep the condition at bay.

THE HALE APPROACH

Orthodox treatment of dermatitis and eczema is geared towards suppression of symptoms, with little time or effort spent in isolating the cause. Provided your skin problem is not spreading rapidly, itching to the point of distraction, bleeding or looking infected (with areas of pus or discharge), then treatment along a complementary line is your first step. Topical steroids may be stopped, but it is better to do this under the care of a complementary practitioner.

As with psoriasis, both nutrition and stress can play a role in precipitating eczema and other skin problems. The Hale Clinic would first recommend nutritional advice to see if any allergies were aggravating the condition – often dairy foods are the culprit. Sugar, saturated fats and alcohol can also contribute to the problem. In fact, any foods which put an excessive strain on the liver should be avoided. For some patients adjusting diet is sufficient to prevent eczema, although the changes may have to be permanent if the problem is to be kept at bay. Others may need to combine nutrition with other complementary treatments in order to be able to return to a less restricted diet.

Homeopathy, Ayurveda and acupuncture are all very effective in dealing with eczema and strengthening a patient's constitution, although with homeopathy the condition often becomes worse for a short period before clearing up. All these treatments will also reduce the patient's stress level, which is often a major contributing factor to the complaint.

Hypnotherapy can be very helpful in treating eczema, particularly where it is stress-related. Often the physical condition disappears completely after a change in the patient's mental attitude. Healing can also be effective, calming the mind and relieving physical symptoms.

The support treatments of aromatherapy and reflexology are also of benefit and trichology can help with any hair problems associated with eczema.

In combination with any of the above treatments T'ai Chi, Chi Kung and yoga will further enhance the healing process.

ACUPUNCTURE

In the main, acupuncturists associate eczema with exposure to heat, damp or wind. Treatment would therefore be based on counteracting the effects of these elements and trying to correct any blood or energy deficiencies that may result. Needles would be inserted along the meridians corresponding to the lungs, large intestine, spleen and stomach. You could hope to see improvement and, in some cases, a total disappearance of the problem in four to eight sessions.

An acupuncturist may recommend a special diet that involves avoiding all alcoholic drinks, coffee, fats and dairy products. A nutritionist may also be involved in helping to work out a specific diet.

HOMEOPATHY

Given that homeopathy treats the body as a whole rather than specific complaints, a homeopath views eczema as an outward sign of an underlying disorder. Obviously, treatment depends on each individual's very personal case and this can be further complicated if they have previously been prescribed steroid creams by an orthodox practitioner. However, in general terms, Graphites are said to be effective, particularly if the eczema oozes a sticky fluid. If the eczema is particularly itchy at night or if it releases a watery discharge, Petroleum is recommended. If the itching becomes intolerable, Sulphur may be suggested, but its effects should be closely monitored as it often aggravates; in these cases Hepar. sulph., Rhus tox. and Ignatia often give good results.

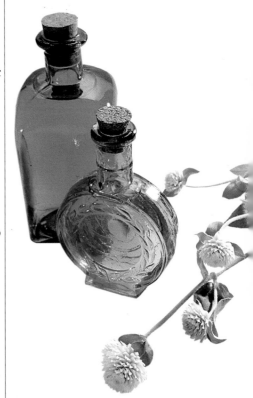

AYURVEDA

As Ayurveda is a holistic system, a dermatitis condition is never treated in isolation. After a consultation in which you will be asked about your private and professional life, your medical history and eating habits, and given a physical examination, a course of treatment will be recommended. The Ayurvedic method is reported to have had particular success in treating eczema.

'This problem could be caused by physical or mental reasons, or simply due to imbalances in the body, or even environmental factors or bad dietary habits,' explains one Ayurvedic physician. Correctly recognizing the cause is imperative in working out the treatment programme. In general, oral preparations are very effective. Including various herbs, according to the individual constitution, may also prove helpful.

'Cleansing is also needed,' continues the physician. 'Maintaining a quality of appetite is an important factor, as are good bowel movements to prevent an accumulation of toxins in the system. *Panchakarma* (detoxification) treatment is essential.'

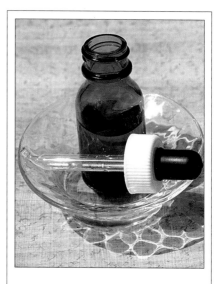

SUPPORTIVE TREATMENTS

There are a number of supportive treatments that can complement, enhance and, in some cases, accelerate the healing effects of the above therapies. Dermatitis patients have successfully combined the beneficial effects of nutrition (dietary advice and investigation of food intolerances), Buteyko (changing breathing patterns can affect eczema), aromatherapy (the use of essential oils for massage, inhalation or bathing), reflexology (stimulation of pressure points on the feet), hypnotherapy (a therapist induces a state of consciousness between wakefulness and sleep during which time the unconscious healing powers of the body and mind are released), healing (the channelled effects of spiritual energy), Chi Kung (a series of exercises described as 'meditation in movement') and trichology (study and diagnosis using the hair and scalp) as supportive treatments to other complementary therapies.

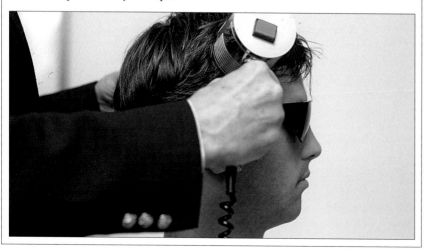

SELF-CARE

Flower Remedies
Depending on the cause of your eczema – does it flare up when you are under stress, for example? – and how you react to the condition, a number of Bach flower remedies might be appropriate. If you are embarrassed by the appearance of your eczema, Crab Apple can decrease these feelings, and Clematis and Mimulus help to combat over-sensitivity. Bach Rescue Remedy cream can bring relief when rubbed on the affected areas.

For the skin condition itself, Lily (Petite Fleur) or Billy Goat Plum (Australian Bush) flower essences may be recommended.

Nutrition
If you notice that your dermatitis is worse or appears after eating certain foodstuffs, these should naturally be avoided. Frequent causes of allergies are milk and milk products, so watch out for these. Other foodstuffs to regard with suspicion are saturated fats, dairy products, alcohol, citrus fruits and, some say, chocolate.

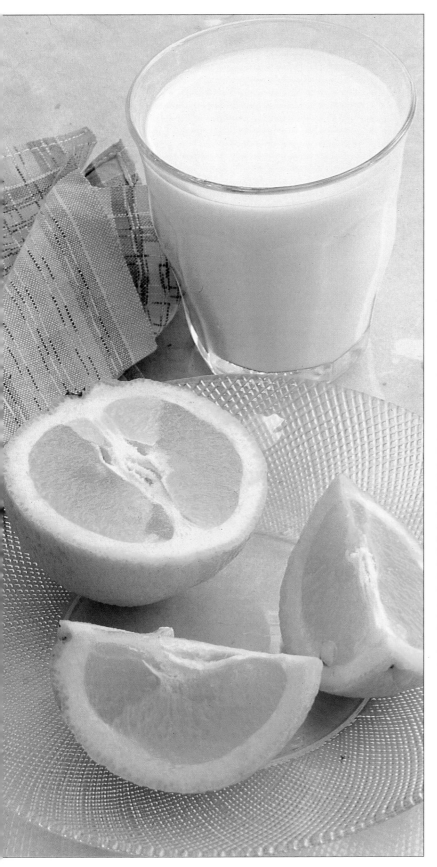

DANDRUFF

Contrary to workplace taunts, dandruff has nothing whatsoever to do with cleanliness or how often you wash your hair. It is a common and harmless condition in which dead skin cells are shed from the scalp, often producing the characteristic white specks or flakes seen on the collar and shoulders of clothes or in the hair. Dandruff can cause great embarrassment but with vigilance it can be controlled, although sadly it is rarely cured.

Although it is possible to treat dandruff, it is far better to take advice on improving your lifestyle and diet, which may be causing the complaint. If you have a tendency to dandruff, a poor diet or stressed living pattern is a good reason for the problem to recur.

Anti-dandruff shampoos should not be used indiscriminately, since they can overstimulate the activity of the oil gland, so you end up swapping one problem for another. Instead, try using a neutral, non-scented, low pH shampoo that is less likely to disturb or aggravate the problem, and keep other styling products right away from the scalp.

If these measures do not clear up the dandruff, or if it recurs repeatedly, take advice from a trichologist or dermatologist.

Two common causes of allergic reactions

Psoriasis

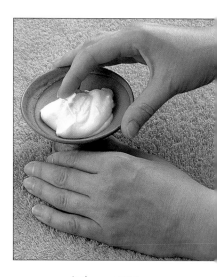

Sufferers from this common skin disease can undergo great discomfort and social embarrassment. It can ruin the summer months – psoriasis victims often prefer to keep their bodies under wraps while others are stripping off around them. The condition is not usually itchy but its appearance often makes a sufferer feel very uncomfortable in unfamiliar social situations. Sadly for those affected, psoriasis is a long-term condition with no permanent cure.

Nonetheless, the good news is that individual attacks can be treated and relieved to a large degree. Although the cause of psoriasis is not known, it tends to run in families, suggesting a genetic link. Somewhere in the region of 2 per cent of Europeans and Americans contract the disease and it is less common in black and Asian communities. Symptoms usually appear for the first time in those in the 10 to 30-year-old age bracket.

Psoriasis sufferers produce new skin cells ten times faster than normal. This causes the patchy, thickened skin effect which may be covered by silvery scales. Recurrent attacks are often triggered by emotional stress, skin damage and physical illness. Symptoms are sometimes accompanied by painful swelling and stiffness of the joints, which can be very disabling.

There are several different types of psoriasis, but discoid or 'plaque' psoriasis is far and away the most common form. It is distinguished by patches of inflamed, scaly skin on the trunk and limbs, appearing particularly on the elbows, knees and scalp. Additionally, a sufferer's nails may become pitted, thickened or separated from their beds. Guttate psoriasis is the form most frequently found in children: small patches appear rapidly over a wide area, often after the child has had a sore throat.

THE ORTHODOX APPROACH

Whatever the form of your psoriasis, if it is a mild case, you may find it helps to expose your skin to the sun or to an ultra-violet lamp, but make sure that it is only in small doses. An emollient (moisturizing cream) can also help. If an attack worsens, it is usually treated with an ointment containing coal tar or dithranol. Other options include PUVA (a type of phototherapy), corticosteroids and other drugs such as methotrexate. Psoriasis sufferers who experience accompanying arthritis may be treated with non-steroidal anti-inflammatory drugs (NSAIDs), anti-rheumatic drugs or methotrexate.

THE HALE APPROACH

While potentially disfiguring and socially disrupting, psoriasis is not in itself dangerous, unless the lesions become secondarily infected by bacteria, which is rare. Psoriasis sufferers may, however, develop severe arthritis and certain bowel problems that can be extremely serious. It is wise to have your condition monitored by a doctor, although most treatment should come from complementary therapists.

Given the key role stress or emotional trauma often plays in the onset of psoriasis, it is vitally important that a patient chooses a complementary treatment that will help relieve stress, such as hypnosis, homeopathy, acupuncture or healing. In addition a self-care programme of relaxation, using self-hypnosis tapes, meditation or flower remedies is recommended in order to prevent a recurrence of the condition.

Nutrition and detoxification play a very important part in the treatment of psoriasis. Trichology addresses the patient's diet as well as providing creams for the external treatment of the symptoms, while light therapy and tangent therapy give useful support.

HYPNOTHERAPY

Some hypnotherapists and psychotherapists claim to have had considerable success using hypnotherapy in treating psoriasis. They believe that the condition can very often be a reflection of repressed emotions. During the course of the initial consultation, a thorough case history would be taken and treatment would be geared to the patient's individual requirements. Role playing while in a hypnotic state may be included.

HOMEOPATHY

One three-point programme used to treat psoriasis includes taking a case history, which lasts about an hour and from which the practitioner decides on the homeopathic remedy that is best suited to the individual patient. Stage two is treatment with nutritional supplements such as algae with acidopholus. The third step involves Neen oil, a rare cream from India, which works by softening the skin. It is an antiseptic and clears up the psoriasis topically. Depending on the severity of the case, the condition may be cleared in as little as three months. The practitioner may then continue to prescribe nutritional supplements so that patients can help themselves at home.

One homeopath reports an 80 per cent improvement in some psoriasis cases, while other cases do not respond at all. If homeopathy is to work for you, you should expect in the region of five sessions to get results. Dietary changes and possibly some supplements may also be helpful, especially zinc and fish oil or linseed oil.

AYURVEDA

According to Ayurvedic medicine, psoriasis is the result of an accumulation of doshas or toxins in the organs of the body, and of an imbalance of the five elements. A course of treatment may vary from six months to two years or longer, according to the individual condition and the extent to which is has spread on the skin. The main purpose of the treatment is a long-term detoxification of every part of the body, especially the organs.

Full treatment consists of *panchakarma*, oral Ayurvedic preparations, external Ayurvedic applications, changes to diet and management of stress through yoga, relaxation and breathing techniques.

ACUPUNCTURE

In acupuncture, diagnosis and therapy are aimed at identifying any imbalance in the body's energy flow and correcting it by inserting needles at appropriate points. For psoriasis, needles would be inserted not only on the meridians dealing with the skin but also on those governing the underlying causes of the condition - stress, anxiety or allergies, for example.

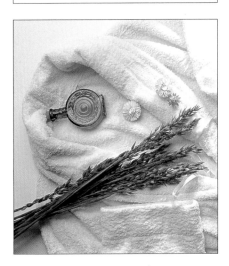

NUTRITION

Psoriasis is characterized by increased cell proliferation and there are certain foods (containing the toxic metabolites collectively known as polyamines) that exacerbate the condition. Such foods include alcohol, all sugars, animal fats (including dairy products), meats and glutens (wheat, oats, barley), and should be reduced or avoided altogether. An increase in oily fish (200g/7oz daily is recommended) has been shown to help the condition, as have the supplements of flaxseed oil, selenium and zinc.

SUPPORTIVE TREATMENTS

Healing
Energy from an outside force is channelled through a healer, not only to clear up the skin condition but also to look deeper at its root causes and deal with those.

Tangent Therapy
As it is acknowledged that stress is a common trigger for psoriasis, relaxing essential oils may be recommended. These may be put in the bath or applied topically as a compress. The best oils for this condition are cajeput, juniper or lavender in a carrier oil of calendula. Oatmeal baths with acidophilus are also helpful.

Trichology
Psoriasis is a complex skin condition which may affect widespread areas of the body or occur on isolated areas alone. It is a condition rather than a disease (i.e. it is a result of altered metabolism). Causative factors vary, but while it is acknowledged that hereditary influence may be the link, the problem, if not a congenital one, may be triggered by both physical and emotional trauma at any age. Direct measures in, around and in addition to shampooing routines may consist of products designed to remove scale (keratolytics), calm skin and counter inflammatory effects. Each case has to be assessed individually in terms of its duration, severity and specific features. Often patients benefit from a combination of home and clinic routine.

Light Therapy
Light therapy treats psoriasis symptomically by concentrating light on the outbreak areas and holistically by improving circulation, thereby providing the body with the nutrients it needs to rid itself of the condition.

SELF-CARE

Stress Management
A person suffering from psoriasis can train him or herself to relax and unwind in a few quiet moments. Relaxation and self-hypnosis techniques can be taught, and patients working by themselves can produce good results in stress management.

Flower Remedies
Bach flowers and the extended range of flower essences work on all levels at the same time – emotionally, psychologically and physically – so, in one therapist's words, 'they are great for getting to the root of the stress pattern which caused the physical symptoms in the first place'. For psoriasis, Vanilla Leaf (Pacific), Aloe Vera (FES), Luffa (Pegasus) and Spinifex (Australian Bush) are particularly recommended.

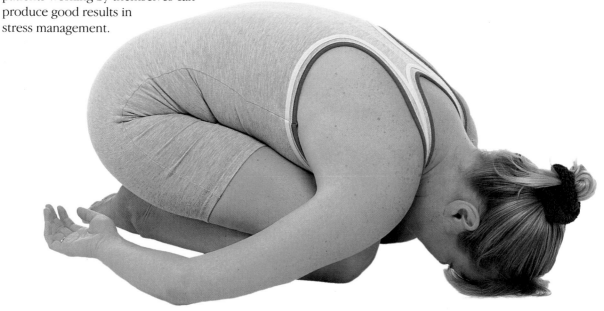

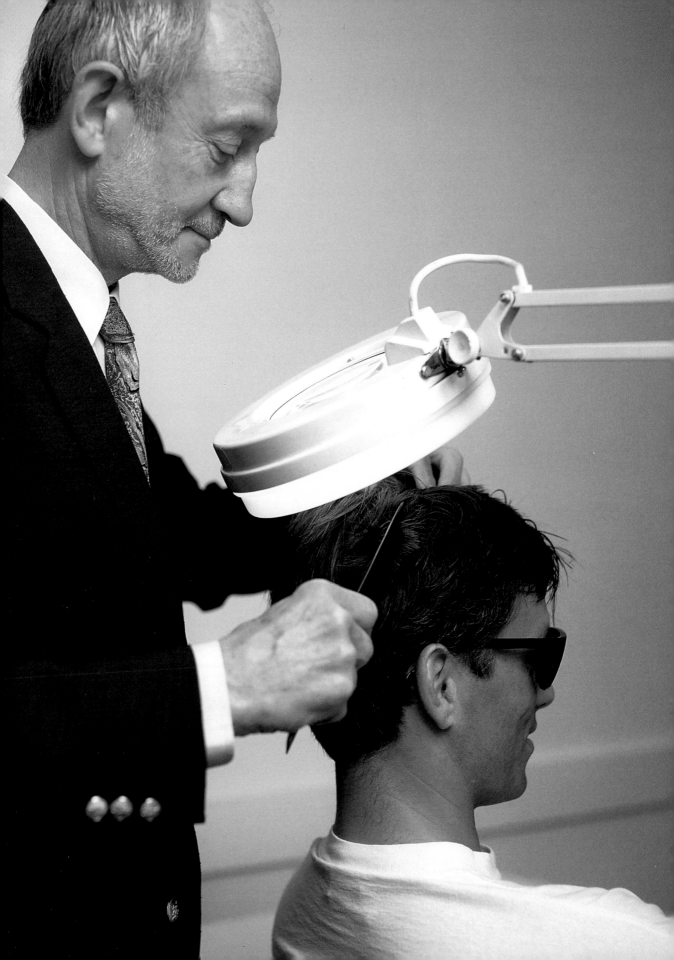

Hair Care

The texture, pattern, density and natural colour of your hair is completely out of your control. That is to say, it depends on heredity, and no amount of wishing for straight hair or blonde locks can change it (unless you resort to the bottle or the hairdresser).

However, the look and condition of your hair lies very much in your own hands since it is largely affected by your general health, hair hygiene, choice of hair products (shampoos, conditioners, mousses, etc.) and grooming equipment (combs, brushes, curling tongs, hair driers, etc.). Almost any illness or emotional stress can result in lifeless, dull hair and so it is a truism to say that healthy hair reflects a healthy body and mind.

On average, hair grows at a rate of about 13mm (½in) a month. Inexplicably, it grows more quickly at night than during the day and faster in summer than in winter. It is the hair's thin coating of sebum (a natural oil secreted by the scalp's sebaceous glands) that keeps it looking supple and shiny, so caring for your scalp is just as important as looking after the hair itself.

If you have no obvious hair problems such as dandruff (see page 77) or any form of alopecia, healthy hair can be maintained by washing hair and scalp regularly and eating an adequate, balanced diet. There are no hard and fast rules as to how frequently hair should be washed – if your hair is particularly greasy, it could be as often as every day, in which case a mild or 'frequent use' shampoo should be used. Those with dry hair should avoid over-washing and could benefit from professional treatment.

In our attempts to improve one of our most striking assets, we can sometimes do our hair more harm than good. Dyeing, bleaching, relaxing and perming can all damage the hair, but even using such apparently innocuous items as plastic brushes, metal combs and rollers can have a detrimental effect. Similarly, strong sunshine, sea water and chlorinated swimming pools can all dry the hair and scalp, so take preventative measures such as wearing a swimming cap, and protecting your hair with a hat in strong sunshine.

To prevent tearing the hair, which leads to split ends, avoid using sharp combs or brushes, and comb it gently when it's wet. Wherever possible, towel dry; if you must use a hair dryer, keep it at least 15cm (6in) from your head and on a medium rather than a high setting.
In fact, hair loss is a process that continues unremarked throughout our lives when the old hair drops out to make way for new growth (a healthy adult normally sheds between fifty and a hundred hairs each day). However, it can become more apparent at certain times – in the case of women, due to hormonal changes after childbirth and during menopause, and, irrespective of sex, after taking some drugs for the treatment of cancer.

THE HALE APPROACH

Orthodox treatment with regard to the care of the hair and scalp is negligible. Complementary approaches are far superior and can be used as first-line treatment. However, sudden hair loss may be associated with underlying medical conditions that are perhaps best dealt with by a doctor. Ask the opinion of your complementary practitioner.

The Hale Clinic approach to hair care looks not only at the external care of the hair, but also at a person's health inside the body, which can have a great bearing on the creation of a healthy head of hair. Trichology treats both scalp and hair, cosmetically and at a deeper level. Nutrition plays a vital part in creating good-quality hair. Ayurveda, Moor treatment and aromatherapy use treatments which treat the hair externally and internally. For specific hair problems such as hair loss, homeopathy can be effective. In certain cases, when a person's mental state has resulted in problems with the hair (because of stress or shock, perhaps), hypnotherapy and healing can be of great assistance.

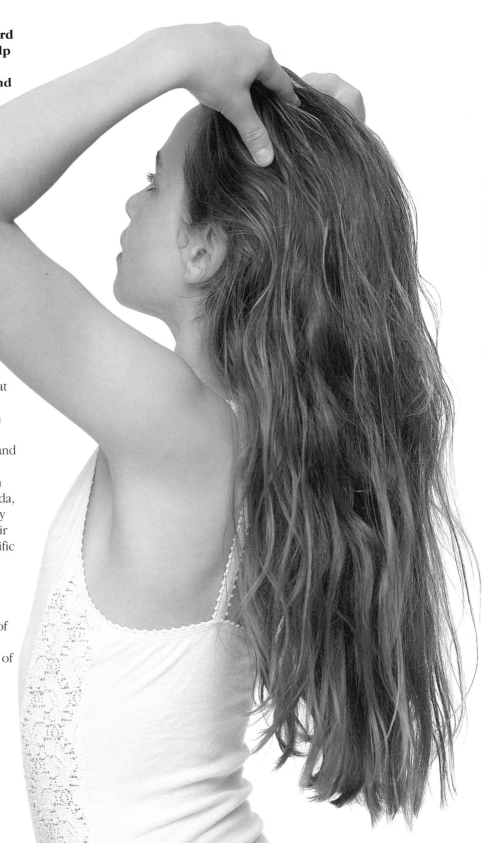

AROMATHERAPY

The vitality of our hair seems to respond well to the stimulating effects on the hair follicles of an aromatherapy head massage. This also relaxes the nervous system, which is of great benefit if lacklustre hair can be attributed to stress and anxiety. A course of treatment may take four to six sessions, supplemented by application of oils at home. After a one and a half hour initial consultation to assess history, duration and triggers to hair loss or condition, a clinical aromatherapist may suggest changes in diet, and recommend vitamins, minerals, phytotherapy or herbs and essential oils; this may be followed by a body and head or just a head massage (depending on hair and scalp condition).

Stress hair loss improves quickly in quantity and the condition of the hair is always improved as a result of this treatment, claims one aromatherapist. As an illustration, she tells of a thirty-year-old woman who regularly lost her hair on one side of her head due to stress. 'Aromatherapy treatment reduced her reaction to stress and the quality of regrowth was good and thick.'

Rosemary, lemon and Scots pine are essential oils which stimulate the circulation in the scalp and are often appropriate for hair care.

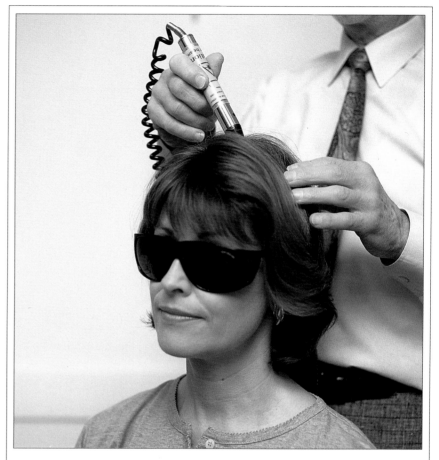

TRICHOLOGY

A trichologist may see patients with scalp and hair problems ranging from various scaling, oily and allergic reactions to many types of hair loss condition, some diffuse, some patchy as in alopecia areata. Most of these reflect metabolic upsets. Any scalp problems will be reflected in the hair. Damaged hair resulting in poor hair condition is a key problem area. Consequently no two patients' cases will be the same, and no one type of product routine can be the answer. Often a combination of treatments is needed.

Hair damage, excess hair loss or scalp changes all demand careful assessment of underlying causes. Once these have been determined, an individual course of action can be recommended.

A minimum of eight to sixteen sessions of 50 minutes each taken over a three-month period (ideally weekly) should be expected. In addition, topical preparations for both scalp and hair are recommended for home use to support clinic treatment. Generally, results start to show during the first few weeks. Response will be dictated by the severity and duration of a problem, but normally over two to three months the improved direction gains momentum. However, trichologists warn that patients must be prepared to persist with their product routines.

A trichologist may work in conjunction with other therapists, depending on any underlying problems that may be determined.

AYURVEDA

Using Ayurvedic herbal medicine, one Hale practitioner was able to halt the premature greying and hair fall of a thirty-year-old male patient. This is just one example of the good results enjoyed by hair care patients using this ancient Indian therapy.

The special oil drip *shiro dhara*, in which warm oil is dripped on to the forehead and massaged into the scalp, is part of scalp therapy. A session of consultation and treatment would probably also involve the application of herbal paste, advice on diet (e.g. avoid acidic food) and yoga exercise. After several of these sessions spread over a two to three month period, your hair should be back to its normal condition. One of the beauties of this holistic therapy is that it is said to be suitable for people of all ages and everyone can benefit.

HOMEOPATHY

Homeopathy is best suited to treating hair problems with a specific cause. For example, if a woman going through the menopause starts to lose her hair or it doesn't look as good as usual, silica with evening primrose oil capsules may be suggested. For premature baldness or greying, lycopodium may be suitable. For hair loss due to shock, aconite works well.

NUTRITION

Hair condition is a good indicator of the state of health as it is often an external reflection of the internal condition of the spleen, pancreas, kidneys and hormones. Fortunately, many cases respond to improved nutrition.

The nutritionist will take a case history, making special note of the hair problems. Holistic treatment with nutrition aims to improve overall health, especially strengthening the immune system. If the misfunction causing the hair problem is corrected, two outcomes are likely: halting the progression of hair deterioration or improving the overall state of the hair, which may include regrowth and improved condition.

SUPPORTIVE TREATMENTS

Acupuncture
Acupuncture can be used successfully to treat hair and scalp problems. A diagnosis is made to ascertain whether the problem is caused by deficiencies or energy blockages, and insertion points are established, mainly on the head.

Healing/Hypnotherapy
'Channelling universal energies into the mind, body and soul of a client' is claimed to produce good results in the treatment of hair problems. Both healing and hypnotherapy are particularly appropriate in conjunction with other therapies when poor hair condition is a result of shock or stress.

MOOR THERAPY

Moor therapy may take the form of a pasteurized drink or a body treatment such as a body wrap or a facial. The aim is to balance up the body and, after an in-depth consultation, Moor therapists choose whatever seems appropriate for the individual patient. 'Even people starting to go grey can go back to their natural colour with Moor,' they say. 'It stimulates the circulation, which nourishes the hair follicles and so the condition of the hair improves.'

SELF-CARE

Aromatherapy, Moor therapy and nutritional advice can all be followed at home after the initial treatment.

Migraine & Headaches

Up to one quarter of the population has a migraine headache at some time in their life and about 10 per cent have them regularly. They usually start in childhood or adolescence, are at their worst in the 30s and 40s and then decline. Very often they run in families. The classic migraine begins with a warning 'aura' – flashing lights in one eye, blurring, blind spots, distortion of vision and tingling of the arms or face. After about 30-60 minutes the headache begins, usually on one side but sometimes all over. It is a pounding, excruciating pain which usually lasts for four to six hours.

The more common 'common migraine' may lack the warning symptoms, and the headache may be far longer lasting, although equally awful. The patient can feel irritable or depressed for hours or even days beforehand. But symptoms vary widely – periods of paralysis, dizziness or even loss of consciousness are all reported.

Attacks may be triggered off by all sorts of things. Common ones include: food – alcohol in general and red wine in particular, chocolate and caffeine; fasting; stress – strong emotional reactions and fatigue; changes in the weather or altitude; hormonal changes such as those caused by menstruation or taking birth control pills. Slightly more women than men suffer with migraines.

Although the cause is not known, the pain and other symptoms seem to be related to changes in the size of the blood vessels feeding the brain.

Other types of headache. The most fearsome sort are the cluster headaches which happen frequently – daily or several times a week – for weeks or months and then stop for months at a time. They are much more common in men, usually young men. They last for about an hour and the pain is almost exclusively on one side of the head, often around or behind the eye. It is so severe that sufferers often run about in despair and may even commit suicide.

The common or garden 'tension headaches' which nearly everyone gets sometimes are caused by involuntary tensing of the face and neck muscles over a long period, usually after concentrating hard or because of stress. The pain is a steady ache, which can last for hours or days, around the back of the head and neck, in the forehead and around the eyes.

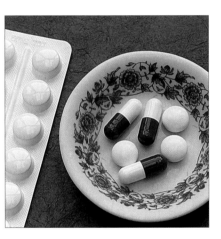

THE ORTHODOX APPROACH

The main treatment for migraine or cluster headaches is with drugs such as ergotamine, which constrict the blood vessels. Taken in the warning stage, they can stop a headache within minutes. But patients who have regular attacks may be put on a course of these drugs, whose side effects include severe blood vessel obstruction and angina. Narcotics may be given to relieve the pain. The latest development is to use calcium channel blockers such as Nifedipine.

Treatment for tension headaches involves hot or cold compresses, relaxation or meditation and simple pain relievers such as aspirin, acetaminophen or ibuprofen.

THE HALE APPROACH

Any severe, protracted or recurrent headache should be reviewed by a doctor with referral to a neurologist if the doctor is not certain of the diagnosis. Once migraine has been fully diagnosed a variety of complementary options are safe, effective and aim at a cure, whereas orthodox treatment tends to alleviate the discomfort by a direct chemical effect on the blood vessels or pain receptors.

As we will see in this section there are many different approaches to migraine – which makes it more than usually difficult for a patient to know which treatment to choose.

The first thing to realize is that migraine symptoms may be similar for many people, but that the aggravating cause may differ from individual to individual. For example, some migraine headaches are the result of a fall or accident which affected the spinal structure, so osteopathy or chiropractic would be the most appropriate therapy. Alternatively, the migraine may be the result of a food allergy, in which case nutrition or naturopathy would be effective. In another case, the

patient may have a blocked meridian in the body, so acupuncture would be the best treatment, or very bad posture, in which case we would recommend the Alexander Technique. Migraine is often exacerbated by hypoglycaemia, poor diet, bad posture and/or hyperventilation.

For stress-related migraines there are treatments aimed at relaxing the patient, such as hypnosis, yoga, Chi Kung and aromatherapy. Patients can be given self-care programmes based on these treatments to alleviate their stress.

At the clinic I would recommend a migraine patient to see our consultant in complementary medicine, for guidance on the right treatment. Where this is not practical, try to choose the treatment on the basis of the information given here e.g. if you had a fall even 20 years ago, see an osteopath or chiropractor; if you notice the headache occurs after you have eaten a particular food, try nutrition therapy or naturopathy; if it is due to other factors, choose one of the relaxation techniques.

HERBAL THERAPIES

The two herbs that have been extensively tested and found to be effective in reducing the number and severity of attacks are ergotamine, now part of conventional treatment, and feverfew. Also very likely to be effective in reducing pain are cayenne pepper and valerian.

In traditional lore the following are also valuable:
• To ease pain, at the first sign of attack take equal parts of black willow, meadowsweet, passion flower, valerian and wood betony.
• For migraine associated with stress, use equal parts of hawthorn berries, lime flowers, wood betony, skullcap and crampbark.

A Migraine Herbal Tea Recipe
Make a cold infusion from:
　6 parts rosemary leaves
　4 parts peppermint leaves
　4 parts lemon balm leaves
　4 parts sweet violet
　3 parts feverfew
　½ part sweet violet flowers

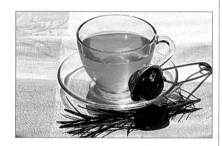

BIOENERGETICS

By testing the patient bio-energetically and prescribing homeopathic remedies, the causative factors of migraine can be treated successfully. This unique approach designs a treatment programme that pinpoints the probable toxic trigger, be it food additives, heavy metals, mercury poisoning, dental materials or toxicity. Additionally attention is given to the circulation, which is supported when necessary, as many congestive headaches are ultimately due to impaired circulation.

ACUPUNCTURE

Migraine may be caused externally by the invasion of wind and damp, or internally by blood stasis. There are different sorts of migraines depending on the meridians involved. For instance, pain in the neck is related to the urinary bladder meridian, while pain in the forehead is related to the stomach meridian. Treatment involves avoiding cold and damp and stimulating the relevant meridians. Sometimes herbs are used as well. Many patients claim that this reduces the number of attacks they suffer and for many the migraines completely disappear. Six to eight sessions are usually sufficient to bring about a marked improvement.

HOMEOPATHY

Treatment can deal with both immediate symptoms and underlying cause, usually stress, but the treatments are very specific because they are related to individual temperament. For instance:
• For a tension headache that feels like a throbbing hammering, especially at the temples – Belladonna.
• For pain that is aggravated by movement and accompanied by constipation – Bryonia alba.
• A hammering pain that comes and goes with the sun, plus a visual disturbance and preceded by tingling of the lips – Natrum mur.
• A sensation of a tight band around the head that is relieved by urinating – Gelsemium.

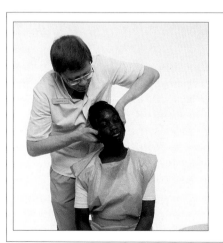

CHIROPRACTIC

Studies have found that restoring normal function to stiff joints by making precise adjustments of the spine can reduce the pain from the associated muscle spasm, but there is controversy as to whether it makes the number of attacks less frequent.

OSTEOPATHY

In considering the treatment of migraine, most osteopaths will take into account not only the more obvious physical causes, but also physiological ones relating to diet and lifestyle. For instance, if the migraine seems to be triggered by food or drink, this will be the first line of treatment. You may be encouraged to cut down on your intake of or completely eliminate certain foods such as caffeine, shellfish, citrus fruits, etc. You will also be advised to eat at regular intervals to reduce the risk of hypoglycaemia.

Bearing in mind the link between low levels of certain neuro-transmitters in migraine attacks, the osteopath will try to facilitate the best possible balance in the neural pathways by encouraging spinal relaxation through deep muscle massage, stretching techniques and manipulation. You may be asked about your work and home environment, as easily overlooked factors such as excessive heat, light or noise may be contributing to the problem. Sleep patterns will also be considered: migraine may be triggered by too much or too little sleep.

Cranial osteopathy – gentle manipulation of the bones and soft tissues of the skull – can relieve tension caused by traumatic events in the past (including birth trauma), head injury or general muscular tension affecting the head. It can also be used to achieve a balance of hormonal activity. An imbalance of hormones – such as that caused by the onset of puberty or by taking the contraceptive pill or hormone replacement therapy (HRT) – is another major cause of migraine.

Visceral osteopathy works on the abdomen to release underlying tension in structures surrounding organs, to improve local blood supply and gastro-intestinal function. This reduces some of the physical stresses which can lead to migraine.

One osteopath also uses electro-magnetic therapy (Empulse Therapy), a safe and non-invasive treatment in which electro-magnetic impulses closely resembling those of the brain's normal activity stimulate responses found to be low in migraine sufferers. 'It has proven to be a very effective tool, used both on its own and with the other treatments mentioned,' he says.

NUTRITION/ALLERGY TREATMENT

The link between food and migraine is well established and in some patients can be completely cleared simply by removing the foods which cause an allergic reaction from their diet. The most commonly troublesome ones are: alcohol, cows' milk, wheat, chocolate, cheese, citrus fruit and shellfish.

How they trigger attacks is not clear. It could be that substances in certain foods have a chemical effect and the levels of the enzyme that normally removes them is low. What is known is that food allergies can affect levels of serotonin – a 'feel good' compound in the brain – and these are low in migraine sufferers. Fatty acids may also play a part, so reducing animal fats and increasing the amount of fish you eat is a good idea.

To identify the source of an allergic reaction you should go on an elimination diet and then, when you are symptom free, gradually reintroduce foods to see which produce the problem. You should also include in your diet foods which reduce the amount blood cells stick together – vegetable oils, fish oils, garlic and onion.

Certain vitamins and food supplements

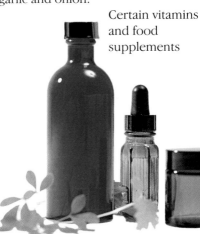

have been found to be helpful in cases of migraine. Bioflavonoids are compounds found in green plants which help in the treatment of many diseases. One, called quercetin, reduces inflammation and may help to combat the effects of food allergies.

Niacin has the effect of dilating the blood vessels and some studies have found it effective in reducing migraine symptoms. It is not recommended for the treatment of cluster headaches.

Magnesium is involved in blood irregularities found in migraine patients; low levels of magnesium are also linked with a collapse of one of the mitral valves in the heart – a condition found in some migraine patients. Magnesium occurs naturally in wholemeal bread and cereals, many green vegetables, nuts and sea-food; it is also available in mineral supplements.

AYURVEDA

In Ayurvedic lore headaches are more common on Sundays and get worse as the sun rises, which is why they are called *Surya* (meaning sun) *Vata* (meaning the force in the body that creates pain). They stem from too much acid in the blood due to eating acidic foods. Treatment involves changing the diet and the use of various detoxifying techniques (known as *panchakarma*) such as enemas, herbal inhalants and *shiro dhara,* dripping warm oil on to the forehead and massaging it into the scalp.

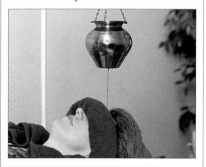

MARMA MASSAGE

There are points on the neck and legs that can be massaged to relieve migraines, but they vary slightly with each individual. Once you have learned where they are you can make use of them to treat yourself.

ENERGY HEALING

By placing his or her hands over the patient, the healer unblocks energy at the back of the neck and relieves stress headaches. Some cases of migraine can clear up in as little as 30 minutes.

SUPPORTIVE TREATMENTS

Hellerwork
The root of the problem is posture. If you carry your head too far forward that is a 4.5kg (10lb) weight in the wrong place, which puts your whole body out of line. The head needs to be over the shoulders, the shoulders in line with the spine and so on (right). Hellerwork gradually brings the body into line through soft-tissue manipulation and movement education. As alignment improves, headaches often diminish in strength and frequency.

Buteyko
Everyone who suffers from asthma over-breathes. One of the effects of this is that the blood vessels that supply the brain go into spasm, causing pain. Once you have learned to breathe correctly, the correct CO_2 levels in the body return the blood vessels to their normal functioning. A few people respond immediately, but generally the effect is not so quick and dramatic as it is with asthma. However, if you persevere with breathing exercises there is a gradual improvement and attacks reduce in severity and frequency.

Hypnotherapy
Severe headaches can be a way of avoiding things, according to one hypnotherapist. Whenever the person is threatened or asked to do something they don't like, an attack is a good, if drastic, way of ducking responsibility. When it has worked successfully once, perhaps by accident, the chances that it will happen again increase. Hypnosis can help people to see the psychological pattern underlying their attacks.

Keeping a 'diary' of migraine attacks often shows a sufferer that these are triggered by tension and anxiety,

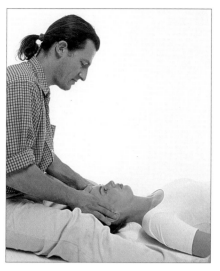

perhaps because the sufferer is unable to deal with problems individually and sees them all as being linked and therefore one and the same. Hypnosis enables a sufferer to separate problems and deal with them one at a time. This avoids the build-up of tension and pressure which results in migraine.

Remedial Yoga
Some causes of headaches centre on negative feelings – anxiety, depression, unrelieved stress. Yoga can help to deal with the way the body tenses up in response to those feelings. Sluggish circulation can cause headaches, and yoga improves blood supply around the neck and shoulders, the route of circulation to the head. The emphasis on breathing can also bring a sense of control over the way you react to events in your life and in your body.

Chi Kung
Special exercises can direct energy to the affected area. There are over 1,500 exercises, and once you have mastered which are most suitable for you, this is an ideal therapy to practise at home.

Light Therapy
Exposure to full-spectrum light can help by dilating the blood vessels and

so improving the circulation. It also greatly reduces stress in the patient by increasing the levels of seratonin (the 'feel good' hormone) in the brain.

BodyHarmonics

This therapy specializes in dealing with severe pain, using the Chinese system of massage called *tuina*. According to this system, migraine is the result of disturbances in the meridians of the gall bladder and the large intestine, so treatment concentrates on them. For some, acupuncture is useful. An Indonesian massage which helps muscles in spasm, often found in the neck with migraine, may also form part of the treatment.

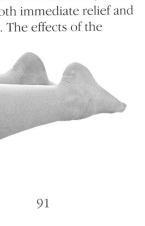

SELF-CARE

Ayurveda
Pressure points: massage the inside of the arm on the side the pain is from the elbow to the wrist. If veins come up, rub them, as this will speed up circulation. For pain on both sides of the head, *shiro dhara* treatment, in which warm oil is dripped on to the forehead and massaged into the scalp, is recommended.

Reflexology
To ease migraine pain the patient will be shown how to massage the reflex point for the head, which is located on the big toe.

Aromatherapy
Aromatherapy massage can help reduce head pain by working over acupressure points, alleviating tension in the head, neck, shoulder and back, and inducing deep breathing and relaxation. Mentha piperita is one oil often used to cool the liver energy, clear the head and settle digestive disturbances. The aim is to create a better blood and energy supply to the neck and head. Six treatments of 45 minutes each are usually enough; essential oils and meditation techniques are given for home use.

Flower Remedies
Plantain(a Pacific remedy) is good for physical toxicity and feverfew (Pegasus) is especially useful in relieving pain.

Acupressure
The points involved are just above the eyebrows in the middle of the forehead. These should be massaged inwards towards the nose and down. Another point is at the top of the nose at the side of the eye socket; the massage should be towards the nose and down. There are also points on the inner side of the big toe, the back of the hand, the wrist and the elbow.

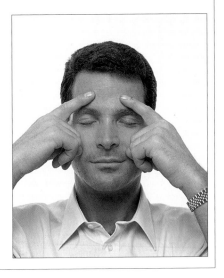

Shiatsu
With cases of migraine and other types of recurrent headache, Shiatsu can offer both immediate relief and prevention. The effects of the massage can be further enhanced by specific diet and lifestyle advice.

Alexander Technique
This therapy is combined with Shiatsu at the Hale Clinic. In migraine cases the balance of the head, the neck and the back is all wrong and needs realigning, since bad posture creates increased tension.

Ears, Eyes, Nose & Throat

The organs of sight, sound, smell, taste and balance are crucial to our reception of information about the world around us. Impairment by injury or disease to any one of these sensory organs can greatly reduce the pleasure that we take in our surroundings and, in some cases, severely curtail our activities. Moreover, these organs are all inextricably linked, so that a condition that affects one may very well have a knock-on effect on the function of another.

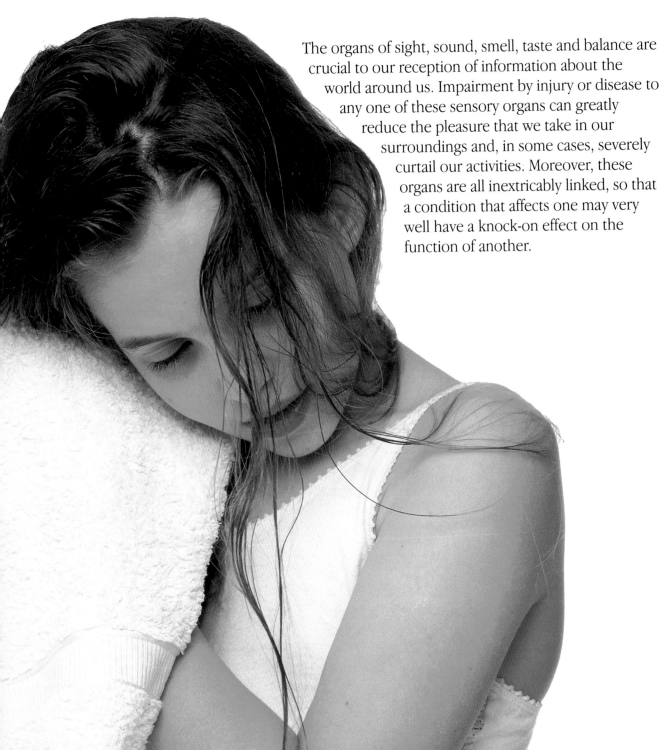

Ears

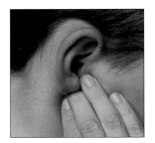

The ear is the organ of hearing and balance. It comprises three parts – the outer, middle and inner ear. The outer and middle ear are primarily concerned with the collection and transmission of sound, while the inner ear is responsible for analysing sound waves and also contains mechanisms by which the body maintains its balance.

Ears are susceptible to many disorders, of which the most common, particularly in childhood, is earache. However, as an example of how the sensory organs are interlinked, pain experienced in the ear may originate there or may hail from a disorder in a nearby structure. Indeed, many people encounter intermittent earache as a 'referred' pain from dental problems, tonsillitis, throat cancer or pain in the lower jaw or neck muscles. This is because the ear and many adjacent areas are supplied by the same nerves.

Although known principally as a childhood illness, earache has been known to reduce the toughest adult to tears. It is an unremitting and intense pain. The most common cause of earache is otitis media (infection of the middle ear), which is particularly common in young children. The accompanying pain is severe and stabbing and may also produce hearing loss and a raised temperature. When otitis media is uncontrolled, it is the most common cause of a perforated eardrum (where the membrane ruptures). However, when the eardrum bursts and the fluid discharges, it sometimes gives immediate relief from pain.

The other common cause of earache is otitis externa (inflammation of the outer ear canal), often caused by infection. Pain may be accompanied by irritation in the ear canal, and by a discharge; there may also be a slight hearing loss.

THE ORTHODOX APPROACH

The doctor examines the ear canal and eardrum with an otoscope and, if necessary, a binocular microscope. Mouth, teeth and throat are also examined. Analgesic drugs may be given to relieve the pain. The treatment, however, depends on the underlying cause of the earache. Antibiotic drugs may be prescribed for infection; pus in the outer ear may need to be aspirated (sucked out), usually as an outpatient procedure; pus in the middle ear may require draining through a hole made in the eardrum – an operation known as myringotomy.

EAR DISORDERS

There is a whole host of disorders to which the ear is susceptible. Although they vary in severity, some can lead to deafness.

Vertigo (the dizziness associated with a disturbance of your balance) can result from some disorders of the inner ear. Similarly, a virus infection of the inner ear may cause labyrinthitis with severe vertigo or sudden hearing loss, or both.

There are also some ear disorders which result from injury. The irresistible urge to poke small objects into the ear that young children experience can result in damage to the external ear canal and perforation of the eardrum. A sudden blow, especially a slap, or a very loud noise may also perforate the eardrum. Prolonged exposure to loud noise or close proximity to a loud explosion can cause tinnitus (noises within the ear) and/or deafness.

Eyes

Whether or not you choose to believe that the eyes are the mirror of the soul, there is no denying that they are extremely complex organs of sight. Many eye disorders are minor, but some lead to serious complications if left untreated. Here are a few of the more common disorders for which you should seek attention.

Conjunctivitis is the most common eye infection, but it rarely affects vision. It is characterized by redness due to widening of blood vessels in the conjunctiva (the mucous membrane that covers the eyeball). It feels rather like the irritation caused by a bit of grit in the eye. Conjunctivitis may be due to viral or bacterial infections, irritants (e.g. chemicals) or allergies. Viral conjunctivitis usually affects both eyes and is mildly infectious.

Corneal infections are more serious and can lead to blurred vision or corneal perforation if not treated early.

Popularly known as red eye, uveitis can be caused by infection or autoimmune disorders. It produces a dull, aching pain, often due to swelling within the front of the eye and spasm in the muscles around the iris. The distinctive redness is caused by a widening of the blood vessels around the iris.

Similarly, glaucoma is distinguished by the whites of the eyes becoming red due to the increased blood flow in the surrounding vessels. This is a result of a sudden increase in pressure within the eyeball, which causes severe pain accompanied by nausea, vomiting, blurred vision and seeing haloes. If untreated, glaucoma can lead to permanent loss of vision.

Finally, a foreign body on the surface of the eye often results in pain and inflammation known as keratitis.

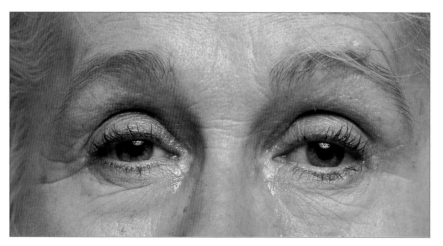

THE ORTHODOX APPROACH

Although the eye is an extremely complex organ, its saving grace is that it is particularly accessible for examination because of the transparency of its structures, so many diseases that affect the eye can be viewed directly. To do this, the practitioner would use an ophthalmoscope and slit lamp.

Nose

Whatever the shape of your nose, it performs a common purpose, namely to filter, warm and moisten the air we breathe, and to detect smells. It is also the nose that gives our voices their characteristic tones by acting as a resonator. Whether it be roman, aquiline, retroussé or snub, the prominent position of the nose makes it particularly prone to injury, while infections and allergic conditions, causing stuffiness, sneezing and sometimes loss of sense of smell, are also common. Most prevalent is the common cold, a virus infection which causes inflammation of the lining of the nasal passages and excessive production of mucus, and hence nasal congestion (better known as a bunged up and/or runny nose). Small boils are also common just inside the nostrils, where they can cause considerable pain.

Fracture of the nasal bones (a broken nose) is a familiar sports injury, while nosebleeds are most common in children. They are primarily caused by fragile blood vessels, an infection of the lining of the nose or a blow to the nose.

You can do irreparable damage to your nose by repeated sniffing of cocaine, which interferes with the blood supply to the mucous membrane lining the nose and can cause perforation of the nasal septum (the cartilage dividing the two nostrils).

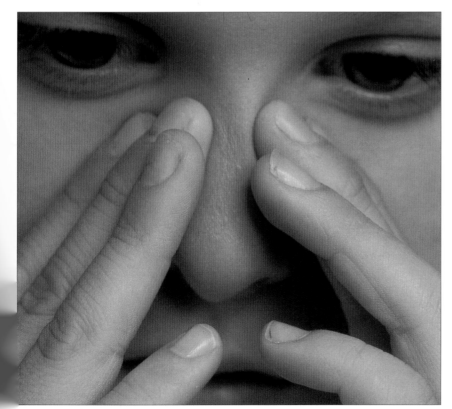

THE ORTHODOX APPROACH

To inspect inside the nose, a doctor uses a speculum to open the nostrils. If a fracture is suspected an X-ray will be taken. For suspected cancer, a nasal endoscopy and a biopsy are performed.

Throat

A sore throat may be the favourite excuse for a day off school but the real thing is very painful and causes great discomfort. It may be the first sign of the common cold, influenza, laryngitis or many of the childhood viral illnesses, including chicken pox, measles and mumps. On the other hand, it could be caused by pharyngitis and occasionally tonsillitis. Strep throat (caused by infection with beta-haemolytic streptococcal bacteria) requires immediate action. Left untreated, it may lead to acute glomerulonephritis or rheumatic fever.

THE ORTHODOX APPROACH

A sore throat can sometimes be relieved by gargling salt water. Adults may benefit from taking aspirin. If symptoms persist for more than 48 hours or a rash appears, consult your doctor. Sore throats due to bacterial infection are treated with antibiotic drugs.

THE HALE APPROACH

All problems involving the eye should be checked initially by an optician and if no obvious problems are viewed then a complementary therapist can be consulted. If the optician has any doubts about the normality of the eye, then referral (through your doctor or complementary practitioner) to an opthalmic surgeon is essential, since eye problems can advance rapidly.

Itching, flaking and blockage of the outer ear is best assessed initially by your doctor. If steroid or antibiotic drops are recommended, see a complementary therapist before using them.

Any persistent or severe ear pain should be examined by a doctor. You should ask if there is any serious visible damage of the eardrum, such as perforation. If there is, then orthodox treatment should be commenced and completed, although complementary treatments may be very effective and even more swift in their efficacy than antibiotics. If the condition will permit a delay, then complementary therapies should be utilized first.

Nasal injuries are best assessed by a hospital casualty department or your own doctor. More chronic problems such as polyps or loss of the sense of smell can be treated by complementary therapy, but if the condition does not respond within two months, then referral to an ENT specialist could be beneficial. As always, with any problem that comes on rapidly, a doctor's opinion should be the first option.

A sore throat should initially be dealt with by complementary methods in all cases except those where a rash appears, breathing is compromised or the pain is substantial. If complementary methods do not work within 48 hours, then antibiotics may be appropriate and you should consult your doctor.

Complementary medicine can be very effective in both the prevention and the treatment of EENT problems. Unlike orthodox medicine, treatments do not focus exclusively on specific symptom areas (e.g. excluding milk from your diet to reduce phlegm), but on the overall situation. Spinal manipulation, for instance, can clear up certain problems with the throat. Marma massage to the back of the head could treat a swollen eye. The Buteyko Method of breath reconditioning treats and prevents ENT problems and is particularly effective with sinus problems and snoring.

Often a good way to start treating EENT problems is with nutritional advice and the identification of any allergic reactions. Buteyko may also prevent the recurrence of allergies that aggravate these problems.

Alternatively the cause may lie with the structure of the spine and the cranium. It is not generally understood what an important role chiropractic, osteopathy and cranial osteopathy can play in the treatment of EENT problems. Marma massage, as part of a general Ayurvedic approach, will address both the structural and the nutritional aspects of the problem as well as providing a range of self-care techniques to prevent a recurrence. Homeopathy and acupuncture are also very effective in treating these problems, with homeopathy and cranial osteopathy being a particularly helpful combination for children.

In this section there is also a range of self-care and support therapies to help the body's ability to ward off EENT problems.

TEETH

The mouth – including the tongue and teeth – is a very important area for diagnosing systemic as well as local disorders. Aware dentists are often the first to diagnose diseases such as oral cancer, AIDS and anaemia. The oral symptoms of any kind of cancer include cracks in the corner of the mouth, changes in the colour of the tongue and lips (sometimes turning blood red) and chronic gum bleeding. Even at the pre-cancer stage gum bleeding can occur, so if treated appropriately this can be reversed.

Holistic dentistry applies prevention-oriented care and understands the impact of good nutrition and natural medicines on the dental and general healing process. Antibiotics are used only as a last resort. Nutritional, homeopathic and natural medicines prevent their being necessary most of the time. Natural mouth washes such as propolis, tea tree oil and extract of grapefruit seed are recommended and in low-disease mouths fluoride-free pastes are suggested as fluoride has been shown to be rather toxic.

Mercury-based fillings and root fillings are avoided as far as possible. The mouth and body can be tested for heavy metal poisoning and cleansed by using special homeopathic remedies and mouth washes. Existing mercury-based fillings are removed under very isolative and protective conditions and the body is prepared accordingly with vitamins and natural medicines.

Holistic dentists are sensitive to the detrimental impact of negative emotions such as stress and fear. Excessive tooth wear, dysfunction of the joints of the jaw and many kinds of migraines and other headaches can be diagnosed and treating by understanding a patient's lifestyle. Dentists may recommend hypnotherapy, cranial osteopathy and many forms of massage, including aromatherapy.

Any dentist should naturally be able to put people at ease. If a patient still feels fearful of visiting the dentist, then a whole host of methods can be applied to calm them – hypnotherapy, the use of essential oils or flower remedies, or energy healing may all help.

OSTEOPATHY

Cranial osteopathy would almost certainly be the answer in treating problems of the ears, eyes, nose and throat. Osteopathy aims to diagnose and treat mechanical problems in the framework and cranial osteopathy extends this principle by applying gentle pressure and/or manipulation to the head, neck and upper back. Success has been reported even with certain forms of blindness and deafness. Spinal manipulation may also be introduced for problems with the throat. Cranial osteopathy tends to be slightly slower in achieving results than structural osteopathy, so several weeks of treatment may be required.

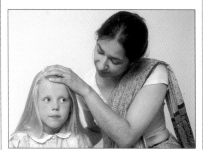

HOMEOPATHY

Most cases of recurrent otitis media and tonsillitis respond well to this method of stimulating the natural healing reaction. In this area homeopathy is especially successful in treating children. The range of remedies that may be prescribed is vast, but some of the more common ones are:

- For earache with a throbbing pain – Belladonna.

- For earache with severe pain – Chamomilla.

- To soothe the irritation of conjunctivitis – Euphrasia.

- In the early stages of a cold – Natrum mur.

- For a flu-like cold – Gelsemium.

- For a sudden sore throat with swollen tonsils – Aconite.

- For a dry sore throat accompanied by hoarseness and a tickling cough – Phosphorus.

- If a child is clingy, whingeing and irritable – Pulsatilla.

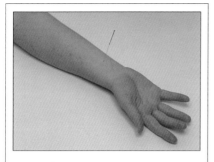

ACUPUNCTURE

Acupuncture is appropriate for most of the conditions affecting the ears, eyes, nose and throat and is particularly successful in dealing with sinus infection. A combination of acupuncture and Chinese herbs would normally produce a total cure of this condition after six sessions.

BUTEYKO

The Buteyko system uses a series of special breathing exercises and lifestyle changes which initially teach patients to overcome their symptoms. Patients generally find an increase in vigour, concentration and the elimination of many symptoms that one would not necessarily attribute to improved breathing. The Buteyko techniques are taught over a minimum of five one-hour sessions on consecutive days, and the method is especially suitable for children aged five and over, who often achieve results more quickly than adults and who are particularly prone to disorders of the ear. It has also been successful in treating those with sinus problems and in reducing snoring!

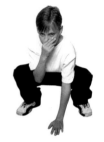

SUPPORTIVE TREATMENTS

The following produce good results when used in isolation but are more effective in association with other therapies.

Nutrition
Investigating allergies is a good starting point for recurrent earache and other problems with the ears, eyes, nose and throat. Secretory earache is more than twice as frequent in allergic children than in non-allergic children, according to one study of 540 patients. The most common culprits in the diet seem to be cows' milk, cocoa, cane sugar, cola, grains, citrus fruit, eggs and nuts, so these should be avoided. Sulphites and monosodium glutamate (MSG), both common food additives, can also provoke earache. Avoiding these and supplementing the diet with molybdenum can improve symptoms.

Airborne allergens such as house-dust components, tobacco smoke, animal dander and fungus spores are linked to infections of the ears, eyes, nose and throat, and should be avoided as far as possible.

Remedial Yoga
One of the accepted practices of Hatha yoga which is particularly useful for conditions of congestion such as rhinitis and sinusitis is Jala Neti (washing the nasal passages with warm salt water). This gently cleanses the nasal and throat tissues, increases the circulation and stimulates healing energy within these areas. A patient can be taught the technique in one 30-minute session and can then use it at home. In addition, breathing practice benefits the nose and throat and is also a good way to clear the head of congestion.

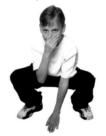

Chi Kung
In conjunction with diet and Chinese herbal treatment, this traditional therapy can be used to identify and overcome the irritants that frequently cause problems to the ears, eyes, nose and throat. Chi Kung exercises stimulate the kidney meridian, which rules these areas. With time, students will learn to tune into their bodies and rectify the energy imbalances that are causing the problems. Once the exercises are mastered, Chi Kung can easily be practised at home.

Healing
For any of the ear, eye, nose or throat conditions, a healer may work in conjunction with other therapists to bring relief. During a treatment, the patient may be asked to sit or lie down and healing energy will be channelled to them through the healer. Some healers lay their hands on the patient, while others work through the aura (the magnetic field around the body). The patient may experience heat, cold or tingling sensations, although these are not necessarily present.

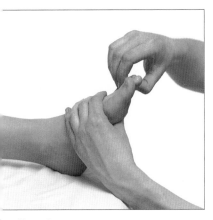

Reflexology

A full reflexology treatment, lasting about 45 minutes, would be followed by treatment of the area connected to the specific problem. For eye problems, these areas would relate to the eyes, kidneys, neck, cervical spine, adrenal glands and upper lymphatic areas; for ears they would relate to the ears, sinuses, Eustachian tube, upper lymph nodes, the side of the head, neck, cervical spine and adrenal glands; for the nose to the face and sinuses; and for the throat to the throat, neck and upper lymphatic areas.

You can treat yourself for eye problems by working along the soles of the feet, just beneath the second and third toe webs and possibly slightly up the sides of those toes; for ear problems in the same position but below the fourth and fifth toes; for the nose the surface of the big toe; and for the throat also the surface of the big toe, around the joint. However, you should attempt this self-help only after you have been instructed by your practitioner and have a clear understanding of what you are doing. Inexpert treatment can overwork a reflex area, possibly upsetting the balance in the body, with unpleasant results.

Auditory Integration Training

Auditory Integration Training (AIT) can be helpful to those with hearing disorders, particularly when used in conjunction with other therapies. It entails listening to electronically modulated music through headphones over a certain period of time. Prior to treatment, the trainee's hearing is evaluated audiometrically and the AIT is adjusted by setting filters so that any frequencies to which the individual is sensitive may be dampened.

Clinical Aromatherapy

Inner ear infections benefit from the twice-daily application of oils such as spice lavender, which is normally used with *Eucalyptus globulus*, niaouli and tea tree to reinforce its strength. Aromatherapy has many splendid immune stimulants to help with sinus, throat and ear infections. The oils may be used diluted in a maceration of echinacea or, in intensive care, applied directly to the feet.

Clinical aromatherapy massage incorporates lymphatic drainage and acupressure to reduce swelling, stimulate drainage, eliminate stagnation and fight off pathogenic factors. Oils are then prepared for the patient's home use.

SELF-CARE

Practitioners of many of the therapies that successfully treat problems of the ears, eyes, nose and throat will give valuable advice on ways in which you might help yourself at home. For example, nutritional advice is always applicable, and an aromatherapist may recommend essential oils that can help to relieve the symptoms of recurrent ENT problems. A combination of *Eucalyptus radiata* and *E. globulus,* rosemary, spike lavender, sweet marjoram, cypress, tea tree, naoili and thyme makes a good inhalation for sinusitis, while eucalyptus is good for a throat infection and could be burned in an aromatherapy lamp by your bedside.

Bach flowers and the extended range of flower essences (there are over 2,000) can be used at home to good effect. Ox-eyed Daisy (Pacific) and French Lavender (Petite Fleur) are excellent for ear problems and, as a generalization, Eucalyptus (Pegasus), Jasmine (Pegasus), Onion (Petite Fleur) and Echinacea (Hawaii) are just some of the essences that produce good results with problems of the ears, eyes, nose and throat.

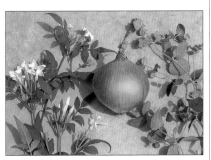

AYURVEDA/MARMA MASSAGE

These holistic therapies aim to teach the patient how to prevent the diseases of the ears, nose and throat as well as to treat existing conditions. Self-care techniques help patients to understand ENT better which, in turn, helps to prevent disease. Improvement should be noticed after the first session and by the end of the course of treatment (about three sessions), a substantial improvement and a knowledge of preventative techniques for the future can be expected.

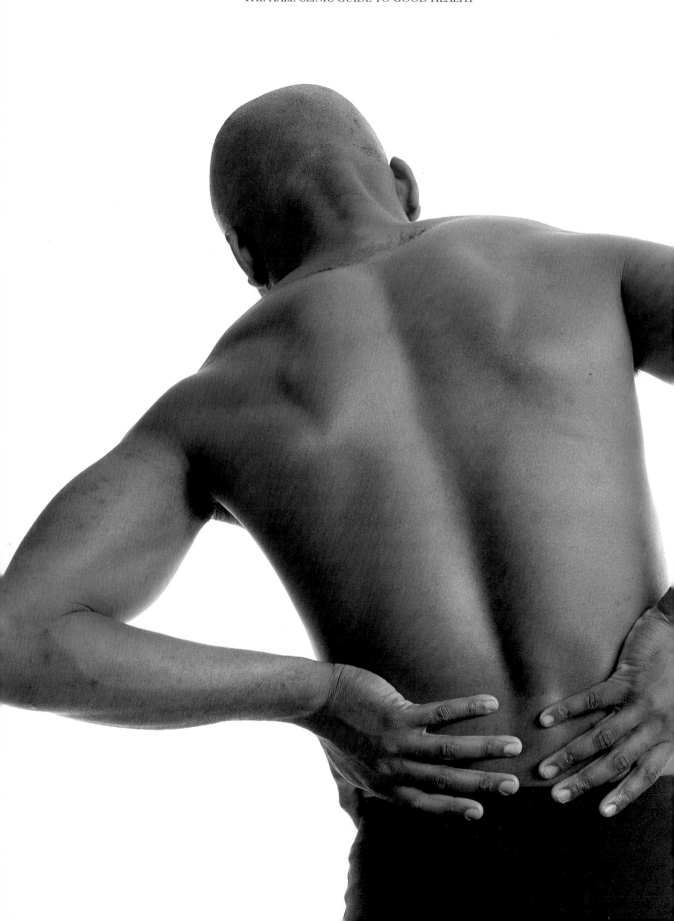

Back Pain

You can count yourself extremely lucky if you manage to get through life without experiencing back pain at some time or another. Very often we can trace the cause to our own over-enthusiasm – perhaps working too hard in the garden in the first warm days of spring, or lifting a heavy chest of drawers to clean behind it. In the main, these back aches and pains get better of their own accord after a relaxing bath, some rest and, on occasion, a couple of analgesic tablets for pain relief. The medical profession refers to such cases as 'non-specific back pain', one of the largest single causes of working days lost through sick leave in the Western world.

In cases where non-specific back pain is not the result of over-ambitious exertion, there are a few categories of people who are more prone to it than most: those who are overweight and those – like nurses and factory employees, for example – whose work involves lifting and carrying. Non-specific back pain is thought to occur as a result of ligament strain, a muscle tear, damage to a spinal joint or prolapse of an intervertebral disc (slipped disc). This is often coupled with spasm in the surrounding back muscles, which causes additional pain and tenderness over a wide area and, in some cases, can lead to temporary scoliosis (abnormal sideways curvature of the spine). A slipped disc and damage to the facet joints of the spine can both cause sciatica (pain in the buttocks and down the back of the leg into the foot). Sciatica is painful enough at the best of times, but if you cough, sneeze or strain in any way during a bout, the pain is excruciating.

Those who suffer from osteoarthritis in the joints of the spine often complain of never being free from pain and, as with sufferers from ankylosing spondylitis (arthritis affecting the spine), they frequently experience stiffness and a loss of back mobility which prevents them from performing many of the simplest tasks, such as tying a shoe lace.

The condition of fibrositis (pain and tenderness in the muscles) can sometimes affect the back without there being any problem of the bones or joints.

THE ORTHODOX APPROACH

An examination of the back may reveal tenderness or a lack of mobility which could indicate several of the non-specific back pains mentioned above. To confirm structural damage, an X-ray would be arranged and there are several specialized forms of X-ray or scanning which may be employed if pressure on a nerve root is suspected. If a specific cause can be found, then the treatment will be appropriate to the situation. Acute non-specific back pain is treated by analgesics and a short period of restriction, if necessary.

Chronic back pain is more difficult – the treatment could include a course of aspirin and related drugs, non-steroidal anti-inflammatory drugs or muscle-relaxants; acupuncture or spinal injections; exercise, spinal manipulation, the wearing of a surgical corset or even spinal surgery. Fibrositis often improves with the use of non-steroidal anti-inflammatory drugs.

THE HALE APPROACH

Most doctors, except those who have taken a specific interest in the subject of back pain, will agree that osteopaths and chiropractors have far more training in this field. Any back injury or back pain is therefore best assessed by either of these specialists, who can make a referral to an orthodox specialist if required.

The causes of back pain are very diverse and I would recommend some patients to see our consultant in complementary medicine to be advised about the most appropriate form of treatment. Where this is not practical, try to choose the most suitable treatment on the basis of the information given here.

The most usual treatments for back pain are manipulative therapies such as osteopathy and chiropractic, which aim to bring the vertebrae back into line, by working either directly or through the muscular system. In cases of muscle spasm or sciatica, however, acupuncture, aromatherapy, massage or reflexology may be more appropriate.

If the back pain keeps recurring, it may be that the treatment should be focused more on the muscles. Osteopathy or chiropractic may still be appropriate, but homeopathy can also be effective in strengthening the muscles in order to keep the vertebrae in place. Equally, working on the muscles with Marma massage or *tuina* massage can be very helpful.

For chronic back pain postural treatments such as the Alexander Technique, Hellerwork or GDS may be more appropriate than constant manipulation. If a patient is receptive to the idea of energy healing, this can be effective, particularly with very serious cases.

The self-care aspect is also important in the treatment and prevention of back pain – try gentle exercises like T'ai Chi, Chi Kung and yoga.

Finally, the possibility of a psychological aspect to back pain cannot be ignored. We once had a patient who suffered from neck pain. Every 'standard' treatment had been ineffective and eventually he saw a psychologist, who asked him which person in his life was 'a pain in the neck'. The patient immediately recognized who that person was, and the pain disappeared within a few hours. Homeopathy can also be of great assistance if there is a strong psychological basis for back pain.

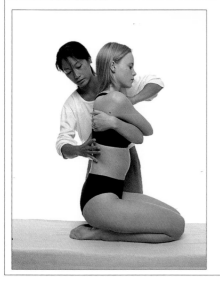

GDS TECHNIQUES

Bad posture, repetitive movements or stress, accidents or injuries can all build up a physical pattern causing long-term articular and muscular limitations, according to GDS practitioners. As a result, pain appears in a different part of the body in reaction to the initial process. For example, a limitation in the hip joints' flexibility due to shortening hamstrings and buttocks will imbalance the position of the pelvis, in the long term inducing a pain in the lower back.

GDS Techniques work on three levels. Firstly, a therapist would analyse your posture and movement, then body awareness would be explained and discussed, and finally there would be a physical treatment to readjust the imbalance. This could involve isometric techniques, gentle stretching, postures, breathing techniques or soft-tissue massage. Between five and ten weekly sessions should produce improvement and/or total disappearance of the problem.

OSTEOPATHY

After taking a medical history and carrying out a detailed physical examination, an osteopath will plan a course of treatment. Each session, which usually lasts about thirty minutes, may involve soft-tissue massage, gentle, repetitive movement of joints and rapid guiding of the joints through their normal range of movements (producing the characteristic clicking that most people associate with osteopathy). There may also be advice on posture, exercise and relaxation techniques. A short spell of perhaps three or four treatments should sort out the majority of back problems.

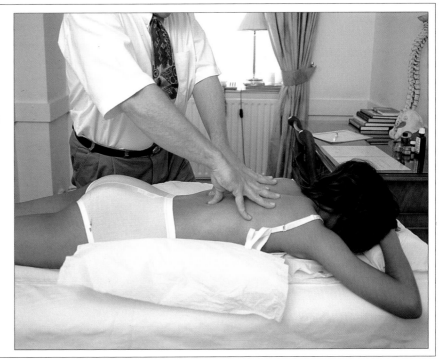

CHIROPRACTIC

Spinal manipulation (chiropractic) is one of the most well-documented complementary therapies in terms of effectiveness and cost effectiveness. Studies suggest that with manipulation the stimulation of nerves (reflexes) can cause the muscles to relax and possibly also have an effect on the vascular system via these nervous reflexes. The majority of cases need an average of five to eight treatments, but chronic back pain will often need more than ten, spread over several weeks or months, in conjunction with exercises, ergonomic advice, stress management and so on.

A first consultation would entail a full physical examination, treatment and explanation of the patient's symptoms; subsequent sessions would comprise treatment and exercises with continuous monitoring of progress. Provided the patient follows the advice and exercises, chiropractic claims a success rate of over 95 per cent in most (uncomplicated) cases. In the case of chronic back pain, patients could hope for a significant reduction in pain medication, and increased mobility and social function. A maintenance programme whereby you might attend a treatment every one to three months may well be recommended following the more intensive course of treatment.

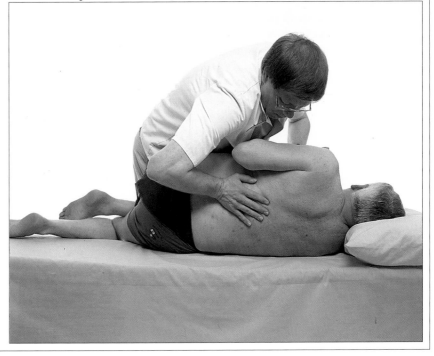

ACUPUNCTURE/CHINESE HERBS

Depending on a patient's condition, a combination of acupuncture and Chinese herbs may be used to regulate the energy balance and get through any blockage in the body's meridians, particularly the bladder and kidney meridians. Most patients will experience some improvement and some will achieve a complete cure after a course of this treatment. Acupuncture has been particularly successful in the treatment of back pain caused by muscular spasm or sciatica.

HOMEOPATHY

Although each case has to be judged individually, there are a number of homeopathic remedies that are commonly associated with the treatment of back pain. The first step is to find the origin of the back pain. Rhus tox is a very common remedy when there is stiffness in the back and particularly if there is stiffness after the first movement of the day which then disappears. Arnica is also useful, especially when there is a sensation of bruising in the back and after mental or physical trauma. Sometimes the problem is weakness in the back rather than pain, and then phosphoric acid is used. Ruta grav. and Hypericum are often indicated when nerve damage is involved.

MARMA MASSAGE

Marma is a form of deep-tissue massage which is used together with yoga and Ayurveda to eradicate muscle spasm and inflammation, and to correct mechanical and pathological conditions of the back. This integrated physical therapy has been ver effective with back pain. The duration of treatment varies with the severity of the case, but as a rule of thumb two or three sessions should be enough to eradicate acute pain; between six and twenty sessions may be needed to relieve chronic pain completely.

According to one Ayurvedic physician and Marma therapist, 'The back maintains a unique pressure. If there is an imbalance of pressure for mechanical or pathological reasons, muscle spasms and inflammation will be created and this results in back pain. Marma therapy can help the back to maintain its normal pressure. In terms of lifestyle changes, diet and exercise are very important for the prevention of back pain. I also recommend no acidic food.'

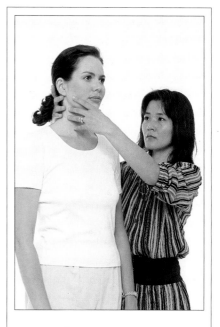

ALEXANDER TECHNIQUE

The Alexander Technique improves posture, allowing the body to work in a more natural, relaxed and efficient manner. To treat back pain, the therapist begins by watching how you use your body. He or she will then guide you to correct any harmful postures you may have acquired over the years and help you regain the habit of using your muscles with minimum effort and maximum efficiency. Good posture and correct use of the body will release tension, alleviate symptoms and prevent further pain.

SHIATSU

Shiatsu and its associated maintenance advice (such as corrective *chi* yoga/exercise) focus on the underlying causes of the back pain. Therapy aims to support and energize the weak areas and relax the tense areas of the back (and indeed the whole body).

Following a series of treatments the individual may not only expect relief from pain, but will also be equipped actively to prevent further attacks.

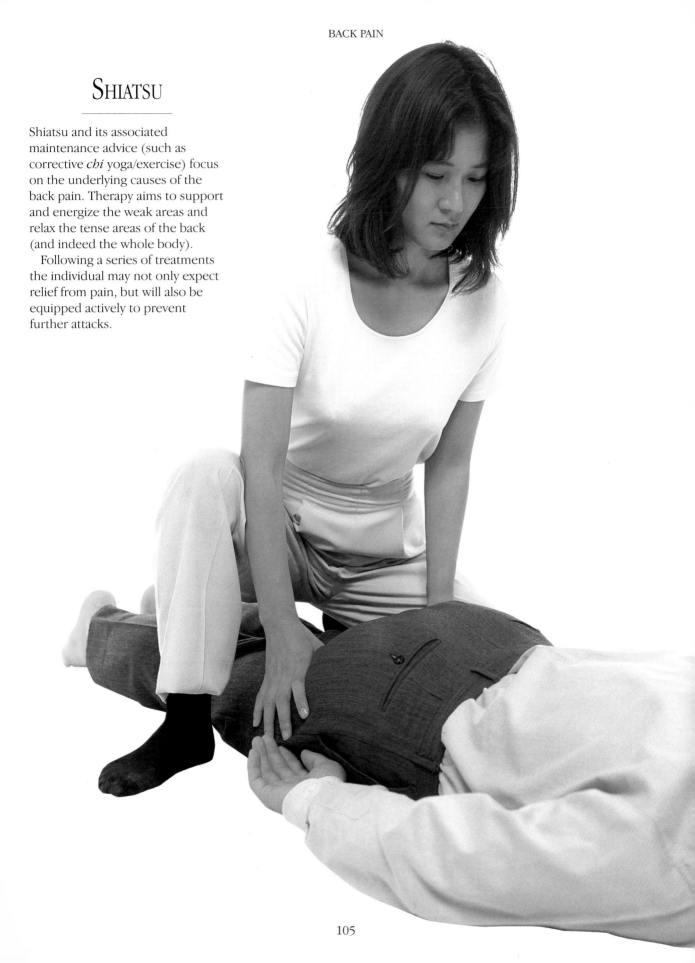

REFLEXOLOGY

Whatever the complaint, reflexologists willgive a full reflexology treatment, based on treating the whole body, before moving on to specific areas relating to the particular problem. With back pain, a full treatment would be followed by extra treatment specific to the area where the pain was being experienced, such as the lower back, and to the neck, adrenal glands and solar plexus.

The duration of treatment depends on how long the problem has been present. Some people who are sensitive and react very quickly may need only three treatments. Others need a longer time, particularly if the problem is deep seated.

You can treat yourself by working along the inner side of both feet, but only after you have been instructed by your practitioner and have a clear understanding of what you are doing. Inexpert treatment can overwork a reflex area, possibly upsetting the balance in the body, with unpleasant results.

TUINA

Tuina (meaning 'push' and 'squeeze') is traditional Chinese massage working over acupoints and meridians, using deep pressure, tapping, clapping or friction to alleviate pain (caused by the stagnation of *chi* energy in the body). This stimulates the flow of blood and is helpful in the treatment of chronic and acute back pain, and sports injuries. The treatment is normally very deep tissue massage, leaving the patient alert and balanced. Chi Kung exercises are also normally prescribed.

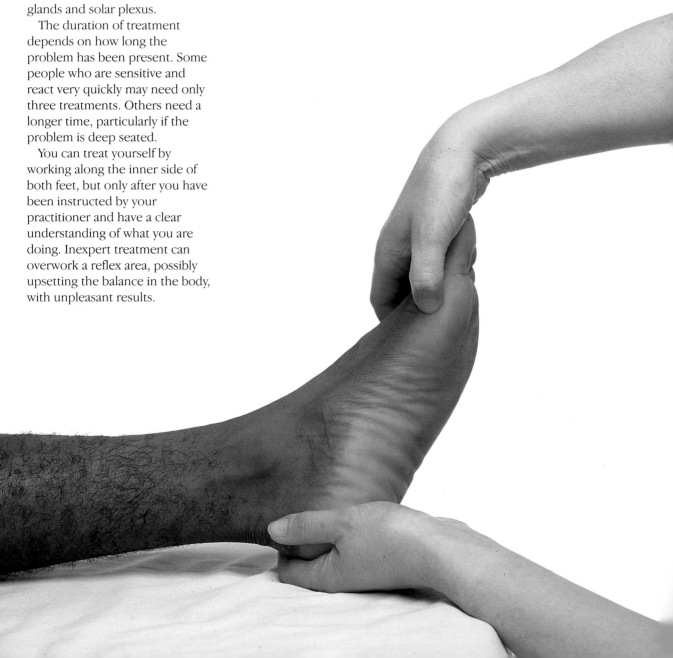

HELLERWORK

Hellerwork systematically treats the whole structure of the body by a method known technically as 'myo-fascial' (including bones and muscles) bodywork. It does this not through a forceful manipulation of bones but by capitalizing on the fact that bone position is determined by the pattern of tension in the soft tissues. When this pattern is normalized the structure can return to a more harmonious relationship with gravity, the single most powerful force acting on our bodies at all times.

Back pain is almost always a result of compression in the spinal structure caused by a less-than-optimal relationship of the body with its gravitational field. If there is a single cause for the virtual epidemic of back pain in the Western world today, says one Hellerwork practitioner, it is this: we do not know how to use our bodies efficiently enough in the field of gravity.

When the back goes out it seems a sudden event, but in most cases we are a case of back pain waiting to happen! Accumulated stress overwhelms the structure in its weakest place. Stress on the body may come from wearing high heels, sitting a lot or habitual asymmetry (e.g. from playing 'one-sided' sports like tennis or golf). Poor design of furniture is a primary contributor.

As an integral part of Hellerwork treatment, movement coaching allows the client to participate intimately in the rehabilitation process, finding new, efficient and non-stressful ways of doing what previously triggered back pain.

ENERGY HEALING

An energy healer's powers of healing are channelled through him or her to help the patient, whom some healers do not even touch. The patient is simply asked to lie down and close their eyes and the healer does the rest. Although frequently dismissed by conventional medicine, energy healing enjoys good results. Back pain is often relieved in one session, although if there is a slight spinal defect, it can take a few sessions to sort out.

The initial stage has been described as 'a psychic diagnosis screening' during which the healer may recognize another complaint and will then treat the whole problem by 'realigning the energies and working through a person's aura'.

Other healers use their energies to treat patients in conjunction with physical adjustment, dietary advice and breathing techniques. Some adjustment to the posture may be performed and better ways of moving are taught. Some exercise 'supplements' may also be recommended. With this form of treatment the situation may be resolved in one session, but if not it is likely that five or six will be required. One woman who had suffered with back pain for many years despite visiting many 'experts', experienced amazing results after one healing session. She says, 'He felt my back and picked up correctly that it had started in puberty. I was actually 15. I had two exercises to practise and a golden light meditation. I am pain free now for the first time in countless years and consequently have so much new energy and drive.'

NUTRITION

In general terms, nutrition cannot be used to treat back pain which is caused by muscular pain or injury. However, some people are sensitive to the tannin and caffeine group of products, e.g. tea, coffee, chocolate, cocoa, cola, red wine, etc., and for them these foods appear to dry out the synovial fluids which lubricate joints. If synovial fluid becomes low, general wear and tear on the joints (and, of course, the back is basically a series of joints), is greater and you are much more likely to experience 'lesser grade' back pain. A good way to identify whether this food sensitivity is present is to eliminate these products from your diet. If you then have a pressure headache for several days and are generally slow and mentally unfocused, you probably do have a sensitivity – you are experiencing withdrawal symptoms, which would be instantly relieved if you were to take half a cup of coffee or tea.

AROMATHERAPY

A massage using specifically chosen essential oils can relax and stretch the muscles, calm nervous activity, stimulate the flow of blood and *chi* (intrinsic) energy and mobilize joints, thereby reducing pain and increasing flexibility. Two to three treatments involving massage, exercises and stretches should be enough to relieve back pain, although this is obviously dependent on the severity of the condition, how long it has been present and your emotional state. In the case of arthritic or stress-related muscle spasm and in sufferers who do not exercise sufficiently or are overweight, improvement is normally immediate; in other cases total cure is often achieved.

As well as the treatments, it is important for exercise to be incorporated into a patient's lifestyle if success is to be long-lived; good posture must also be maintained. Advice on these subjects would be given during the treatment sessions.

The essential oils recommended for your condition can also be used in moderation and under direction at home to relieve early symptoms of back pain through muscle relaxation. Rosemary is good for muscular pain, while eucalyptus, citriodora, juniper, ginger and orange are deeply relaxing.

TANGENT THERAPY

Tangent therapists first diagnose the condition by assessing the patient's posture from head to toe; they also look at lifestyle, any ailments associated with the back pain, and any weakness arising from former accidents. Tangent therapists believe that back pain may be caused by sitting or standing too much and by general bad postural habits. During the course of the hour-long session (sometimes one and a half hours depending on the condition), a combination of the following treatments may be used: essential oils, passive stretches, food herbs, aromatherapy massage, shiatsu pressure points and breathing techniques. Corrective exercises are often given for patients to do at home.

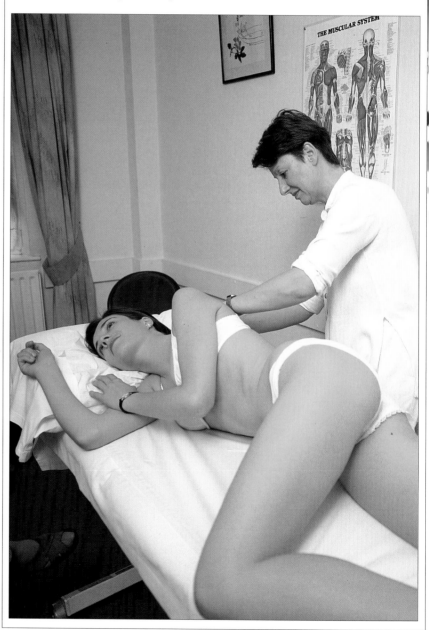

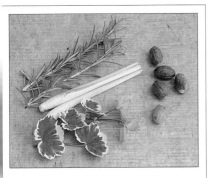

HERBALISM

This is a useful complementary therapy in cases of acute back pain such as lumbar strain, when a patient is consulting an osteopath or a similar therapist.

Anti-inflammatories such as devil's claw or turmeric extracts taken internally can be helpful. Arnica tincture applied to unbroken skin and various arnica creams are useful for any external strain. Very dilute concentrations of various essential oils which have anti-spasmodic and analgesic qualities and which increase blood flow might be recommended as the base for a vegetable oil. Suitable oils include rosemary, peppermint, lemon grass, geranium and nutmeg.

If the back pain is related to a bone problem such as osteoarthritis of the spine, an external treatment with an anti-inflammatory such as devil's claw and willow bark is still useful. Certain herbs, including capsicum and prickly ash, improve blood flow, which helps osteoarthritis. In addition, horsetail, which contains silica, can help to reconstruct the joints.

In some cases, back pain may be a symptom of depression and this can be treated quite effectively by herbal medicine. The main herb for this situation is hypericum (St John's wort).

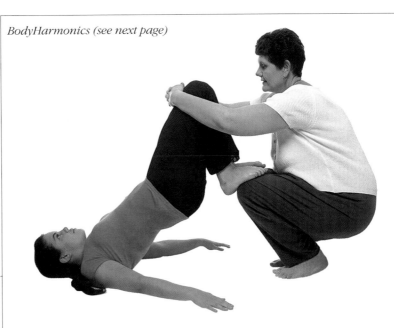

BodyHarmonics (see next page)

SELF-CARE

If you overdo it and back pain is the result, or if you just tend to 'suffer with your back', make sure you sleep on a firm orthopedic mattress or put a board under the mattress. Use only one pillow.

Once you are aware that you are prone to back pain or have a weakness in that area, it is wise to examine ways in which you might prevent a recurrence of the pain or in which you might relieve the pain yourself before the condition escalates.

Osteopathy
When the pain is acute rest is the most beneficial treatment. Listen to your body and rest in whatever position is the most comfortable. The application of heat or ice may also be of help. Heat is used in the relaxation of tight muscles and to restore the blood supply; ice helps to reduce inflammation. In an acute case there will usually be tight muscles supporting and protecting an inflamed area, so 'contrast bathing' (alternating applications of heat and ice) may help most.

In a more long-term case there may have been repetitive strain of the same area. This area can be helped by maintaining good mobility of the joint by gentle repetitive stretching and support of the affected joint with toned muscles. Often posture will play a large part in this (e.g. back muscles are tight, but there is no support from the abdominal muscles). This collapse of the posture into 'swayback' will put more strain on the affected lower back pain or disc. Keep the back flexible and stretched.

Flower Remedies
The original Bach flower remedies and the extended range of over 2,000 essences from around the world are ideal for helping yourself to combat back pain. Although there are a number from which to choose, and a consultation with a practitioner would pinpoint the most appropriate for your specific condition, in general terms the Australian Living essence Menzies Banksia is particularly recommended for back pain.

SUPPORTIVE TREATMENTS

Certain alternative therapies enjoy good results with back pain but are even more effective when combined with other types of complementary treatment.

BodyHarmonics

This therapy works by clearing blockages in the meridians (lines of energy) on the same theory as acupuncture. Using *tuina* (see previous page), the treatment for neck, shoulder and back pain works deeply on the bladder and gall bladder meridian. Thai stretching and, in extreme cases of lumbar pain and sciatica, acupuncture may be used to complement *tuina*. Depending on the severity of the

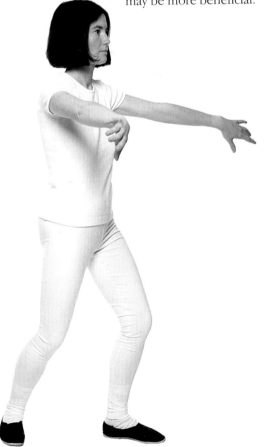

case, about five sessions should be sufficient to bring about an improvement. According to this system it is recommended that more exercise, specifically swimming, be incorporated into a patient's lifestyle.

Colonic Hydrotherapy

According to colonics therapists, back pain may be caused by toxicity of the muscles, kidneys or a congested colon or spasms. Where this is the case, colonic hydrotherapy (gently flushing out the colon to remove any unbeneficial material) can alleviate and even remove the condition. In these situations, colonics combine very well with massage to remove back pain. However, if the pain is due to poor posture, spinal misalignment or serious spasms, colonics is not really appropriate and massage alone or in conjunction with another therapy may be more beneficial.

Remedial Yoga

Before attempting to alleviate back pain through yoga it is important to determine if the condition is due to an acute injury – misplacement or whiplash, for example. Once this is established, yoga can be highly beneficial. Retained tension and overworked muscles bring a lot of pain to the upper spine. You can overwork muscles by the way you use them. In Hatha yoga therapy, you can learn through the *asanas* (postures) to relax the spine, which makes it supple and avoids further problems in the spine itself.

In cases of whiplash or after surgery, yoga can help renew the tone and suppleness in the spine once you are on the way to recovery.

Yoga also brings strength back to the muscles and helps to build confidence in the affected area (confidence can be lost after experiencing pain), so that the back and body can once again be used fully. Shock needs to be worked through. One of the ways to break through these blockages is to ensure that breathing is complete and not limited. Breath awareness helps to release the body of blockages.

Chi Kung

The seven basic exercises of Chi Kung and the eight fundamental T'ai Chi exercises form the basic reference point from which treatment begins. Both philosophies treat the person as a whole by using and balancing the *chi* (intrinsic) energy in the body. The underlying purpose is to bring the patient back to his or her 'tantien' centre, thereby strengthening lower back muscles. Gentle exercises, stretching and affirmations are used to release tension in the back and bring relief from pain. Once mastered, Chi Kung can be used as a preventative therapy for back pain.

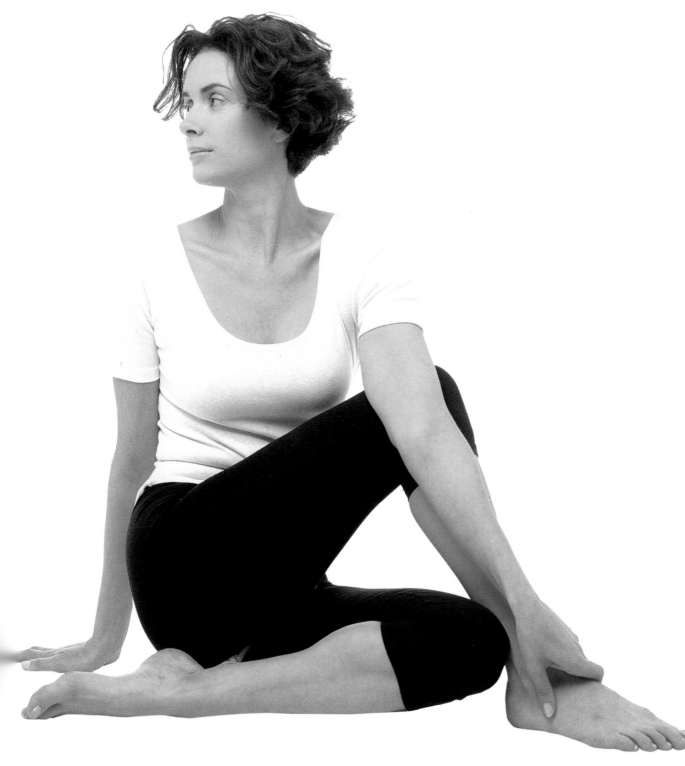

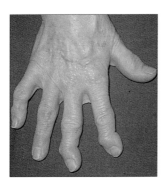

Arthritis

There are several types of arthritis. Osteoarthritis develops with age, often where there have been old injuries or in joints that have been overused, perhaps because of the type of work a person has done. Rheumatoid arthritis is a disease of the immune system which occurs when the lining of the joints becomes inflamed and swollen. There are also rarer forms which come from virus or bacterial infections. Rheumatism is a general term for muscular aches and pains that may be the forerunners of rheumatoid arthritis or due to a virus infection.

In osteoarthritis the cartilage covering the surface of the joint breaks down and the underlying bone becomes thickened and distorted, making movement difficult and painful. The joints most commonly involved are the hips, knees and spine. Being overweight or taking too many laxatives makes things worse. It is most common in the elderly – some surveys says that 80 per cent of those over 50 have it. Before the age of 45 it is much more common in men and after that point much more likely to affect women.

Described as a disease of the immune system, rheumatoid arthritis, besides affecting the joints, can also involve the skin, lymph nodes, heart, lungs, blood and nervous systems. Joint pains are combined with a low-grade fever. It affects people of all ages, although three times as many women as men get it. It is still not clear why rheumatoid arthritis develops. Blood tests show a special antibody which acts against the normal antibodies in the blood. The pain and swelling happen because the body's white blood cells respond to this intruder by attacking the joints.

THE ORTHODOX APPROACH

The first line of treatment for both types of arthritis is ordinary painkillers, such as paracetamol, or a group of drugs, which includes aspirin, called non-steroidal anti-inflammatory drugs (NSAIDs). These reduce joint inflammation and pain but the amounts used are quite large – two to four grams per day – and side effects may include irritation of the stomach and tinnitus. There is also evidence that NSAIDs actually speed up the rate at which cartilage degenerates - the key effect of osteoarthritis.

In severe cases of rheumatoid arthritis more aggressive treatments with potentially severe side effects are used, such as gold salt injections, d-penicillamine and corticosteroids, which may be used to reduce inflammation.

There are also a number of mechanical treatments. Splints may be applied to prevent deformities, fluid can be drawn directly off from a joint and anti-inflammatory drugs injected straight in. Physiotherapists have a programme of exercises to keep joints mobile and they also make use of heat treatment or exercise in a warm pool. Other techniques, none of them very effective, include paraffin wax baths and infra-red lamps. In severe cases surgeons can replace damaged joints with artificial ones made of metal or ceramic. There are also operations to fuse joints, which relieves pain but leads to a loss of movement.

THE HALE APPROACH

A sudden onset of joint pain needs to be taken to your doctor in case there is an infective element, which could rapidly

destroy the joints. A more slowly progressive development of arthritis can be tested by certain blood tests, again through your doctor. Once a diagnosis has been made and the form of arthritis is clear and non-aggressive, then complementary treatments can be very effective and keep you drug free. If drugs are required, then complementary therapies should be used alongside them, to help the curative process as well as diminishing the side effects of the drug treatment.

The effectiveness of complementary medicine in the treatment of arthritis varies considerably from individual to individual, from a dramatic improvement to some relief of painful symptoms.

Diet is a key factor in arthritis, so I would first recommend seeing a Western nutritionist or following an Ayurvedic diet as part of a general Ayurvedic treatment.

Once diet has been addressed, homeopathy, acupuncture and light therapy can bring an improvement to the condition and contribute to the relief of pain, as can osteopathy, chiropractic and aromatherapy.

The supportive treatments can all be of benefit, not in effecting a complete cure but in the relief of symptoms.

ACUPUNCTURE/ CHINESE HERBS

The causes are wind, cold and dampness which cause the blood and the *chi* energy in the body to become stuck. Needles are usually inserted near the affected area, mostly to relieve pain. Sometimes herbs are also given to relieve pain and promote circulation.

NUTRITION

In general, a diet of complex carbohydrates (instead of sugars) and lots of cod liver oil and cold-water fish is recommended. One specialized diet involves cutting out all consumables from the nightshade family, which includes tomatoes, potatoes, aubergine (eggplant), chillies and tobacco. The idea is that some people are genetically susceptible to the alkaloids found in this family. Eating ginger may be beneficial. Certain mineral and other supplements have also been found to be useful in repairing damaged cartilage, including: bromelain, niacinamide (this can sometimes have a harmful effect on the liver), methionine (an essential amino acid), Vitamins C and E, and pantothenic acid. The herbs yucca, *Boswellia serrata*, devil's claw, *Curamia longa* and *Withania somnifera* have been shown, in controlled experiments, to improve osteoarthritis.

Many sufferers from rheumatoid arthritis have bowel problems which allow bacteria out of the gut and into the bloodstream and this may be what lies behind the auto-immune response. Certainly the disease is rare in societies that don't eat a Western diet. Food allergy also seems to contribute, so besides cutting out foods from the nightshade family, wheat, corn, dairy products, sugar and beef should also go.

A vegetarian diet is useful because arachidonic acid, which makes inflammatory conditions worse, is made from animal products. Inflammation may be further reduced by increasing the intake of eicosa-pentaenoic acid (EPA), which comes from cold-water fish such as mackerel, herrings, sardines and salmon. Supplements are also advised; in addition to those for osteoarthritis, they might include the antioxidant selenium, some manganese and flavonoids. Liquorice, turmeric (right) and ginseng would also be liberally included in the diet.

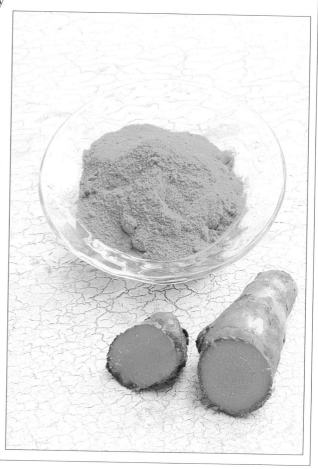

AYURVEDA

According to Ayurvedic practitioners, arthritis stems from eating the wrong sort of food. If we eat the foods that don't fit in with our type (*dosha*), then toxins build up and are stored in the joints. In general our Western diet – in which meat, dairy products and foods high in acid, such as alcohol and certain fruits, predominate – are the cause of the problem, since they affect the *Vata dosha*, which controls the central nervous system.

Patients need to switch to a more alkaline diet with rice, fruit, grains and vegetables. A complete *panchakarma* detoxification is essential and will use such methods as enemas, laxatives, herbal steam inhalation and oil massages. Patients will also be advised to take some exercise and to find the right activity for the mind such as meditation.

LIGHT THERAPY

Placing people under full-spectrum lights suspended from the ceiling dilates the blood vessels, which in turn boosts the rate at which the body can repair itself via improvement in blood circulation. In the case of arthritis this helps to reduce swelling and pain. Treatment may be once a week or once a month, depending on the severity of the case.

OSTEOPATHY

Treatment for osteoarthritis varies according to the stage the disease has reached. In acute, recent-onset cases, the osteopath's first job is to reduce pain through muscle manipulation and deep muscle massage to ease pressure on the affected joints. This treatment also improves blood supply to the joints as part of the body's natural healing process. Ice or cold water therapy may be used to reduce swelling, and advice would be given on how this can be done at home.

In chronic cases, a X-ray may be necessary to establish whether there is any problem such as osteoporosis or a fracture, in which case the spine would be treated very delicately. If there is no such problem, treatment concentrates on mobilizing joints. Soft tissue manipulation improves the condition of the muscles and blood vessels around the affected joints. Treatment of the nerves in the spine through pressure techniques improves neurological supply to joints and muscles.

Diet is absolutely crucial with arthritis and most osteopaths will give advice, first testing saliva and urine to assess the body's pH balance. Bad diet may lead to excess acidity, which the body can eliminate only at the cost of its reserves of alkaline minerals such as calcium and magnesium. Loss of these minerals can lead to osteoporosis and many arthritic conditions.

For rheumatoid arthritis, treatment centres on lifestyle, diet and control of the problem. Good nutrition can support glandular function, reducing stress. Manipulation to relieve pressure on the spine also relieves pressure on the immune glands.

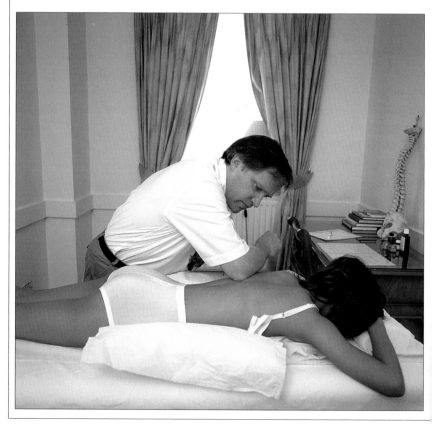

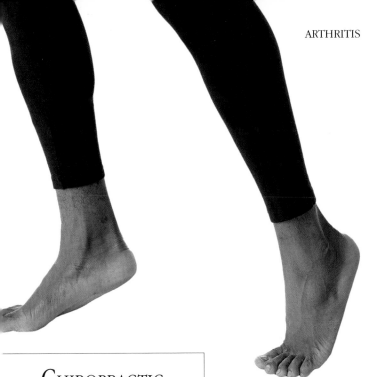

SELF-CARE

Indian Medicine
If the knee joints are affected walk on tip toes every day.

Avoid all acidic foods such as citrus fruits and seafood.

Make a paste of ginger powder and turmeric in equal parts and put it on the affected part for 30 minutes. Alternatively rub in arnica balm or tiger balm.

Nutrition
An alkalinizing diet – cutting out acidic food – may be recommended, because a poor digestion doesn't break down toxic acids properly; they therefore accumulate in the joints, where they cause inflammation and pain. Do not stay on this diet for more than a month – after that others foods should be introduced gradually. Full details are available from a naturopath, but the foods to avoid include red meat, dairy products, wheat products, sugar and coffee. Instead go for the likes of white fish, pulses, chicken, goats' milk, oats and vegetables. Foods said to be especially beneficial include green-lipped mussel, devil's claw and kelp. You will also be recommended vitamin and mineral supplements.

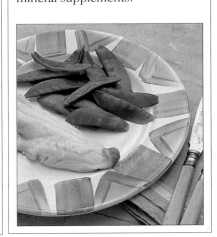

CHIROPRACTIC

The term arthritis (from the Greek *arthros*, a joint, and *itis*, inflammation) is a generally used description for joint disease, of which there are about 200 different types. A more appropriate name for what many people suffer would be *arthrosis*, in which the joint is not inflamed and may not itself be painful. This problem is also commonly called 'wear and tear' and can happen to anyone over the age of about 30. Pain comes not just from the joints but more often from the tight and tender muscles associated with the worn joints, which no longer function with optimal movement.

Chiropractic does not claim to be a cure for arthrosis, but it can relieve the symptoms in the joints. By locating the problem area and freeing up stiffened joints and muscles, mechanical correction usually improves joint function and significantly reduces pain and discomfort. Often this means a reduced intake of medication and a more enjoyable lifestyle.

HOMEOPATHY

When cases of osteoarthritis flare up there are a number of specific remedies, depending on the particular case, such as:

• When the pain is relieved by heat but aggravated by cold and damp, is worse when resting and in the morning but gets better with movement and as the day wears on – Rhus tox.

• Severe pain made worse by heat and movement, helped by cold applications – Bryonia.

• Heat and warm rooms make pain worse, patient feels weepy – Pulsatilla.

For rheumatoid arthritis the treatment generally aims at strengthening the whole system and pays special attention to diet.

SUPPORTIVE TREATMENTS

Tangent Therapy

The special treatment here for rheumatoid arthritis is to use compresses of hot ginger to ease the pain. These wouldn't be used with osteoarthritis. Otherwise the two conditions are treated similarly. Acupressure points are stimulated in massage, using special oils such as cypress, juniper and rosemary. When the arthritis is cold, hot ginger is good; when hot, witch hazel is soothing. Cajaput mixed with peppermint may also be used. Stretching exercises help to mobilize the affected joints.You are also put on a detoxification diet which avoids acidic food such as red meat, salt, tea, coffee and tomatoes.

Healing

Improvements from healing take longer with arthritis than with many other conditions, but the treatment does reduce the pain and dramatically increases mobility.

Moor Therapy

The ancient peaty material, containing over 300 recognized medicinal herbs and plant matter, as well as vitamins and minerals, is applied to the affected part of the body. It soothes inflammation, strengthens the tissues and restores the mobility of the joints.

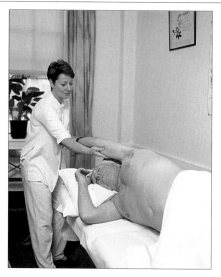

Remedial Yoga

When patients are in acute pain and joints are inflamed, yoga is not appropriate, but when the inflammation is under control yoga can be useful to improve circulation and help to relax muscles that have been tense for a long time. Long-term pain can unbalance the body and make you lose confidence; yoga can rebalance the body and give you a greater feeling of control.

Chi Kung

Special exercises, also know as 'chi massage' can direct energy to the affected area.

Reflexology

A reflexologist would give a full treatment, then concentrate on the points on the foot relevant to the location of the pain. The reflex area for the shoulder, for example, is on the top and sole of the foot just below the little toe. For the hip, it is across the top of the foot just below the ankle bone. In either case, the right foot refers to pain on the right-hand side of the body and the left foot to the left-hand side.

Hypnotherapy

According to hypnotherapists, the outlook of someone with arthritis is ossified and stuck. The sufferer tends to be entrenched in one view and stuck on their path in life. Under hypnosis they are likely to say that they can see no way out of their present plight. Even the part of the body affected can be significant – arthritis in the right hand suggests problems with practical, worldly matters; in the left hand it represents problems with the female, nurturing side. Dealing with the underlying emotional issues brings great relief.

Clinical Aromatherapy

Massage using analgesic, anti-inflammatory, anti-arthritic oils helps reduce pain and inflammation and improve mobility. Acupressure, lymphatic drainage and neuro-muscular techniques are used in the massage. Oils for use at home include rosemary, yellow birch and juniper. A low acid/low toxin diet, including herbs and food supplements, is recommended. Exercises will be prescribed for self-care.

Facing page: Rosemary and juniper

TIPS

Take light exercise where possible – swimming is especially good. Rest occasionally during the day and sleep on a firm bed.

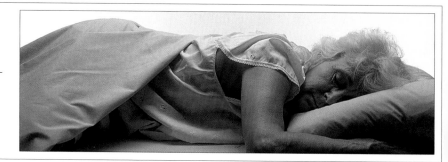

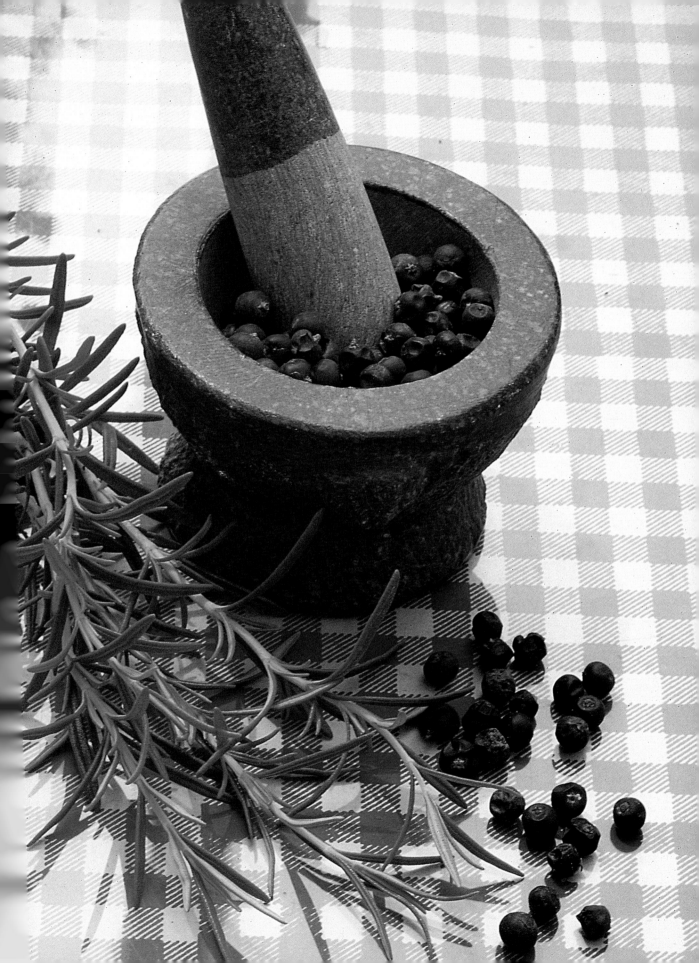

RSI

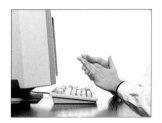

The jury is still out on what is popularly known as repetitive strain injury (RSI) and the medical profession is split. Anyone who has suffered the debilitating effects of this complaint needs no convincing of its existence, but the British government is still hedging its bets. The legal profession, on the other hand, has no such doubts and, in 1993, a learned judge in a court of law decreed that RSI did not exist.

Whichever side of the fence you fall, there can be no disputing the fact that the number of people exhibiting the symptoms of RSI has recently reached epidemic proportions. It is also true to say that the epidemic appears to have increased roughly in proportion to the rise in the use of word processors and desk-top computers. Public awareness has been fuelled by trades unions concerned for the wellbeing of their members since, in its extreme form, RSI can mean its victims have to give up a particular line of work.

The condition features disabling hand and arm pain, stiffness and an inability to continue to perform a particular function, especially the use of a computer keyboard.

THE ORTHODOX APPROACH

The quandary for the medical profession is that RSI excludes any diagnosable cause of symptoms such as tenosynovitis (inflammation of the tendons), because, if such a condition is found, then that is what is treated and there is no need to call it by any other name. The usual advice to patients presenting RSI-type symptoms is to cease the repetitive action that is causing the problems. If this is impossible due to economic necessity, your doctor may suggest looking at any underlying factors, such as anxiety, that can be corrected.

Occasionally, a mechanical support may be suggested and, in extreme cases, antispasmodic or sedative drugs may be used.

THE HALE APPROACH

As with most structural problems, osteopaths and chiropractors are generally better trained than doctors. Initial assessment should be made by specialists such as these, and only if the condition does not respond to initial treatment should an orthodox opinion, perhaps from an orthopaedic specialist, be obtained.

Once a correct diagnosis of RSI has been made, the Hale Clinic would advise using Marma massage, acupuncture combined with Chinese massage (*tuina*), Shiatsu or osteopathy and, where appropriate, the support of clinical aromatherapy.

When the course of treatment has finished, self-care exercises to relieve the constant stress to the muscles involved in repetitive movement can be done at home or at intervals during the patient's day.

TUINA/ACUPUNCTURE

One practitioner of these ancient Chinese therapies uses a combination of 20 minutes of acupuncture and *tuina* (a Chinese deep-massage technique whose name means 'push' and 'squeeze') to treat RSI sufferers. *Tuina* rates equally with acupuncture and herbal medicine in the Chinese system and is used for the control of chronic pain and the maintenance of good health. Like acupuncture, it achieves its effects by balancing the intrinsic energies of the body. It is a robust, vigorous and deep treatment that contributes strongly to the 'feel good' factor.

MARMA MASSAGE

According to the Hale Clinic's marma therapist, when muscles are overused, they produce lactic acid and eventually go into spasm more and more quickly. He gives RSI sufferers a marma (Indian deep-tissue) massage to relieve the pain, but also teaches them how to massage themselves so that they can drain off lactic acid and stimulate the essential marma points. He says, 'If the lactic acid is draining effectively, then there is no muscle spasm and no RSI.' He would use either almond or mustard oil plus a mix of Indian herbs to improve circulation and to promote the elimination of lactic acid.

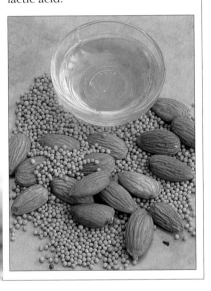

SHIATSU

According to Shiatsu practitioners, the colon meridian is usually blocked in cases of RSI, indicating that poor elimination of waste is affecting the movement of the muscles. Specific techniques are used to relieve the build-up of toxicity which results.

OSTEOPATHY

The osteopath will always check for postural problems in the RSI sufferer. Determining how a person sits, stands or moves at the time the strain is occurring can be crucial in formulating a recovery programme. The position of the neck vertebrae in sitting can affect the nerves that serve the arms and hands of the computer operator, for instance, and if RSI is diagnosed, osteopathic treatment will be given to those parts of the spine.

A build-up of lactic acid in the muscles in the arms can also aggravate RSI. An osteopath would advise on reducing your intake of acidic foods, and specific manipulation techniques would be used to reduce toxicity. In some cases the use of supports and strappings would be advocated.

SUPPORTIVE TREATMENT

Clinical Aromatherapy
RSI is a multi-factorial muscular and joint dysfunction, according to one aromatherapist. Deep massage and mobilization of the joints using anti-arthritic and detoxifying essential oils in combination with anti-inflammatory essential oils and base oils greatly reduce pain and discomfort. The massage, using acupressure and neuromuscular techniques, helps to relax the muscles and calm the nervous system, at the same time stimulating the flow of blood and *chi* (intrinsic) energy. Diet is assessed to eliminate allergens which may be causing the symptoms and to improve nutrition to aid tissue repair.

SELF-CARE

Marma Massage: Once mastered under the guidance of a professional, the marma massage movements can be used at home to prevent and relieve the symptoms of RSI.

Aromatherapy: Rosemary, eucalyptus, citriodora, juniper and yellow birch may be used for home massage treatments.

Hellerwork: Experienced Hellerwork practitioner Sharon Butler has written a book, *Conquering Carpal Tunnel Syndrome and After Repetitive Strain Injury*, on the self-treatment of RSI, including gentle stretching techniques. Good ergonomics and use of the body are essential to prevent this kind of injury.

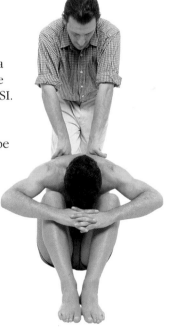

Circulation Problems

The heart and blood vessels are collectively responsible for maintaining a continuous flow of blood through the body, known as the circulatory system. This provides all the body tissues with a regular supply of oxygen and nutrients, and carries away carbon dioxide and other waste products. The circulatory system consists of two main parts: the systemic circulation, which constitutes the blood supply to the entire body except the lungs; and the pulmonary circulation, which carries blood to and from the lungs where its supply of oxygen is replenished.

On its journey from the heart to the tissues, blood is forced along the arteries at high pressure. On the return journey through the veins back to the heart, it is at low pressure, kept moving by the muscles in the arms and legs compressing the walls of the veins and by valves in the veins preventing the blood from flowing backwards. Lack of exercise or a sedentary lifestyle may therefore be at the root of circulatory problems.

Poor circulation may also be the result of, or indeed the cause of, some disorders of the arteries or veins such as an abnormal narrowing (reducing blood flow and possibly causing tissue damage) or abnormal widening and thinning of the walls (increasing the risk of rupture). Symptoms of poor circulation can range from chilblains on exposure to the cold through varicose veins to chest pains and leg pains in cases of severe arteriosclerosis (thickening and loss of elasticity of the artery walls). Poor circulation is particularly prevalent in those who are overweight or who drink too much alcohol. Heavy smokers are advised to cut down, because nicotine reduces the blood circulation in the skin.

THE ORTHODOX APPROACH

Conditions associated with poor circulation such as arteriosclerosis, aneurysm (thinning and ballooning of the artery wall), thrombosis (a blood clot within an artery) are all treated by a combination of drugs to reduce high blood pressure and sometimes surgery to replace blocked sections of artery with pieces taken from healthy veins. Some veins can be stripped altogether. Doctors agree that not smoking, switching to low-fat diets, taking moderate exercise and leading a less stressful lifestyle will help many people with arteriosclerosis.

THE HALE APPROACH

Poor circulation can affect any part of the body and a decision whether an orthodox opinion is required is rather dependent on what the symptoms are. Any symptoms that involve arteries must be dealt with initially by a doctor, since these high-pressure tubes can bleed rapidly or cause serious problems if they clog. Capillary and venous circulation problems are less likely to cause an emergency and can therefore be treated with less aggression.

Acupuncture, homeopathy, Marma massage and herbalism are all effective treatments for circulatory problems, as are the support treatments of Moo therapy, aromatherapy and reflexology. These treatments 'jump start' the circulation so that it functions normally. However, to *maintain* good circulation in the long term it is important to look at your nutrition and exercise programmes. T'ai Chi and yoga are some of the more gentle exercises; more vigorous exercise can also be of great benefit.

ACUPUNCTURE

According to acupuncturists, poor circulation usually results from an energy blockage related to the heart meridian, so treatment would concentrate on this meridian. A course of six to eight sessions of acupuncture is recommended.

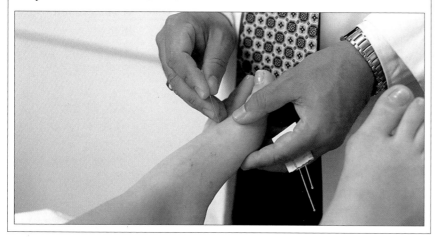

HOMEOPATHY

A common remedy for poor circulation is Hamamelis, but any number of remedies could be suitable, depending on the individual symptoms. For varicose veins which appear during pregnancy, Pulsatilla may be recommended; for arteriosclerosis in an elderly person also suffering from high blood pressure, Baryta carb. may be suitable. If chilblains burn and itch and the skin is red and swollen, Agaricus may be prescribed; if the skin is weepy Petroleum may be more appropriate.

HERBALISM

The main herb for treatment of poor circulation is capsicum, but it is very strong and is used only in small quantities, perhaps as a tincture. Prickly ash is also good for poor peripheral circulation and ginkgo is particularly effective for impaired cerebral circulation. (It reduces the viscosity of the blood and prevents the platelets from sticking together, so it is often used in Europe as an alternative to aspirin.) Another important herb is garlic, which can lower blood pressure and have a protective effect on the arteries. For problems of varicose veins and varicose ulcers, horse chestnut is frequently used, but bilberry is also a good tonic for veins in general. Witch hazel in tincture form or as a dry extract can also be helpful.

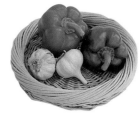

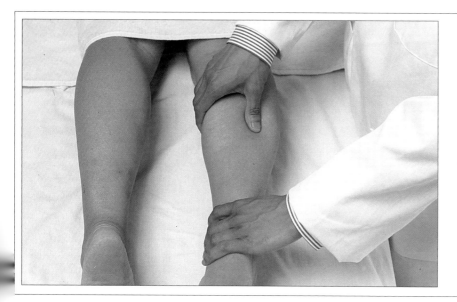

MARMA MASSAGE

This Indian deep-tissue massage is used to cleanse the cells using almond or mustard oil, which helps the blood to flow normally. It is used in conjunction with Ayurvedic medicine and anything between one and ten sessions may be required to bring the condition under control.

AYURVEDA

According to traditional Indian medicine, poor circulation or venous congestion is due to problems of *Vata*. *Vata* is one of the three basic elements or *doshas* in the body and is likened to the workings of the wind, i.e. constantly on the move. It controls the central nervous system. The main treatment for circulation aims to improve the efficiency of *Vata* and various Ayurvedic preparations would be prepared according to the individual needs of the patient, with multiple decoctions required in some cases.

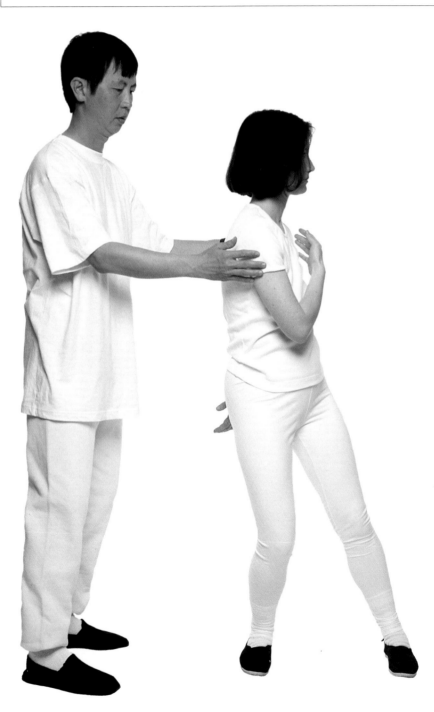

SUPPORTIVE TREATMENTS

The following therapies are especially effective when combined with other treatments.

Chi Kung

In Chinese medicine circulation includes the flow of blood in veins and arteries and the flow of *chi* (intrinsic) energy through the body. Practising exercises and correct breathing redirects the flow of *chi*, rights the body's balance and helps with circulatory problems.

Moor Therapy

After an in-depth interview and an examination of a patient's emotional, spiritual and physical symptoms, a combination of treatments may be chosen. These could include a pasteurized moor drink to be taken internally, a body massage with moor oil or putting on a body wrap. All are aimed at rebalancing the body and promoting self-healing.

Aromatherapy

Aromatherapy massage using essential oils such as lemon in a base oil to stimulate the blood flow is particularly beneficial to sufferers from poor circulation and oedema. By combining the therapeutic effects of the oils, an aromatherapist is able to address the multi-faceted problems causing the condition. A combination of angelica (a blood-cleansing oil), rosemary (generally strengthening) and juniper (good for varicose veins) is a useful massage oil or may be added to your bath.

Nutrition

Nutritionists recommend a detoxification programme as the first stage of a treatment because any 'rubbish' in the system makes it sluggish. They also test for allergies, as these can cause circulation problems, and look for dietary deficiencies. Many patients need additional Vitamins A, C and E and selenium; vegetarians may lack the Omega 3 oils found in fish oil or linseed oil. A diet that was high in these nutrients would be recommended and, if necessary, supplements would be suggested. Advice may also be given on exercise. Seeing a nutritionist three or four times over a period of three or four months should be adequate to counter poor circulation problems, but patients should start to feel better as soon as they have begun treatment.

Remedial Yoga

Yoga therapy concentrates not only on the heart for circulation problems; the diaphragm is also very important, since changing the pressure in the chest has an effect on moving the blood back to the heart from the extremities. Moreover, circulation is improved by the movement of soft tissue (muscles), so the *asanas* (yoga postures) – sequences of pressure, restriction and release – are chosen to stimulate specific muscle groups. Flexing and relaxing encourage the free movement of circulation and the benefits begin to be felt straight away.

Reflexology

Reflexology can be very successful in treating circulation problems, but is not advised for patients suffering from associated illnesses such as phlebitis or thrombosis. The duration of treatment depends on how long the

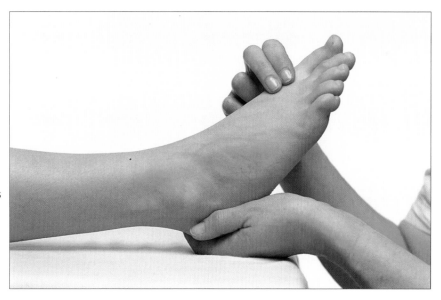

problem has been present, but is normally somewhere between three and eight treatments.

A session would begin with full treatment, covering all reflex areas on both feet, followed by extra massage of the areas relating to the heart, intestines, liver, adrenal glands and lymphatic areas. Self-treatment is not advisable for circulation problems.

TIPS

• Massage the stomach clockwise as soon as you wake up in the morning. Massage the inside of the thigh, hand and both sides of the neck with sesame oil for 2-5 minutes.
• Eat a cooked red apple at breakfast time – it increases the oxygen level in the blood, which promotes good circulation.
• Soak your feet in hot water for 10-20 minutes while covering your upper body with a blanket.
• Rub the side of your (dry) body from the armpit to the hip with a towel.

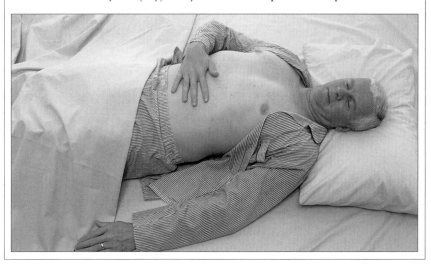

Stroke

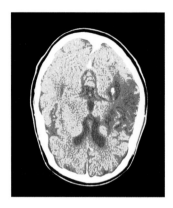

The human brain, awesome in its intricacy and power, is still largely a mystery to modern science. With more than ten million nerve cells it is the home of all that we know and feel, the generator of every physical action and response. Yet, unlike other cells in the body, brain cells once damaged are not good at repairing themselves. And they can be damaged quite easily – by infection, injury or oxygen starvation. Should any part of the brain go without oxygenated blood for more than a few minutes the affected cells will pack up permanently – the body has suffered a stroke.

The signs of a stroke vary a great deal, depending on which part of the brain has been damaged, but symptoms range from a sudden loss of speech or movement to dizziness, blurred vision, confusion and unconsciousness. They may last only a few hours: this is called a transient ischaemic attack (TIA). If the symptoms don't disappear, this is a full-scale stroke.

There are various ways that the flow of blood to the brain can be slowed or stopped. Sometimes a clot (thrombosis) forms, blocking the flow of oxygenated blood. Or a blood clot (embolism) which formed somewhere else in the body breaks free and ends up blocking an artery to the brain. In other cases, blood bursts through the wall of a weak artery into the brain (haemorrhage), eventually building up into a clot.

The good health of our arteries is crucial in avoiding strokes. Anything that makes them fur up or harden – such as smoking or high levels of cholesterol (caused by eating animal fat, lack of exercise and stress) can make a stroke more likely. These are not risks to be taken lightly: a third of first strokes are fatal.

Luckily, our brain cells have so many connections between them that healthy cells can often take over the function of damaged cells so that we hardly know that anything has gone wrong. Half of stroke survivors return to full health, but much depends on how much damage has been done to the brain, as well as on the aftercare provided.

THE ORTHODOX APPROACH

Orthodox care and rehabilitation includes speech therapy and physiotherapy to help with recovering language and mobility. Sometimes doctors also prescribe anticoagulants (a range of medicines which includes aspirin) to stop other blood clots from forming. Surgery may be necessary to remove any remaining obstructions from arteries.

THE HALE APPROACH

Any neurological symptoms such as visual disturbance, loss of balance or power, confusion, etc., must be assessed initially by your doctor, who may refer you to a neurologist. Complementary treatments have more to offer for neurological problems, including stroke, than orthodox treatment, although rehabilitation including speech therapy and physiotherapy are found in both camps. As always a holistic approach is best. If while you are undergoing complementary therapy the condition in any way worsens, ensure that your doctor or neurological specialist is aware and assesses you further.

The Hale Clinic sees certain complementary medicine treatments playing a key role in stroke recovery. The most important thing to remember is to start treatment as soon as possible after the stroke occurs. However, some treatments, such as marma massage, are of benefit to patients who have had a stroke as much as three or four years earlier.

Immediately after the stroke, homeopathy and cranial osteopathy can be of great assistance, although it may not be possible to have these treatments in a hospital. In addition a course of acupuncture combines well with marma massage twice a week over about a three-month period (depending on the severity of the stroke) – see below under *Marma Massage* and *Acupuncture/ Chinese Herbs* for details of research into these treatments for stroke patients. Clinical aromatherapy will help support the patient emotionally through these changes and the massage will stimulate the blood and relax muscles in the affected limbs, speeding up the recovery process.

Special exercises are very important to enhance and maintain the benefits of this treatment. They can be combined with healing, a good diet, reflexology and the use of essential oils.

MARMA MASSAGE

The knowledge of vital points in treating injuries has been used for thousands of years by Ayurvedic physicians. In 1995 a pilot study was held at Hammersmith Hospital in London to see how Marma could help chronic stroke patients. For six months one Marma practitioner gave treatment twice a week to a dozen elderly people who were bedridden and too ill to go home after suffering strokes. After he had massaged the Marma points to promote healing in related parts of the body, his patients showed 'modest but definite improvement' concluded the report.

'Physiotherapy is generally not very effective in such cases,' it went on, but Marma massage is 'very promising'.

The practitioner in question sees stroke damage in terms of lack of co-ordination between body and mind. Marma therapy for a stroke normally consists of 24 half-hour sessions once or twice a week, together with intensive exercises to practise at home (see below). 'Marma therapy can clear away obstructions between muscles, nerves and the brain, explains the practitioner, 'so that the brain can relearn how to control and co-ordinate the body, helping you to get back to a normal life.'

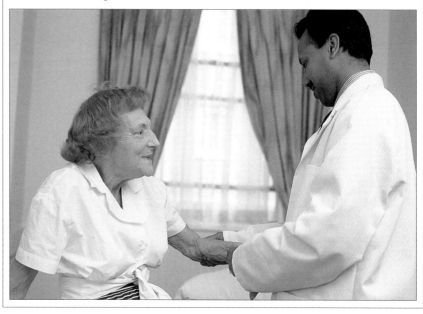

AYURVEDA

In this ancient Indian system of health care, the body's active energies need to be balanced and maintained in order to stay well. Powerful oils and herbal medicines may be used to treat people who have had strokes. Treatment concentrating on the *Vata dosha*, which controls the nervous system, can correct obstructions to the nerve pathways, believes one Ayurvedic practitioner. '*Panchakarma* (revitalizing) methods are highly successful and should be given regularly.' He also prescribes exercises, according to the condition of the individual. A course of treatment can take months or even years, with consultations once a month.

This practitioner has recently treated a 69-year-old solicitor whose right side was weakened by a stroke in 1995: 'After an eight-month-long course of ayurvedic treatment he is now able to walk with no more than a slight limp. These methods have proved highly successful in India and Sri Lanka, where almost all cases of stroke are treated by specialist Ayurvedic physicians.'

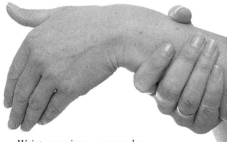

*Wrist exercises – see under
Self-Care opposite*

CRANIAL OSTEOPATHY

In this very gentle and subtle form of manipulation, which works to re-establish a normal cranial rhythmic impulse (CRI), cranial osteopaths work with the skeletal system and its supporting tissues to take the body to a point of balance.

Practitioners work with the structural supports of the skull as well as working with the cerebral spinal fluid through the CRI. 'The aim of all cranial osteopathy is to restore normal function,' explains one, 'assisting the body's self-healing mechanisms. After a stroke, I would work to restore the normal function of the blood supply, especially to and from the head.'

The therapy varies according to the type of stroke and its causes, 'but it is always a gentle technique using very small movements'. This makes it especially suitable for those of us who can't bear to be physically pulled about. The number of treatments needed after a stroke can vary depending on the response of the patient. Ongoing maintenance may also be recommended – further 'fine tuning' is always possible with cranial osteopathy. Depending on the seriousness of damage to the brain 'stroke patients have responded very well indeed'.

HOMEOPATHY

Aconite x30 is a remedy which – by stimulating your adrenal gland – can help the body to repair itself very swiftly. 'If this is given early, it could make a major difference to recovery from stroke,' according to one homeopath, who recommends taking it at ten-minute intervals until medical help arrives.

After a stroke a constitutional remedy will usually be prescribed to bolster your general health, and beyond that there are many homeopathic remedies – depending on your symptoms – which can support other treatments. Amongst them are the snake and spider poison remedies which relate to paralysis and bleeding. Agaricus may be helpful in the relief of pain, but as with all homeopathic remedies, accurate prescription by an experienced professional is very important.

HEALING

Some healers use a 'hands on' technique; others stay a short distance away from clients, in a process which one therapist describes as 'the channelling of incredibly high energy'.

In her perception, strokes have the effect of 'forcing people out of their physical bodies, with the result that they come back into the body on one side or at an angle' – hence the one-sided weakness or paralysis that accompanies strokes.

''Through healing I work to realign a person's energies so that – amongst other things – the blood circulates properly and the nervous system functions again.'

ACUPUNCTURE/CHINESE HERBS

In Chinese medicine, health is maintained when *chi* (vital energy) is well-balanced throughout the body. A combination of acupuncture and Chinese herbs may be used to help people suffering from the after-effects of a stroke. 'These therapies regulate the energy balance of the body and can get through blockages in the meridians,' explains one acupuncturist. Stroke treatment would concentrate on the stomach meridian. Within about a dozen sessions of treatment he would expect to see 'some improvement in some patients, complete recovery in others'.

This treatment should ideally be started within six months of the stroke. A recent research study in Sweden showed that acupuncture achieved better results than physiotherapy in the treatment of those who had suffered strokes.

SELF-CARE

Anything that helps keep your blood circulating in a healthy way can help recovery from a stroke. A whole food diet, low in animal fats and high in fresh fruit and vegetables, together with exercises (such as those taught as a part of marma therapy, see below) are crucial. It's also important to stop smoking and to learn to relax in order to combat stress.

Exercises

Simply daily exercises based on marma therapy which stimulate the nervous system and the marma points can aid recovery from a stroke. The theory is that information from your brain can become blocked at the joints; to remedy this, you rotate your ankle, knee, hip, wrist, elbow and shoulder joints twenty times in each direction (clockwise and anti-clockwise). You can learn these exercises in one session in order to practise them at home on a daily basis.

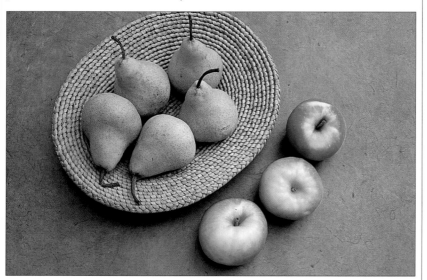

SUPPORTIVE TREATMENTS

Reflexology
'Reflexology treats the whole system,' according to one reflexologist, 'countering the feelings of exhaustion, debility and disorientation which often follow a stroke and encouraging the body's own healing mechanism to get into gear.'

In addition, by concentrating on stimulating the circulation of the blood, a reflexologist can help the colateral circulation which develops to circumvent blood clots in the body.

Perhaps most important of all, reflexology is a deeply relaxing and very pleasant therapy, making it a 'wonderful adjunct' to treatment for stroke.

Aromatherapy
This treatment can work powerfully on mind and body to help with relaxation. Oils such as rosemary, lemon and lavender help to improve blood circulation and oedema and induce relaxation.

Flower Remedies
Cherokee Rose (Petite Fleur), Fortunes Double Yellow (Petite Fleur) and Fireweed (Pacific) are useful aids to relaxation.

Colonic Hydrotherapy
This treatment can be very beneficial for paralysis of the bowel caused by stroke.

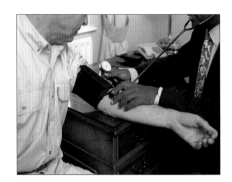

Blood Pressure Problems

Taking the blood pressure is one of the most common and useful ways of measuring variations in someone's health. It forms a standard part of an orthodox medical examination and is widely accepted as a barometer of stress. By measuring blood pressure, it is possible to tell how hard the heart has to work to pump blood round the body.

The measurement is taken by placing an inflatable cuff around the upper arm. This is then pumped up until it exerts enough pressure to stop the flow of blood in the arm's main artery. As the cuff is gradually deflated and the blood begins to flow again, readings are taken on a gauge at two points of the heart's pumping cycle. The first reading, of the systolic pressure, is taken at the moment when the heart actually beats (peak pressure); the second, called the diastolic pressure, is measured between heart beats (lowest pressure). The two readings are combined as a fraction with systolic pressure over diastolic pressure.

A normal measurement for an adult is about 120 over 80 (though blood pressure varies slightly throughout the day depending on what you are doing). However, systolic pressures of 100-140 and diastolic measurements of 60-90 are usually considered within normal bounds. Indeed, most doctors now regard a systolic reading of 100 plus a patient's age as acceptable and would not necessarily be concerned by 60-year-old with a systolic blood pressure of 160.

Abnormally high blood pressure is known as hypertension; low blood pressure is called hypotension. Both conditions may require treatment, although hypertension is usually regarded as the more serious. High blood pressure is most common among the middle-aged (about one in ten is affected), particularly men. It is an invisible disease and many people are completely unaware that they have it, although others experience symptoms such as headaches, dizziness or ringing in the ears.

Most cases of hypertension result from a combination of factors. Any one or more of the following can cause high blood pressure: being overweight, drinking too much, eating too much salt, insufficient exercise, hardening of the arteries, taking the contraceptive pill, smoking or hereditary factors. In rare cases, the cause may be a kidney disorder, and some pregnant women develop dangerously high blood pressure. If high blood pressure continues unchecked, it can contribute to serious conditions such as angina, heart attack, stroke (see page 124), haemorrhage or kidney complaints.

Low blood pressure can be as hard to detect as the opposite extreme. It mostly affects elderly people and is usually temporary. The symptoms, if there are any, include momentary giddiness or fainting on standing up suddenly after sitting or lying down.

When low blood pressure is persistent, it may be due to an underactive adrenal gland.

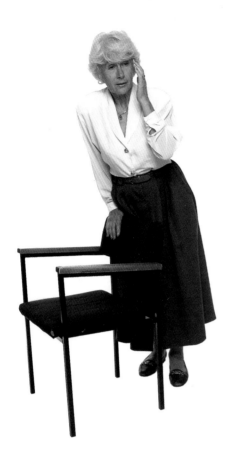

THE ORTHODOX APPROACH

Before prescribing any medication, most doctors will offer advice on some necessary changes to your lifestyle in order to reduce hypertension. These might include reducing alcohol consumption, stopping smoking, losing excess weight, cutting down on salt intake, trying other methods of contraception instead of the pill, taking more regular aerobic exercise such as walking, swimming or cycling. If these measures fail to reduce your high blood pressure, drugs such as beta-blockers (which lower the heart rate), diuretics (which increase production and excretion of urine) or vasodilators (which enlarge blood vessels) may be prescribed. Nevertheless, these treat only the symptoms and not the underlying causes, so, unless the reason for the hypertension is cured by some other means, you will have to take the drugs indefinitely to be free from the symptoms.

THE HALE APPROACH

High blood pressure is a potentially dangerous condition leading to strokes and heart attacks. A systolic blood pressure above 180mmHg or diastolic blood pressure above 90mmHg may need drug treatment. However, unless your doctor is very concerned, you may try complementary therapies, as they are often very effective and are drug free. Persisting high blood pressure or a persistence of symptoms associated with high blood pressure should be discussed with your complementary therapist so that potentially necessary orthodox drug treatment may be started. These symptoms include visual disturbance, persistent headaches, dizziness or altered consciousness.

Complementary medicine can play an important role in reducing blood pressure. The Hale Clinic approach is to do this in conjunction with orthodox medicine. If high blood pressure is diagnosed, it is initially necessary to take pharmaceutical drugs in order to lower it, as in certain cases this can be a life-threatening illness. However, complementary treatments are also effective in reducing blood pressure and once your doctor can see that the blood pressure is returning to normal, the orthodox medication can be reduced.

The Hale Clinic would first advise Buteyko breathing technique as a very useful tool the patient can use in everyday life to reduce blood pressure. Any of the following treatments can also be used, in conjunction with Buteyko or separately from it: homeopathy, healing, acupuncture, hypnotherapy and Ayurveda. These can be combined with the supportive treatments mentioned below, with particular emphasis on nutrition.

Homeopathy, again in conjunction with the supportive treatments, is also effective for low blood pressure.

HOMEOPATHY

High blood pressure rarely responds well to homeopathy alone: making changes in diet, taking more exercise, supplements and adopting relaxation exercises are essential if treatment is to work. Low blood pressure, however, can respond well after three to four sessions. Treatment would be constitutional and would depend very much on the individual case.

HEALING

One spiritual healer at the Hale Clinic who works through a person's aura (the electro-magnetic field that surrounds us all) claims to be able to reduce high blood pressure in one session and to normalize it in about six. However, she points out that high blood pressure should not be treated in isolation; a number of other factors such as fluid retention, heart problems, stress, etc. may also need attention.

ACUPUNCTURE

This ancient Chinese therapy regulates the balance between yin (the passive force) and yang (the aggressive force) in the body; an imbalance is believed to cause illness. In acupuncture theory, hypertension is caused by too much yang. A course of about six sessions should regulate the blood pressure, rebalancing yin and yang by tonifying yin and eliminating excess yang.

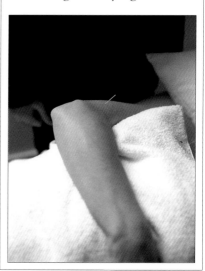

SELF-HYPNOSIS

Hypertension is a classic symptom of stress, but hypnotherapists believe that a person suffering from hypertension can train themselves to relax in a few moments of quietness or meditation and to bring their blood pressure back under control. 'I would certainly teach a patient suffering from high blood pressure relaxation, stress management and self-hypnosis techniques,' says one hypno- and psychotherapist. 'The trick is to adapt the techniques to a person's character and lifestyle. As we work together, very often people react favourably to a certain concept that I might use and they can take that and adapt it for themselves at home. The best work occurs in the time between sessions as they learn how to use these techniques and gain confidence in their ability to control their blood pressure.'

AYURVEDA

According to the teachings of this traditional Indian medicine, high blood pressure is often caused by an excess of *Vata*, one of the three elemental forces, in the head. This presents itself in the early stages as insomnia, restlessness, anxiety or headaches. 'Ayurvedic treatments are very successful in treating high blood pressure,' according to one practitioner. 'Sarpaganda is a proven Ayurvedic plant. Many years ago, drug companies produced the tablet Serpasil using the alkasoid of this plant.'

After consultation, Ayurvedic preparations will be prescribed, and dietary and lifestyle advice will be given. *Panchakarma* (revitalization) therapy can be highly successful. This may involve massage, a herbal steam bath and detoxification, and may be used in conjunction with *shiro dhara* oil therapy, in which warm oil is dripped on to the forehead and then massaged into the scalp.

BUTEYKO

All people who have blood pressure problems overbreathe or chronically hyperventilate. Correcting dysfunctional breathing with the Buteyko Method has consistently been shown to re-establish normal blood gas values, increase oxygenation and reduce smooth muscle constriction and spasms. Patients can usually safely cut down on their medication as their blood pressure normalizes. This generally begins to happen within a few days of treatment.

SUPPORTIVE TREATMENTS

Nutrition

As with a circulatory problem, a nutritionist's first aim is to undo the damage to the arteries, caused by cell proliferation, which causes narrowing of the arteries and in turn attracts calcium and cholesterol. To do this, the nutritionist would recommend foods and supplements rich in anti-oxidants, particularly Vitamins A, C and E and selenium. He or she would also use fish oils and Vitamin E to make the blood thinner so that it flowed better. However, if a patient is already

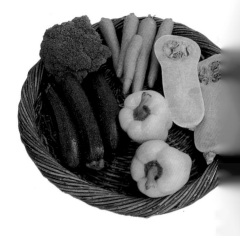

taking blood-thinning drugs, the nutritional treatment must be co-ordinated with their doctor and taken slowly so that the blood is not thinned too dramatically or too quickly.

Tangent Therapy
To reduce high blood pressure a tangent therapist would call upon a combination of Chi Kung movements and aromatherapy treatments. A detoxification and nourishing diet would also be suggested, and sufferers would be recommended to adopt Chi Kung and meditation into their daily lifestyle.

Moor Therapy
Moor therapy aims to balance the body in general. It works with the kidneys, helping them to function better and, as a result, balancing out the blood pressure as well. Moor therapy is also good for the nervous system and, since high blood pressure is a symptom of those prone to nervous anxiety, it seems to produce beneficial effects in that way too.

The Moor herbal drink is the starting point for treatment. The body cannot heal itself until it is detoxified. With Moor the healing comes from within and symptoms start to subside before the application of any topical treatment such as a body wrap.

Chi Kung
This traditional Chinese exercise system is ideal when combined with other therapies. Practitioners report that those with high blood pressure get excellent results from adopting the principles of Chi Kung, because the exercises slow a person down, enabling them to achieve more with less effort.

Flower Remedies
Both high and low blood pressure can be treated successfully with the Bach flower remedies and the extended range of over 2,000 flower essences. Fireweed (Pacific) is good for both conditions, Periwinkle is beneficial for hypertension and Kapok Bush (Pacific) or Penta (Petite Fleur) for hypotension.

Remedial Yoga
If you suffer from hypertension you should ensure that you do yoga with a qualified teacher and inform your doctor. That said, both high and low blood pressure can benefit from yoga's *asanas* (postures) and breathing practices. According to one teacher, 'The system can relax and allow the body to balance or centre itself. More balanced breathing means better use of the diaphragm and that helps all functions of the body.' Yoga has a direct effect on the circulation of the blood, encouraging a free flow both to and from the heart.

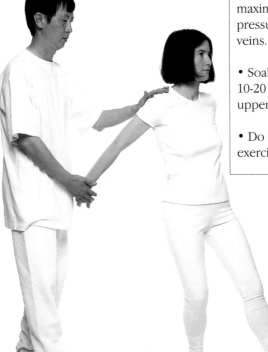

Asthma

Fifty years ago asthma was comparatively rare and caused a handful of deaths every year. Today, despite, or possibly because of, a wide variety of drug treatments, the numbers have soared and it now affects three million people in the UK, 750,000 seriously, and kills about 2,000 a year.

The symptoms, which often appear in early childhood, are wheezing, coughing, shortness of breath and difficulty in breathing. During an asthma attack, the airways of the lungs narrow because their walls go into spasm. Breathing is often made even harder because the airways can also become blocked with thick plugs of sputum.

The attacks happen because the airways are especially sensitive and so the spasms can be triggered off by all sorts of irritants that are harmless to most people - pollen, house-dust mite, cat hairs, even cold air. In many cases this seems to be an allergic response because sufferers have a high level of the white blood cells which are involved in an allergic reaction. Also, asthma patients often suffer from other allergic diseases such as eczema (see page 74) or hay fever.

In non-allergic cases the culprits include certain types of drugs (for example beta-blockers, aspirin and its relatives such as ibuprofen) and the fumes produced by some industries such as vinyl manufacture. An extraordinary range of activities is said to make asthma worse, including colds, laughing, talking too much, stress and passive smoking.

Doctors faced with a wheezy cough that seems to vary with the seasons and be affected by pets or certain chemicals would probably diagnose asthma and confirm it with a test that measures the volume of air breathed out. If this is not as large as it should be then the patient is given a drug to relax the air passages (the bronchioles) and the test is repeated. An improvement indicates asthma.

THE ORTHODOX APPROACH

Patients are advised to avoid all the things that might trigger an attack – house mites, etc. – and a few seem to be helped by allergy injections, but for the majority treatment consists of inhaling two different types of drugs – bronchiodilators to relax the constricted airways and steroids to reduce inflammation.

The emphasis is on catching sufferers early – a recent programme, for instance, has been targeting schoolchildren. However, drug side effects can be severe – increased sensitivity and shaking hands from the dilators, and decreased resistance to infection, stomach problems and osteoporosis from steroids – and despite huge resources allocated to research, orthodox treatment has presided over an enormous increase in mortality, morbidity and incidence of the disease.

THE HALE APPROACH

Asthma is a life-threatening condition which can develop very rapidly. The diagnosis of asthma is currently on the increase and doctors are very quick to label children especially with this condition, when in fact the problem is no more than a wheeze. But true asthma is particularly aggressive in younger people and children, and all asthmatics should be under the care of a general practitioner, if not a hospital specialist. Once life-saving drug treatment has been established and is available to the patient or his

or her parents, comple-mentary treatments can be utilized safely and with great efficacy.

Please note the following as differentiating signs for a serious attack:

1 An inability to move.

2 A persisting pallor or blueness of the skin and lips.

3 Obviously, an inability to inhale or a respiratory rate (the number of breaths) greater than 30 per minute.

4 A pulse or cardiac rate of greater than 120, persisting for more than five minutes when at rest.

Any of these signs should alert the asthmatic to the need for drug treatment or to call the doctor.

Our experience at the Hale Clinic has shown the great results of the Buteyko breathing system in preventing asthma attacks – up to a 92 per cent success rate in one research study. The advantage is that, once trained, the patient has a tool to prevent further attacks occurring. However, it does involve a lifelong commitment to changing your pattern of breathing. If it is difficult to find a Buteyko practitioner in your area, the following treatments can be helpful.

Nutritional therapy has helped eradicate asthma completely in some cases but not in others. These approaches may also involve a restricted diet for most of the patient's life, whereas with Buteyko you can return to eating what you like after the completion of treatment. Homeopathy, Ayurveda, acupuncture and herbalism can all be effective in treating asthma.

If attacks have a strong psycho-logical basis – if, for example, you notice that they come on after periods of stress or emotional outburst – it may be advisable to choose homeopathy or psychotherapy or hypnotherapy. If using other therapies you get rid of the asthma but the underlying emotional cause remains, it may subsequently manifest itself in another disease pattern.

BUTEYKO

Although asthma sufferers feel that their problem is not getting enough air this radical approach – developed by the Russian professor of physiology Konstantin Buteyko – is based on the idea that asthma is caused by breathing too much.

'All asthmatics breathe two, three, four times more than the healthy norm,' says one Buteyko practitioner. To understand why this is harmful you need to understand a few unfamiliar facts about respiration. Although most of us think of carbon dioxide (CO_2) as the waste product from breathing, we actually need about 6 per cent CO_2 in the body for maximum oxygen absorption.

The problem is that CO_2 makes up only 0.03 per cent of the atmosphere, so our lungs actually store CO_2. Over-breathing is a problem because it dilutes that CO_2 store. Closing down the airways is the body's way of saying, 'Stop breathing so much!'

The Buteyko Method involves learning to breathe within the medically recognized norms of tidal volume, during a week-long course comprising five one-hour lessons. Bona fide Buteyko practitioners have a policy to refund tuition fees to any asthmatics who do not achieve substantial benefits.

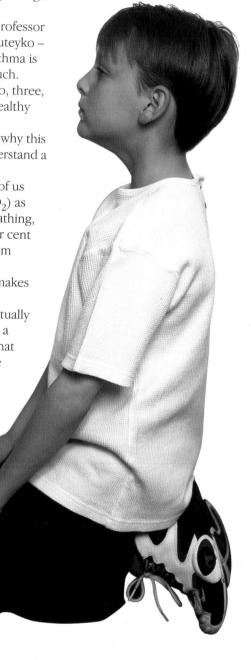

ACUPUNCTURE/ CHINESE HERBS

Acupuncture classifies asthma into three types. The most common is a physical type known as 'overheating mixed with damp'. The second stems from a deficiency in kidney and lung energy – in Chinese medicine the lungs are just bellows controlled by the kidneys. The third is 'windy cold' and is caused by living in a cold environment, so cold drinks and raw food should be avoided.

Treatment, which normally takes eight sessions, involves needles in the relevant meridians as well as the use of about ten herbs, including balloon flower root, lepidum feet and bitter almond.

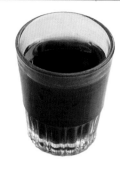

AYURVEDA

According to the Ayurvedic system, the body is controlled by three forces or *doshas*. Asthma is the result of an excess of *Kapha* (the *dosha* which controls the lymph system) in the lungs, although *Vata* (responsible for the central nervous system) can also be involved. Using diet, lifestyle changes and massage, the *doshas* are brought into balance again.

A full course of treatment, which includes Ayurvedic oral preparations, may take from three months to two years, with a session once a month.

HOMEOPATHY

If the attacks are caused by an allergy, the patient may be given a homeopathic dose of the trigger, such as cats' hair. What is prescribed for an acute attack depends very much on the individual case but here are some examples:

• For an attack that comes on between midnight and 2 a.m., when the patient is very anxious, restless and chilly and feels better sitting up – Arsenicum.
• For an attack which involves small amounts of phlegm, nausea and the chest feels as if there is a heavy weight on it – Ipecac.
• For an attack between 2 and 4 a.m. when the person gets up and sits with face on knees and looks pale and tired – Kali carb.
• For an attack that makes the patient feel exhausted, with mucus in the lungs that cannot be coughed up and pale, clammy skin – Antimonium tart.

NUTRITION/ALLERGY TREATMENT

Some cases of asthma, especially in children, can clear up when certain foods are removed from the diet. Eggs, fish, shellfish and nuts are most commonly linked to an immediate reaction, while the following are likely to have a delayed effect: milk, chocolate, wheat, citrus fruit and colourings, especially tartrazine (orange), sunset yellow, amaranth and coccine (both red). One study found that 80 per cent of asthmatic children had low stomach acid; this has to be corrected or fresh allergies may develop. Buteyko treatment (see previous page) can also be helpful here, by correcting acid/alkaline balance in the body.

Eliminating all animal products from the diet – no meat, fish, eggs or dairy products – has also proved effective. This is because many asthmatics have an imbalance in their fatty acid metabolism which makes them produce more leukotrines – the body chemical involved in the sort of inflammatory reactions found in the airways. The point is that leukotrines are made from arachidonic acid, which in turn is only found in animal products.

The vitamins B_6, B_{12}, C and E have all been found to be useful, as have the minerals selenium and magnesium.

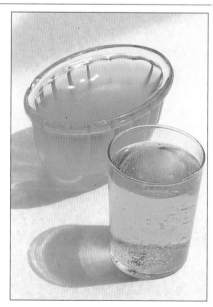

Some food colourings have been linked with asthma

HERBALISM

Ephedra has long been used in treating asthma, hay fever and colds, and the alkaloid ephedrine is often found in prescription drugs for asthma. The plant has other anti-inflammatory ingredients, but can be damaging if used for a long time because it weakens the adrenal gland. Consequently ephedra is usually given together with liquorice, which strengthens the gland. Liquorice has another beneficial effect, which is that it increases the time the anti-inflammatory hormone cortisol stays active in the body, while at the same time reducing its side effects.

Another anti-inflammatory herb is Chinese skullcap. Its effect is similar to that of aspirin, but while aspirin has been linked with asthma attacks, Chinese skullcap has no adverse effects. Angelica has been found to be effective in cases where there is an allergic reaction to pollen, dust, etc., by reducing the amount of allergic antibodies in the blood.

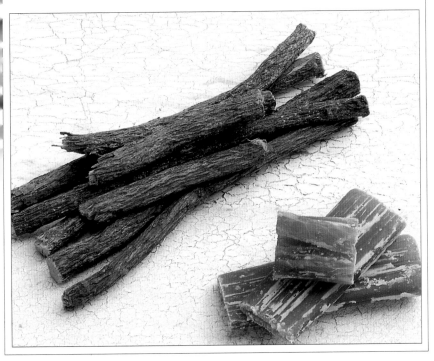

HYPNOSIS

According to hypnotherapists, the problem asthmatics often have is that they can't get their breath out. The underlying psychological message is that some thought or feeling is not being expressed. Under hypnosis patients can be helped to discover what the events are that have led to these feelings and then to let them out. Once they have been expressed, the asthma improves and often clears up completely.

One hypnotherapist says that once asthmatic's symptoms occur, conditions can worsen through expectation and repetition. Through hypnosis, the patient can be assured that this need not necessarily be the case, and that by reducing anxiety and tension attacks can be controlled and drug usage contained to the prescribed level.

SUPPORTIVE TREATMENTS

Healing
Healing relieves stress and calms the patient down. Then it is easier to reduce or stop the inflammation by going into the lung area of the aura and dilating the airways to allow freer breathing.

Alexander Technique
This postural therapy brings the body into better alignment, reducing tension in the thoracic area and making breathing easier. After a course of treatment, which may consist of as many as 20 or 30 sessions once or twice a week, you should know enough about the techniques to practise them yourself and incorporate them into your daily life.

Reflexology
For asthma sufferers, this entails working on the balls of the feet, which are linked to the chest, lungs and shoulders.

Osteopathy
This can help a lot by gently releasing the tense ribcage and the soft tissue dysfunction of the pleural dome, diaphragm and thoracic cavity, as well as concentrating on the respiratory centres and the nervous system in general. Osteopathy is normally a long-term treatment, but with children the results can be seen very quickly. In most cases the frequency and intensity of the attacks are significantly reduced. Parents and partners can be taught how to do massage as well.

Chi Kung

A number of the 1,500 special exercises are relevant here, depending on the individual. These slow patients down so they can begin to listen to their own pulse, learning to concentrate their *chi* (intrinsic) energy and sending it to the affected areas. The exercises help to open up the lung meridian, alleviating and preventing symptoms.

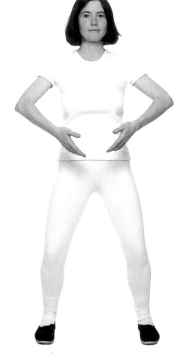

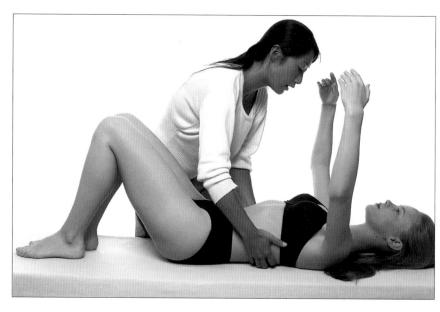

Remedial Yoga

One effect of an asthma attack is that tension, a spasm, occurs within the muscles of the chest. This tightening adds to the sense of shortness of breath, disrupting breathing rhythm. Yoga teaches us to relax and extend the muscles of the chest, helping breathing to relax. Within the lungs, yogic breathing helps bring a healthy flow of air and circulation to the lungs, encouraging the healing of inflammation. This results in us developing a deeper, more relaxed rhythm of breathing, and a sense of confidence in our breathing is restored.

GDS Techniques

Asthma patients have a limited ability to expand the chest fully while breathing in, due to excessive tension in the muscles used for breathing out. Therefore they compensate by using the muscles connected with the spine, the shoulders and the upper chest while breathing in. This process of compensation affects the posture of the trunk, in the long term inducing tension in the back, shoulders and upper chest.

In such cases GDS Techniques work to stretch the muscles used for breathing out and to relax the muscles used to compensate. The techniques can help asthma patients improve their quality of life by teaching them optimal breathing patterns as well as correct posture for the whole body.

An hour-long GDS Techniques session comprises an interview, assessment of posture and movement, establishing a link between the problem and its cause, and finally treatment, which could include soft-tissue massage, stretching, isometric exercise, breathing techniques and instruction in body awareness. You should expect to attend anywhere between five and ten sessions before achieving a marked improvement in your condition. Your therapist will also recommend a programme of movements and breathing techniques which you can continue on your own for the rest of your life.

Aromatherapy

The treatment aims to relax the patient and reduce the histamine reaction, using antispasmodic oils such as lavender. Advice will also be given on lifestyle changes and diet. Massage concentrates on the neck, chest and abdomen, making use of acupressure points.

SELF-CARE

Aromatherapy
Marjoram has a soothing, fortifying and warming effect and is very good for use in steam inhalation. Other helpful oils are amber, cedar wood, eucalyptus and peppermint.

Indian Medicine
As a breathing exercise, breathe in for two counts and out for three. Repeat ten times.

Pressure points: press between the big toe and the next, on the under side rather than the top, for thirty seconds (below). Repeat on the other foot. There is a spot, known as lung 7, on the inside of the wrist in the crease just below the thumb; pressing it for thirty seconds during an acute attack brings relief.

Yoga postures: there are specific yoga postures that can help, but what is best varies from individual to individual. One generally helpful one is the cobra (left) – lie face downwards on the ground and raise the head, shoulders and chest.

Diet: avoid mucus-forming foods such as milk and cheese.

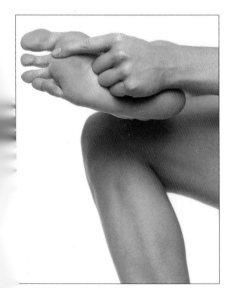

TIPS

- Keep your bed dust free.
- Practise shallow breathing.

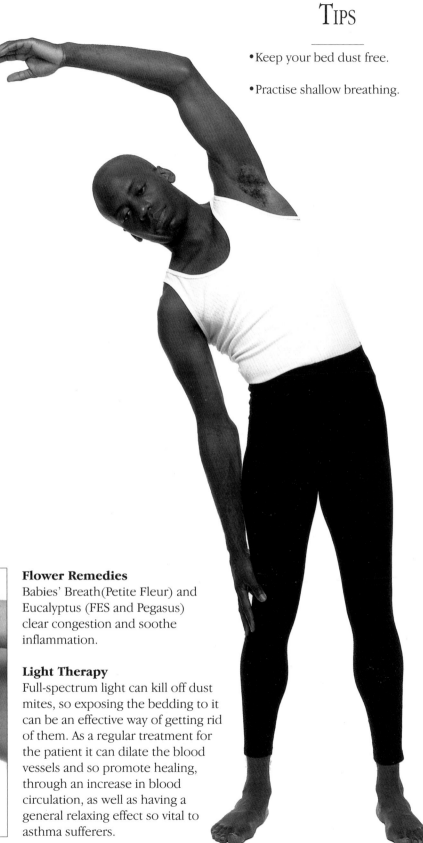

Flower Remedies
Babies' Breath(Petite Fleur) and Eucalyptus (FES and Pegasus) clear congestion and soothe inflammation.

Light Therapy
Full-spectrum light can kill off dust mites, so exposing the bedding to it can be an effective way of getting rid of them. As a regular treatment for the patient it can dilate the blood vessels and so promote healing, through an increase in blood circulation, as well as having a general relaxing effect so vital to asthma sufferers.

Emphysema

Despite being largely associated in former days with miners who inhaled coal dust from primitive pit conditions, nowadays many cases of emphysema would appear to be caused by cigarette smoking. Atmospheric pollution is sometimes still a predisposing factor and, in rare cases, emphysema is inherited, but in the main this painful and often fatal disease is attributed to inhaling tobacco smoke. However, many sufferers have never smoked and many heavy smokers do not develop emphysema. This may mean that there is another primary cause of the disease.

Emphysema is a disease in which the alveoli (tiny air sacs) in the lungs become damaged. This, in turn, leads to shortness of breath and, in severe cases, to respiratory failure or heart failure. In order to understand the progress of the disease, it helps to know a little about the mechanics of breathing. Firstly, the role of the all-important alveoli: inhaled oxygen is passed into the bloodstream and carbon dioxide is removed from capillaries to be breathed out through the walls of the alveoli which line the lungs. Tobacco smoke and other pollutants provoke the alveoli to release chemicals that damage their walls. As the damage gets progressively worse, so the oxygen and carbon dioxide exchange is impaired, making the lungs progressively less efficient. Eventually, the level of oxygen in the blood falls, with one of two effects. Either pulmonary hypertension develops, leading to cor pulmonale (enlargement and strain on the right-hand side of the heart) and subsequently to oedema (accumulation of fluid in tissues), particularly in the lower legs; or patients compensate for the loss of oxygen by breathing faster. Unfortunately, however much a sufferer tries to compensate by breathing more rapidly, if the condition is left untreated and/or a patient continues to smoke, they will find it increasingly difficult to breathe.

Emphysema is often accompanied by chronic bronchitis, which is also brought on by smoking and air pollutants.

THE ORTHODOX APPROACH

The characteristic symptoms of emphysema for which a doctor will be looking include shortness of breath, first noticed on exertion but eventually present even at rest; bluish lips; possibly a barrel-shaped chest; a chronic cough and/or a slight wheeze. From these signs, a chest examination and various other tests, emphysema may be diagnosed. The tests may include a blood sample from an artery to measure blood gases; a venous blood sample to establish levels of alpha-antitrypsin (present in the rare cases of inherited emphysema); a chest X-ray to exclude other causes and determine the extent of the disease's spread; and pulmonary function tests to assess breathing capacity and the efficiency of the alveoli.

Emphysema is incurable, so any treatment will only control the disease. First and foremost, the patient must stop smoking completely. Bronchodilator drugs are given to widen the bronchioles and ease breathing. Occasionally, corticosteroid drugs, taken by an inhaler, are used to reduce inflammation. If oedema is present, diuretic drugs are prescribed to reduce the volume of fluid. In extreme cases, oxygen therapy may be used.

THE HALE APPROACH

Emphysema, being a loss of lung tissue, can lead to episodes of severe shortness of breath, often worsened by overrriding infection. Modern drugs may be necessary and therefore emphysema should initially be diagnosed and monitored by your doctor. However, no orthodox treatment has methods of recuperating damaged or destroyed lung tissue, whereas complementary therapies aim at just that.

Complementary medicine cannot yet offer a cure for emphysema; however, it can not only relieve the severe symptoms, it can also considerably delay the onset of the disease.

The Hale Clinic would highly recommend the Buteyko breathing technique as a tool which the patient can use to relieve symptoms.

Also of assistance are osteopathy or the GDS Technique combined with acupuncture and healing.

GDS TECHNIQUES

GDS Techniques is a preventative as well as a curative physical treatment. One GDS Techniques practitioner and physiotherapist explains, 'GDS Techniques can improve the quality of someone's life and their breathing. Emphysema patients tend to over-expand the chest and exhaust the muscles used for breathing in as they fight for more and more breath while neglecting the muscles for breathing out. I have to determine, by observing their ribcage and back, how they use their muscles; then I use techniques like massage and breathing exercises and posture to relax them. I focus on the breathing, but I must check posture as well. If you have a tense spine, you cannot breathe in and out properly.'

An hour-long GDS Techiques session comprises an interview, assessment of posture and movement, establishing a link between the problem and its cause, and finally treatment, which could include soft-tissue massage, stretching, isometric exercise, breathing techniques and instruction in body awareness. You should expect to attend anywhere between five and ten sessions before achieving a marked improvement in your condition. Your therapist will also recommend a programme of movements and breathing techniques which you can continue on your own for the rest of your life.

GDS Techniques combine exceptionally well with the other therapies that are suitable for emphysema patients.

ACUPUNCTURE

In less advanced cases of emphysema, where the lungs are not too badly damaged, acupuncturists have been able to ease a patient's breathing and improve blood circulation in the lungs, so bringing some relief to the sufferer. They do this by applying needles on the acupuncture points on the lung meridian, and, depending on the cause and effect of the emphysema, other meridians as well. For example, many emphysema victims suffer badly with mucus, so this problem would also be addressed using the appropriate acupuncture points.

OSTEOPATHY

Some emphysema sufferers have gained relief from their symptoms using osteopathy. 'There are certain osteopathic moves that help to empty the congested pockets of the lungs,' explains one osteopath. 'The upper dorsal region of the spine supplies the heart and lungs, so we would loosen up that area in particular. Emphysema sufferers are often afflicted with congested gall-bladder problems, so a little work on the abdominal area can help. I would certainly also give dietary advice and probably treat them with herbs as well.'

As this is a chronic, long-term illness, a sufferer would probably need an initial course of treatment to improve their condition and then perhaps a monthly consultation to keep things in order.

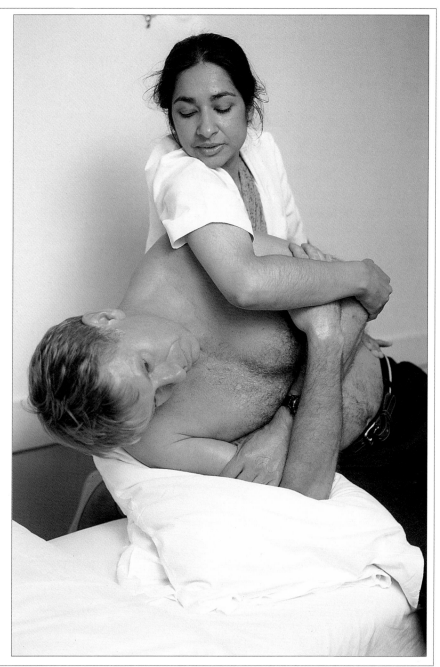

BUTEYKO

According to the principles of the Buteyko Method, some 200 diseases are linked to dysfunctional breathing, emphysema being one of them. Buteyko can recondition and normalize the breathing and restore the body's most important function, using a series of special breathing exercises and lifestyle changes which initially teach patients to overcome their symptoms. 'Patients with emphysema (who generally take the same drugs as asthmatics) will quickly find they can walk further before becoming breathless,' says one Buteyko practitioner. 'Patients are usually delighted to find an increase in vigour, concentration and the elimination of many symptoms that one would not necessarily attribute to improved breathing.' Buteyko cannot claim to cure emphysema, but it can relieve symptoms and delay the onset of the disease. With the application of Buteyko techniques, most patients can reduce their reliance on symptomatic medications and reverse their symptoms.

The Buteyko techniques for emphysema are taught over a minimum of 10 one-hour sessions on consecutive days. Some patients will require more than 10 sessions, depending on their individual condition.

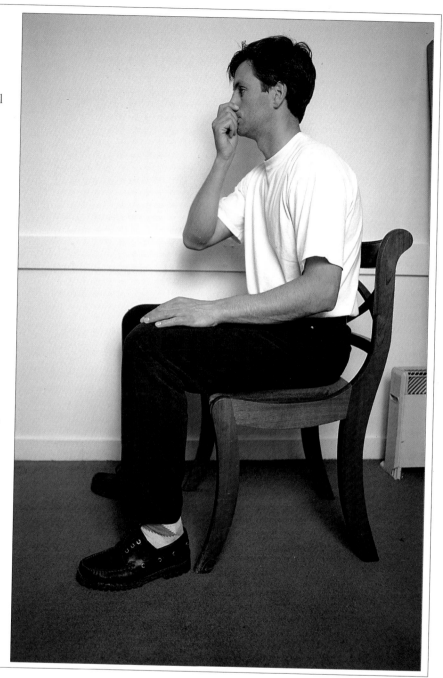

SUPPORTIVE TREATMENTS

Energy Healing
For a condition such as emphysema, healers will work in conjunction with other therapists to bring relief of symptoms and to help improve the patient's breathing. Healing is a completely non-invasive therapy during which the patient lies down while the practitioner channels healing energy through to them. Some patients experience heat, cold or tingling sensations, and the treatment will almost certainly be a powerful experience for them.

Cancer Support

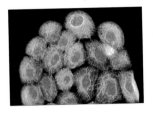

Cancer is a word that strikes fear into the hearts of most people. Because of the terror that surrounds this illness, we are loath to talk about it, and so the myths and misconceptions are perpetuated. In reality, cancer is a blanket term for many different symptoms, some of which are almost invariably curable. Discussion and learning more about this so-called modern scourge can contribute a great deal towards giving patients a positive and determined approach to their illness. Cancer occurs when abnormal cells develop. Body cells are constantly reproducing with over 90 per cent replaced every six months. Occasionally, a dividing cell (which is how they replicate) produces abnormal (mutant) cells which do not have the correct genetic coding. These then multiply uncontrollably and a cancer is formed. Mutant cells can also travel in the body and start other cancers known as 'secondaries' in other parts of the body. In the normal course of events, the body's white blood cells kill off these abnormal cells, but sometimes the regulating system breaks down or is swamped by the sheer volume of mutant cells. In this way, cancer is able to develop and take hold.

Depending on the form of cancer presented, its treatment and the likelihood of a cure will vary greatly. For example, 98 per cent of people with skin cancer survive, while only 7 per cent of lung cancer victims live longer than five years. However, statistics should not always be taken at face value. Death rates generally take no account of the stage at which the condition was diagnosed and when treatment started. It is generally true that early diagnosis greatly improves the chances of survival. Moreover, as more and more killer diseases of previous generations, such as TB and diphtheria, are eradicated, so people live longer but eventually succumb to something else, often cancer. Indeed, over 70 per cent of all new cancers are diagnosed in people aged 60 years or more.

Something between a quarter and a third of the population is now likely to contract cancer of some sort. Of these, about 14 per cent will be men with lung cancer; approximately 10 per cent of cases will be breast cancer in women and 12 per cent will be skin cancer in both sexes. Almost half of those who die of cancer have the disease in the lung, breast, prostate or bowel.

To a certain extent, heredity can affect the likelihood of your getting cancer. The chances of a woman getting breast cancer are four times higher if her mother, aunt or sister has had it. However, more important still are environmental factors. Smoking, heavy alcohol consumption, excessive fat or protein in the diet, inhaling asbestos particles, overexposure to sunlight or radiation from nuclear waste or

leakage (such as at Chernobyl), or contact with benzopyrenes (dry-cleaning chemicals) are all known to increase the likelihood of developing cancer. It has been observed that people in parts of the Himalayas can live to the age of 120 and do not develop degenerative diseases such as cancer, but do succumb to them if they adopt a Western-style diet.

Psychological factors can also contribute. It appears that people who are prone to bottling up their feelings are at greater risk than those who give vent to their emotions. Depression, grief and mental stress can increase the chances of a person getting cancer. Research at King's College, London University, has shown that cancer patients are less able to cope with loss such as bereavement, job loss or a broken relationship.

THE ORTHODOX APPROACH

None of the orthodox treatments for cancer constitutes a complete answer in itself, but a combination of surgery to remove tumours, radiotherapy to kill cancer cells by radiation and chemotherapy to stop the multiplication of mutant cells with drugs is considered effective. However, there are certain restrictions and drawbacks with all of these treatments. If the cancer is well established before treatment begins, it may already have spread to other parts of the body, in which case surgery may not remove all the cancerous tissue. Nevertheless, removal of the cancer is sometimes essential to relieve symptoms caused by obstruction as well as to control local spread.

Although techniques have improved considerably in recent years, radiotherapy treatment is still very often accompanied by unwelcome side effects such as tiredness, nausea and depression. Chemotherapy uses a cocktail of drugs, and some have recently been developed which attack the cancer cells only. This reduces the level of side effects but it is still an unpleasant form of treatment during which a patient may experience nausea, tiredness and hair loss.

Most orthodox doctors accept that any positive steps to increase a person's belief in their power to recover are a good thing; as a result they generally condone psycho-logical support and complementary therapies that address a patient's mental attitude. Several major cancer hospitals in Britain now use aromatherapy, hypnosis and relaxation techniques with cancer patients.

THE HALE APPROACH

All cancers must be monitored by the orthodox profession. Modern-day technology is very advanced and can tell the state of the tumour effectively. When treating cancer it is necessary to know if the problem is worsening, improving or staying the same so that adjustments can be made to the treatment.

The orthodox approach can be very effective with many types of tumour, but sadly most are not cured. Surgery can cut out a tumour, but has no effect on the underlying cause, while chemotherapy and radiotherapy are toxic in themselves. Very few oncologists talk about cure and prefer to discuss the effectiveness of their treatment by looking at two, five or ten-year survival. Any course of treatment that can offer only a low-percentage two or five-year survival rate may also be experimental, since the orthodox world is trying to improve the outcome. It is always worth considering the use of complementary medicine alongside, if not instead of, an orthodox treatment if the chances of success are low or the treatment is liable to be more poisonous than the tumour.

The Hale approach is a very broad and holistic one which will support the correct orthodox treatments while working with the best of complementary care.

Once the initial shock of being diagnosed with cancer has subsided, for many people the question immediately arises, 'What is the best course of treatment for me to take?' This is where questions about the role complementary medicine can play in cancer arise. Orthodox treatment is not pleasant by any stretch of the imagination, and many people ask if they can avoid it.

The Hale Clinic approach at this time is to encourage patients to continue with the orthodox treatment when it is of benefit and use complementary medicine as a valued support at the same time. It is advisable to keep your oncologist informed of the complementary medical treatment you are receiving.

We recommend an approach working with the body, mind and emotions. The treatment given by our consultant in complementary medicine uses nutrition and homeo-pathy combined with healing and Chi Kung. This can help strengthen the patient so that the cancer has more difficulty in taking hold. It can also reduce the side effects of chemotherapy and radiation.

Hypnosis and psychotherapy, autogenic training, visualization and meditation are recommended as means of strengthening the mind and emotions in order to make it more difficult for the cancer to take hold and to reduce the side effects of orthodox treatment.

In addition there will be nutritional therapy using some of the anti-cancer diets. The bio-resonance machine with detect deficiencies in vitamins, minerals and trace elements, as well as testing for food intolerances and providing the patient with a special diet.

The hormonal pathological test can be used to identify cancer at early stages, by looking at blood samples through a computerized microscope and comparing them with thousands of other blood samples. The blood pattern changes in the early stages of cancer, so any problems can be picked up.

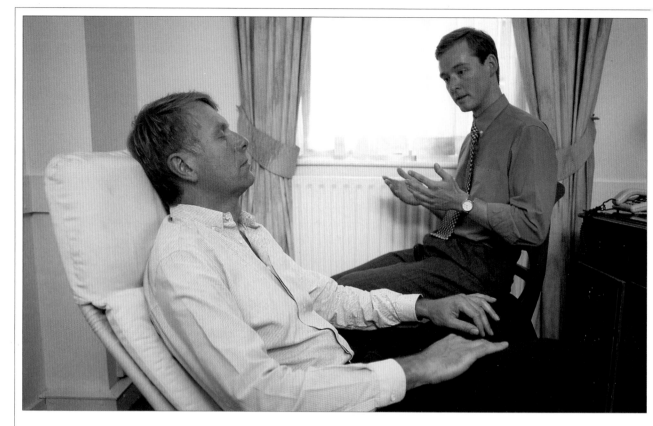

PSYCHOTHERAPY/ HYPNOTHERAPY

Since it is commonly accepted that psychological factors can cause cancer to develop, it seems a logical assumption that they can also play a part in a patient's chances of survival, and there is now a body of evidence to support this theory.

Psychotherapy and hypnotherapy can be used to help cancer patients focus their attention on improving their mental and emotional state. Positive attitudes and a belief in one's wellbeing are now believed by immunologists to enhance the ability of the body's defence mechanisms to destroy cancer cells. One psychotherapist and hypnotherapist agrees that 'imagery and visualization techniques can be used to help people actually to slow down the cancer. Hypnotherapy can

be used very successfully for pain relief and pain control. However, I often find that many people are quite content to allow conventional medicine to treat the cancer and use a complementary therapy to treat the emotional trauma that comes from it.'

In cases of terminal cancer, psychotherapy and hypnotherapy can be beneficial in helping the patient to cope with the trauma of their diagnosis and deal with their impending mortality. The same therapist says, 'In this case, my role is to try to help them to come to terms with their illness and to make peace with themselves. We would concentrate then on more spiritual aspects as we were working.'

Another hypnotherapist adds that it has long been suspected that a major trauma could possibly trigger a cancer. Psychotherapeutic techniques (including hypnosis) can help a patient 'to work through any

lingering effects of a past trauma and reframe their attitude into a positive and progressive one, looking forward to the future. In this way the patient can create conditions in which it is more difficult for the cancer to spread.' It is possible to suggest to a patient in deep trance that he or she has control over hundreds of thousands of operations within the complex system of the body. 'It is well accepted that individuals have the ability to slow or increase their own heartbeat, raise or lower their body temperature and influence other bodily functions normally considered the province of the unconscious self. It would therefore be a tragedy to ignore the capability of individuals to heal themselves, and hypnosis can be used in conjunction with conventional medicine to achieve this.'

ENERGY HEALING

The presumed effect on the immune system of belief in one's power to recover seems to account for instances of 'spontaneous regression' (reduction in the tumour) by spiritual healing. One healer tells of a case where a patient who was in great pain with a large skin melanoma was not only relieved from pain, but the cancer shrank until it was gone. She believes that healing can be beneficial whether the patient is undergoing radiation or chemotherapy or if the tumour is very small.

NATUROPATHY

Not only can a healthy diet and lifestyle reduce your chances of contracting cancer, but, for those who already have the disease, a healthy body can lessen the side effects of orthodox treatment and increase the body's own ability to fight cancer cells. One consultant in complementary medicine has reviewed, used and assessed many of the treatments currently being used to defeat cancer: 'My choice is to select from the following specific anti-cancer medications used in conjunction with suitable orthodox treatments and high-dose anti-oxidant therapy. The medications are Iscador, which has been run through clinical trials; Yeastone, which has been with a British university and undergone trials, and Native Legend Tea, which is only supported by anecdotal evidence.'

The Hale Clinic has a specific programme supervised by our complementary medicine consultant, under which cancer patients come to the clinic over a one to two week period and are given a specific cancer support programme to follow. They are then put in touch with relevant practitioners in their area so that the programme can be followed in the medium to long term.

SELF-CARE

Flower Essences
There are quite a few flower essences that you can use at home which may be helpful and your choice will vary depending on the kind of cancer. However, as a generalization, Lilac (Petite Fleur) and Nani Ahiahi (a Hawaiian essence) are recommended. Lilac, Babies' Breath and Jasmine (all Petite Fleur) are particularly relevant to breast cancer.

Visualization Techniques
One self-help version of this technique, advocated in a book entitled *Getting Well Again* by Dr Carl Simonton, asks the patient to see in their mind's eye a battle in which powerful immune cells hunt down and kill weak, confused cancer cells. Many patients say they have felt better after this treatment and have learned to cope with their illness well enough to improve the quality of their life to a significant extent.

SUPPORTIVE TREATMENTS

Aromatherapy
The beneficial effects of aromatherapy are becoming increasingly widely recognized and many hospitals now offer it as an additional treatment, particularly on oncology wards.

Oils such as neroli (orange blossom), patchouli, lavender and rose, which have a relaxing, calming effect on the body and mind, are used to soothe the patient, together with anti-tumeral oils such as angelica. Often uplifting oil such as benzoin or bergamot may be used.

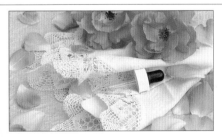

Lavender, rose, Roman chamomile, ylang ylang and patchouli are particularly good for depression.

Massage helps to relax the patient, reducing pain, uplifting, increasing feelings of self-worth and improving sleep. Touch is very important in these cases.

In addition, reflexology, Shiatsu and acupuressure can soothe and relax a patient during orthodox treatment.

Chi Kung
When coming to terms with a serious illness such as cancer, peace of mind is an essential ingredient. Chi Kung, in conjunction with other treatments, can bring inner harmony and relaxation to a cancer sufferer. Generally speaking the redirection of *chi* (intrinsic) energy can restore the balance in the body, relieving pain, helping recovery from operations and supporting the patient through chemotherapy treatments. In the early stages of cancer, according to one Chi Kung teacher, specific exercises can remove 'cancerous *chi* energy' from the body altogether.

Gastro-Intestinal Disorders

As the main gateway into our body, the gastric system, which includes 8m (26ft) of intestine, is susceptible to a range of problems. All of them share the common symptoms of nausea, stomach pains, vomiting and diarrhoea.

When there is an infection in the stomach, it is known generally as gastro-enteritis. This can range from a mild tummy upset, caused by bacteria in contaminated food, to full-blown dysentery. Similar effects can be produced by poisonous foods, large amounts of alcohol, aspirins or laxatives.

Bacteria can also cause a sudden flare up of inflammation of the lining of the intestines. In severe cases the bowel can be perforated and need emergency treatment. When the inflammation is chronic it is called either ulcerative colitis, which affects only the large intestine, or Crohn's disease, which can affect the whole gut. The cause of both of them is unknown, although various sorts of infection may be involved. Both conditions run in families and are more common among Jewish people and in Western societies. Symptoms include an almost constant urge to go to the toilet, blood in your stools, cramps after eating in the case of Crohn's and pain on the left side in the case of colitis. Ulcerative colitis is also associated with skin rashes, arthritis and, in long-term sufferers, cancer.

Crohn's can affect a person at any age, although the peak periods are adolescence and early adulthood, and after the age of 60. In the young the most common site of inflammation is the ileum (part of the small intestine), which causes spasms of pain in the abdomen, diarrhoea, loss of appetite, anaemia and weight loss. In the elderly, Crohn's is more commonly found in the rectum and is the cause of rectal bleeding. In both age groups the condition may also affect the anus, resulting in chronic abscesses, deep fissures (cracks) and fistulas (abnormal passageways). It may also attack the colon, causing bloody diarrhoea, and in rare cases the mouth, oesophagus, stomach and duodenum (the upper part of the small intestine).

The additional distress and discomfort of forming a fistula occurs in about 30 per cent of cases. This can be internal (between the loops of the intestine) or external (between the intestine and the skin of the abdomen, or around the anus), often following an operation or the rupture of an abscess, and this may cause leakage of faeces to the skin. Thankfully, abscesses form in only 20 per cent of cases.

Further complications to look out for may include inflammation of parts of the eye, severe arthritis, ankylosing spondylitis (inflammation of the spine) and skin disorders.

One of the most common forms of gastric problem is irritable bowel syndrome (IBS), also known as spastic colon. Patients have the usual gastric symptoms – pain, gas, diarrhoea or constipation and indigestion – but it is different from Crohn's or ulcerative colitis although the cause is also unknown. IBS is a disturbance of involuntary muscle movement in the large intestine, but there is no structural abnormality of the colon so the patient need not experience weight loss or malnourishment. IBS seems to be linked with stress, is more common in women and often starts in early adult life. Some 10-20 per cent of adults suffer from IBS and although symptoms may subside and even disappear for periods of time, the syndrome is usually recurrent through-out the patient's life.

IBS sufferers sometimes find temporary relief from pain on passing a bowel movement or wind, but are often left with a sense that they have been unable to empty the bowels completely. Additional effects may include heartburn, back pain, faintness, a tendency to tire easily, agitation, reduced appetite and palpitations.

See also *Constipation* (page 154) and *Peptic Ulcers* (page 162).

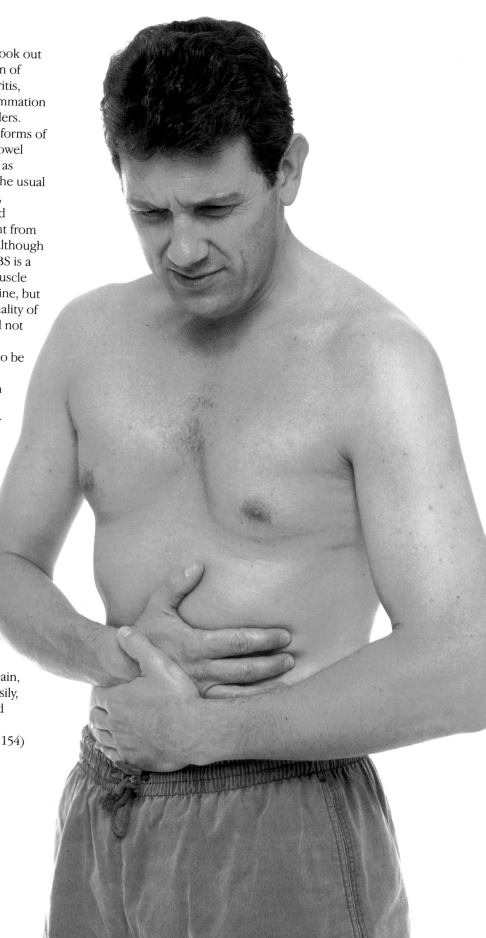

THE ORTHODOX APPROACH

Diagnosis for most gastric conditions involves blood, urine and stool tests, as well as X-rays taken after barium, which outlines the intestines, has been swallowed. For closer examination colonoscopes are inserted via the rectum. If symptoms suggest Crohn's disease, a physical examination may reveal tender abdominal swellings, which may be due to a thickening of the intestinal walls. In this instance a blood test revealing protein deficiency, anaemia or evidence of inflammation is another aid to diagnosis.

Where there is a definite infection antibiotics will be used, plus rest and replacement of lost fluid, vitamins and minerals. Acute cases of colitis may also respond to antibiotics. Treatment for chronic ones begins with Sulphasalazine – a compound that includes aspirin; if that fails steroids are used. The last resort is surgery to remove the colon.

A high-fibre diet is generally suggested. Sufferers from IBS may be recommended to eat bulk-forming agents such as bran or methylcellulose. Short courses of antidiarrhoeal drugs such as loperamide may be given for persistent diarrhoea, as well as antispasmodics to relieve muscular spasm. However it is usually the case that these treatments relieve the symptoms of IBS rather than cure the disorder.

Acute attacks of Crohn's disease may require admission to hospital for a blood transfusion, intravenous feeding and intravenous administration of corticosteroid drugs. In extreme cases a surgical operation may be necessary to remove damaged portions of the intestine, to deal with an abscess,

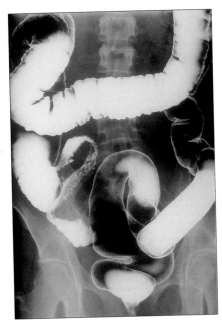

obstruction or perforation (rupture), or in cases of severe bleeding.

Stress and emotional problems are recognized as a factor in many gastric problems, so some doctors may suggest psychological help as well.

THE HALE APPROACH

Any abdominal pains that are severe or persistent must be reviewed by your doctor. Many complementary therapies are far more effective than orthodox medicine in the treatment of a number of abdominal complaints, but it is important to differentiate between an appendix that is about to burst and an irritable bowel syndrome. You should follow through with any advice given by an orthodox practi-tioner until a complementary practitioner can come forward with a better treatment. As always, if you intending to stop orthodox therapy, ensure that your doctor is in agreement, or at least aware.

Gastro-intestinal disorders of one kind or another affect a large proportion of the population and complementary medicine can play an important role in treating them. The Hale Clinic would firstly suggest looking at your nutritional and possible allergic responses to food, which could be aggravating the condition. Homeopathy, acupuncture and Ayurveda will also address nutritional aspects, as well as giving other specific treatments. In addition, colonic irrigation can be very helpful with certain gastro-intestinal disorders, though not for stomach ulcers.

We would also strongly advise a training in the Buteyko breathing method - this will give the patient an effective self-care tool that they can use in the case of nutritional gastro-intestinal disorders.

If the patient is known to be suffering from Crohn's disease, we would specifically recommend a treatment of biological medicine, moving on to homeopathy, acupuncture or Ayurveda once the diet has been stabilized.

Although the above treatments will have a beneficial effect on a patient's stress levels and emotional state generally, the mind and emotions do have an important influence on the wellbeing of the stomach. Hypnosis can therefore play an important role in treating gastro-intestinal problems. For example, many people would see irritable bowel syndrome as an illness with clearly defined physical symptoms, but a recent research programme showed a clear improvement with hypnosis.

There are a whole range of supportive self-care programmes for gastro-intestinal disorders. Many people are unaware of the importance of the full-spectrum light in the absorption of food, but light therapy can be a very beneficial aid to the digestive process.

NATUROPATHY

Many of the gastric diseases, especially irritable bowel syndrome and Crohn's disease, are linked with a typical Western diet – refined foods, etc. – and with food allergies. It also seems that a bran-rich diet, offeed as conventional treatment, can make colitis worse. In one study 45 per cent of patients put on a placebo treatment went into remission, as opposed to only 20 per cent of those who had been given steroids. Many Crohn's sufferers discover for themselves that certain foodstuffs aggravate their condition and a naturopathic consultation would be an extension of this discovery, giving advice on foods to avoid and recommending herbs, vitamins, minerals and a diet that will alleviate symptoms, and possibly cure the illness completely.

The nutritional approach takes account of factors generally ignored by conventional medicine: for instance the bacteria flora of the intestines, disturbed in both colitis and Crohn's. All patients also have difficulty absorbing enough nutrition and may need up to a 25 per cent increase in protein intake. Certain drugs commonly used to treat colitis and Crohn's may make the loss of minerals and nutrients worse.

Some patients may be put temporarily on an elemental diet which contains all necessary nutrients and protein in a pre-digested form. An alternative approach is to use IgG4 and IgE testing (analysis of the immune system's reaction to various substances) to look for food allergies and remove them from the diet. It is best to avoid carrageenin – produced from red seaweed and used in the food industry as a thickener in such products as ice cream and milk chocolate – which has been found on occasion to produce colitis when the gut flora has been disturbed. Meat must also be cut out because the biochemical processes it triggers are linked with increased inflammation. Fish oils do not have this effect.

IBS sufferers are usually recommended a wholefood (but bran-free) diet to maintain regular bowel action. Potential irritants such as alcohol, coffee and strong spices should be avoided, as should grain-related foods such as breads and cereals, and Grade A proteins such as meat. If a laxative is required, use a natural, gentle one such as linseed to restore regularity.

BIOLOGICAL MEDICINE

'Since hidden food sensitivities play a vital role in the development of Crohn's disease, an attempt at identifying the offending food items should always be made,' explains one therapist. 'Elimination provocation diets, cytotoxic food tests and IgG4 antibody food tests are reliable identifying tools, while subsequent diet adjustment will generally produce considerable improvement in a patient.' A stool test for parasites should be carried out, since parasitic intestinal infestation can promote food sensitivities.

The next step is to eliminate the food sensitivities altogether. The most effective treatment for this is Enzyme Potentiated Desensitization (EPD), whereby a minute amount of a food vaccine, mixed with the enzyme beta-glucuronidase, is injected into the skin. This causes a gradual adjustment in the tolerance level of the immune system, curing existing food sensitivities in the course of time. (EPD is not suitable for pregnant women or children under the age of two and a half.) Nutritional supplementation is often useful.

The length of treatment by biological medicine varies but, after initial consultation and starting the diet, you can expect approximately three follow-up appointments (one a month) to monitor progress. EPD involves a minute intradermal injection once every other month, the number of which is determined by the speed of progress (the normal range is about 5-10 injections). As a generalization, therefore, treatment may take anything from six months to one and a half years. Depending on the severity of the case, biological medicine normally produces considerable improvement and, in some cases, total cure.

As testimony to the success of the treatment, the therapist tells of a 29-year-old woman who had suffered from Crohn's disease for over 14 years. She experienced constant stomach ache and diarrhoea, accompanied by fatigue and joint pains. 'Diet adjustment based on cytotoxic food test results produced a disappearance of stomach ache, fatigue and joint pains after one month, and normalization of stools after two months. The patient has now discontinued conventional oral medication and has recently received her first EPD treatment.'

HOMEOPATHY

Treatment is given to strengthen the constitution generally and then there are specific remedies for particular symptoms. For instance:

• Pain suddenly stops and starts as if the abdomen is squeezed by a hand, face red and hot, abdomen tender and sensitive – Belladonna.

• Cutting pain causes the person to double up and cry out, abdomen distended with wind, attack may follow angry outburst – Chamomilla.

• Pain so violent that the person cries out, relieved by warmth, friction and pressure on the abdomen – Magnesia phos.

• Scanty, odourless brown stools which seem to burn skin around the anus, especially after cold drinks, ice creams, ice lollies or over-ripe fruit, small sips of hot drink are soothing – Arsenicum.

• Copious and offensive stools the colour of pea soup and the consistency of batter, with a lot of wind and colic, urgency early in morning, empty feeling afterwards – Podophyllum.

Homeopathy has had some success in treating Crohn's disease, and in the case of IBS one practitioner reports more than 80 per cent improvement in symptoms in some patients and general improvement in most others. This is usually achieved in three or four consultations, although long-standing cases may require three-to six-monthly follow-ups.

BUTEYKO

This method involves teaching people to breathe more shallowly in order to increase the amount of carbon dioxide in the lungs. There is a direct relationship between the amount of acid secreted in the stomach and the levels of carbon dioxide in the body. So if you are over-breathing, getting your breathing right can balance your acid secretions. Bona fide Buteyko practitioners offer a money-back guarantee of substantial improvement for any patient they have agreed to treat for gastric problems.

Although successful in the treatment of a number of gastric complaints, the Buteyko method has yet to be shown to be effective in the case of Crohn's disease.

ACUPUNCTURE

Many sufferers have found acupuncture helpful in the relief of symptoms of Crohn's disease. Treatment would concentrate on the stomach and large intestine meridians, to improve digestion and remove any blockages that were causing imbalance.

A combination of acupuncture and Chinese herbal treatment is reported to have improved some cases a good deal and brought total relief to others. In order to see good results, you should expect to attend six to eight sessions and to follow advice on dietary changes.

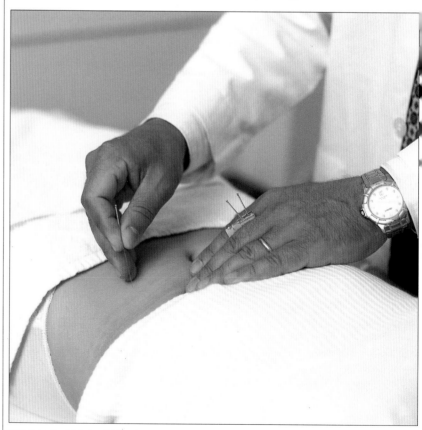

AYURVEDA

The digestion and diet lie at the heart of the Ayurvedic system, so it is a very useful approach for any gastric problems such as nausea, pain, vomiting, accumulation of gases and colic. Herbal remedies may be prescribed depending on individual needs. Also commonly used is *panchakarma* – various methods of detoxifying the body.

According to the Indian system of medicine, irritable bowel syndrome is cause by gas and fermentation of food, which are governed by the mind. A combination of Ayurvedic and marma therapies aim to stop the production of gas and fermentation, and also to balance the mind.

Crohn's disease, known as *Grahani* in Indian medicine, is the result of an imbalance in the *vata* of the gastro-intestinal tract. *Vata*, which is one of the three basic life forces or *doshas* in the body, is likened to the wind (constantly on the move) and controls the nervous system. One Ayurvedic physician calculates that a course of treatment – which would include *panchakarma* and dietary recommendations tailored to the patient's individual needs - will take anywhere from three months to a year, or even longer. Monthly consultations are essential, but improvement and in some cases total relief of the problem can be expected.

COLONIC HYDROTHERAPY

The gentle flushing of the colon with warm, salty water can bring great relief from the symptoms of IBS. As one practitioner explains, 'Colonics takes away the muscle spasm and removes the wind, mucus and bloating. A good flush-out gives the colon a chance to clear itself and the correct mucosal lining is re-established.'

Requirements vary from individual to individual, but three treatments at three-weekly intervals would be about average and you could expect some improvement after the first session. 'People sometimes have quite strong reactions,' warns the therapist, 'because they are detoxifying at quite a deep level. Sometimes they feel tired or get a headache. Others feel euphoric and light-headed.' In cases of indigestion there may be a back-up of bile which can be relieved with irrigation. This treatment should always be combined with supplements to strengthen the liver and the gall bladder. Colonics are not relevant to stomach ulcers.

HYPNOTHERAPY

The stomach is an area very much associated with feelings – 'I can't stomach it' is how people describe something they can't bear. So if there is no obvious organic cause for a gastric complaint, a hypno-therapist would look at the effects emotions could be having, especially with reference to the way the patients feel about themselves. People with stomach problems are often generous but they are also anxious about the way they are seen by others. They expect high standards and when they don't achieve them their anger can be turned inwards. Hypnotherapy can help to unravel these feelings. Particularly in cases of IBS, once the reason for a problem, distressing though it may be, is found and diagnosed, the illness is likely to disappear.

'You can introduce suggestion and visualization to help control and manage the physical symptoms themselves,' explains one hypnotherapist who is also a psychotherapist. 'I believe IBS can be treated successfully and I have seen people at the very least helped enormously so that their lives can be better managed.' If the patient is enthusiastic and keen to be helped, results can be achieved in three or four sessions. 'Hypnotherapy is a short-term treatment. We are trying to investigate the subconscious mind and suggest ways in which it might like to behave in the future.'

Once the illness has been brought under control, the hypnotherapist may well teach a client how to carry out self-hypnosis, so that they can reinforce the results of their treatment at home.

SUPPORTIVE TREATMENTS

Healing

Indigestion can be cleared up relatively quickly, says one healer. You need to clear the blockage that is preventing the right amount of acid from being produced and generally relax the stomach.

Shiatsu

This Japanese pressure-point massage works by stimulating and balancing the body's energy flow. In treating IBS a therapist concentrates on the meridians relating to the colon and other relevant parts of the gastro-intestinal system, thereby relaxing intestinal spasm and stimulating elimination.

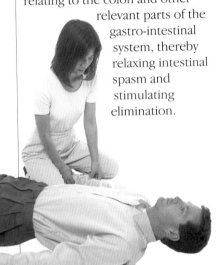

Moor Therapy

The products of the Austrian Moor are taken as a herbal drink to work on the inside. used as a thick paste the Moor may be applied directly to the stomach, where the nutrients are absorbed.

Chi Kung

Some of the many exercises can be taught to patients to show them how to channel energy to the affected area. Once learned, this is an ideal therapy for use at home.

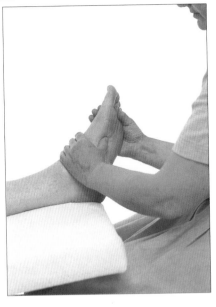

Reflexology

The area linked to the stomach is to be found on the arch of the left foot just below the ball of the foot. A much smaller area in the same place on the right foot affects the duodenum. A key area for the intestines is the one that controls the area where the small intestine empties into the large colon. This is found on the little toe side of the right foot, just before the heel.

Light Therapy

We need light for processing food, so the stomach is exposed to full-spectrum light while the patient lies on a couch. This can be done once a week or once a month depending on need. In serious cases it can also be done at home under supervision.

Remedial Yoga

People with gastric problems are often very stressed, feeling tension, anxiety and worry. These feelings increase the flow of acid in the stomach and may cause problems there. Stress also increases tension in the abdomen, which reduces circulation. Yoga, as well as being generally relaxing, can deeply relax muscles in this area and increase blood supply.

The pelvic area is also where unresolved emotions are held and yoga can concentrate on these areas to relax the mind, body and spirit, as well as bringing emotions to the surface in order to free them. This is particularly effective in dealing with the root causes of IBS.

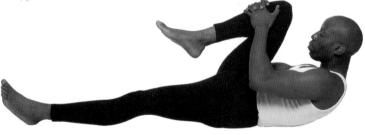

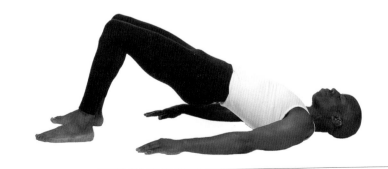

Chamomile, sage and chamomile tea

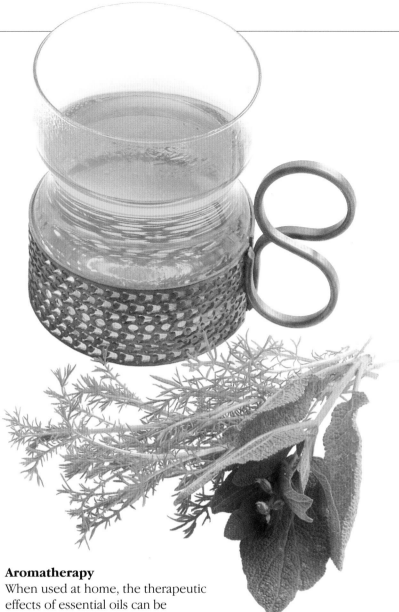

SELF-CARE

Indian Medicine

Pressure points: Bring your hands together as if you were praying and look at the little fingers; if one is shorter than the other, massage the back of the neck on that side of the body. The acupressure point known as 'stomach 36' is four fingers' width below the knee. Press for 30 seconds on each side of the bone there on both legs. It should feel tender. You can also massage both sides of the thumb on the lower joint.

Diet: Avoid drinking liquids while eating a meal.

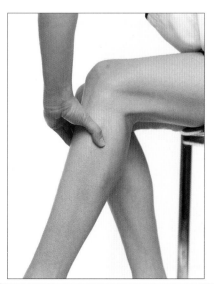

Aromatherapy

When used at home, the therapeutic effects of essential oils can be garnered in several ways: by adding a few drops to the bath, by inhalation, compresses or self-massage.

Orange, more usually used for insomnia in children, is surprisingly helpful for treating indigestion. It is warming, cheering and a confidence builder. Peppermint is the traditional remedy for digestive upsets, colic, diarrhoea, indigestion, vomiting and stomach pain. Thyme is a good digestive stimulant and an intestinal antiseptic.

For IBS commonly used oils include basil, fennel, lavender and lemon grass.

Flower Remedies

In cases of indigestion Chamomile (Petite Fleur, FES) and Sage (Pegasus) affect the stomach and are good against stress. A mixture of Castor Oil plant (from India) and Pink Seaweed (a Pacific essence) should give relief from symptoms of Crohn's disease. For IBS Bamboo (Petite Fleur) and Green Rose (Pegasus) are generally considered useful, although consultation with a flower essence practitioner will determine what best suits your particular condition.

Constipation

As we in the West eat an increasingly more refined, over-processed diet and take less and less exercise, we pay the price with our health. There are many ailments brought on by poor diet, but one of the most common and often the first indication that our diet is inadequate is constipation. It is the direct result of not taking in enough fibre to help the body rid itself of waste products. Moreover, the strain of trying to pass the ensuing small, hard motions from the bowel can lead to further complications such as bowel disorders, piles and, in some cases, appendicitis.

According to received medical wisdom there is no standard frequency that denotes 'normal' bowel movements – it varies considerably from person to person, with some regularly passing three movements a day and others one every three days. However, nutritionists and colonics experts agree that everyone should pass a motion at least twice a day.

Everyone is prone to occasional constipation as, for whatever reason, our environment, diet or drinking water change – if you are visiting friends in a different part of the country, for example, you could be constipated for a few days until your body adjusts or until you return to your customary eating habits and drinking water. This is perfectly normal and nothing to worry about. A better indication of constipation is if, during the normal course of events, your stools are small and hard and you pass them only infrequently. Moreover, if your constipation lasts more than three days, it is worth seeking advice from a doctor. In rare cases, constipation, particularly if there is blood in the stools when you do finally pass a motion, can signal cancer of the bowel.

Apart from the most common culprit of not enough fibre in our food, other causes of constipation include eating too much meat or dairy produce, not drinking enough fluids (fibre needs water to form soft motions), food allergy, lack of exercise, ignoring the need to pass a motion, dependence on laxatives, the side effects of some medicines, pregnancy (the pregnancy hormone progesterone relaxes the muscles of the intestine, which slows down bowel movements, making you more likely to become constipated), anxiety, stress and tension.

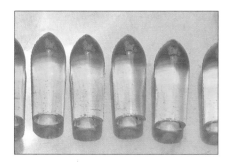

THE ORTHODOX APPROACH

Doctors are now inclined to recommend bran for constipation as well as a diet high in fluids and fibre. Laxatives and suppositories are sometimes prescribed to help retrain the bowels, and an enema may occasionally be needed. If your constipation is the result of taking iron tablets, perhaps due to anaemia or pregnancy, it is advisable to take any supplements on a full stomach, with plenty of fluid, as these tablets can irritate the stomach and exacerbate constipation.

THE HALE APPROACH

Constipation can be treated very effectively by complementary therapies without the use of drugs. Visiting a complementary practitioner initially is therefore perfectly acceptable, although a problem that persists or worsens should be investigated by orthodox means through your doctor. Any sudden change of bowel habit lasting longer than a week should be presented to your doctor, since this is a common early sign of a treatable bowel cancer.

When constipation has been present over a long period and impacted faeces have become embedded in the colon walls, colonic irrigation is highly recommended and can give very quick relief. However, it is not suitable for everyone – see page 241 for contra-indications. Ayurveda, homeopathy and acupuncture, supported by reflexology, are also effective in treating constipation.

These treatments will all require some dietary modification, with Ayurveda and colonics in particular placing great emphasis on the change of diet if the treatment is to be effective.

Nutrition is very important in treating constipation and maintaining a healthy diet is crucial in preventing a recurrence.

Surprisingly, stress figures largely in the causes of constipation for some patients, and relief from stress through hypnosis or flower remedies can help with treatment. Exercise has an important and long-term role not only in relieving stress but in keeping constipation at bay. T'ai Chi, Chi Kung, yoga and aerobic exercise are all recommended.

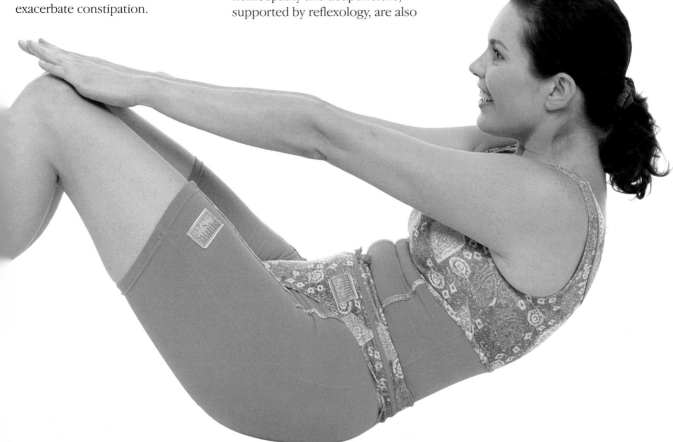

HYPNOSIS

'If you can discover any particular situation which causes an attack or if there is a pattern to the constipation, then it can be investigated under hypnosis,' explains one hypnotherapist and psychologist. He and the client work together on the problem, often using suggestion and visualization to control the physical symptoms. Hypnotherapy is particularly successful where anxiety or stress are the underlying causes of constipation.

AYURVEDA

This holistic, traditional Indian medicine is 'highly successful in the treatment and management of chronic constipation', according to one of its practitioners. 'Various factors may be involved in causing constipation. After initial consultation, Ayurvedic preparations such as herbs will be given orally. *Panchakarma* (revitalizing) methods are most useful in sustaining improvements.' Emphasis would also be placed on dietary and lifestyle advice: 'Every case is improved with proper treatment and maintenance therapy.' *Vasti* (enemas) and *vireka* (laxatives) are an important part of regulating bowel rhythm.

COLONIC HYDROTHERAPY

This gentle process of flushing out the bowel exercises the muscles of the colon and can re-establish muscle tone in a very out-of-shape colon. It also helps to correct or re-introduce normal bowel habits. Treatment lasts about 40 minutes and may include an abdominal massage. Diet is discussed and sticking to a follow-up diet is very important. There is an immediate sensation of relief as the waste is passed.

'Colonics works by rehydrating the bowel,' explains one colonic therapist. 'If the body is dehydrated, it extracts every bit of liquid from the large intestine and so the stools become hard and very difficult to pass. By taking in enough fluid in our diet and introducing water into the bowel, we can retrain the bowel muscle. The bowels need to be exercised like any other muscle. Colonics does this, as does a diet high in fibre and water.'

Colonics can also help to produce the right environment for the correct bacteria to grow in the bowel. Probiotics (beneficial bacteria that live naturally in the body) may be given during a treatment. In severe cases of constipation, there can be a connection with a toxic liver and colonics will also help to flush the liver through.

NUTRITION

Attention to diet is paramount in defeating constipation. One nutritionist recommends that we eat lots of vegetables, brown rice, whole grains, millet and that we drink lots of water but not with food. Contrary to popular belief, wheat should be avoided, especially wheat bran, since this irritates the bowel. In addition, you should cut out diuretics such as coffee, salt, sugar and alcohol. Supplements may also be recommended, particularly if you have been taking laxatives, which increase the risk of vitamin and mineral deficiency. Two teaspoons of linseed washed down with lots of water first thing in the morning are excellent for constipation.

ACUPUNCTURE

Constipation may be due to dryness and a shortage of liquid in the body, or it may be due to overheating and energy blockages. More yin may be needed. An acupuncturist will work on the stomach, liver and spleen meridians and four to six sessions are likely to be needed to 'break through the blockage'. Dietary advice and a recommendation to take more exercise would also be given during these treatments.

HOMEOPATHY

When there is no desire to pass a motion for some days, Alumina can be beneficial. However, if you feel the call to move the bowels but nothing is forthcoming, or if constipation is as a result of laxative abuse, Nux vomica is recommended. For those with piles or particularly hard stools, Collinsonia canadensis can be helpful and Plumbum metallicum is good for long-term constipation with stomach pain. Constitutional treatment is recommended in long-standing cases.

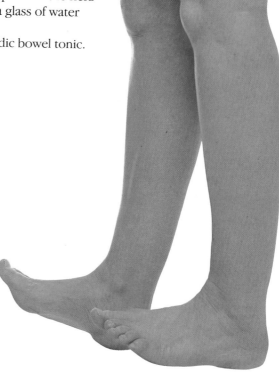

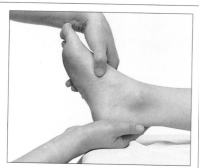

SUPPORTIVE TREATMENTS

Reflexology/Healing

These treatments complement the beneficial effects of other therapies mentioned in this section and work in harmony with them. In the case of reflexology, the areas massaged relate to the small and large intestines, the adrenal glands, solar plexus, liver and lower spine.

Shiatsu

This Japanese pressure-point massage is good for most gastric problems, especially constipation. There is always a knot on the left side of the belly button in these cases that must be massaged away. Patients should avoid cold drinks late at night or first thing in the morning; they should also eat more fibre and cut out sweet things and eating between meals.

Remedial Yoga

Yoga encourages the natural flow in the alimentary canal, enhancing digestion, encouraging absorption of life-giving energy and nutrients and freeing up blockages within our system.

Buteyko

Application of Buteyko shallow breathing techniques guarantees fast and immediate relief from constipation.

TIPS

- Drink two to three glasses of water as soon as you wake up in the morning.
- Walk on your heels for two to five minutes first thing in the morning: this helps to synchronize the intestines.
- Eat a high-fibre breakfast.
- Take one tablespoon of the herb isphaghula with a glass of water before bedtime.
- Take an Ayurvedic bowel tonic.

SELF-CARE

Nutrition

You can apply the tips given above or those gleaned from a nutritional consultation during your daily routine. Good diet with plenty of fluids and exercise will keep constipation at bay.

Flower Remedies

Flower essences can be most beneficial in treating constipation. One expert recommends poppy (Petite Fleur), cedar (FES) and Pink Seaweed (Pacific) in particular.

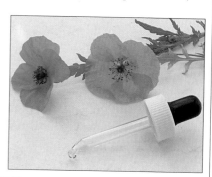

Detoxification

THE ORTHODOX APPROACH

Although conventional medicine is aware of the problems inherent in modern Western life, there is little that can be done to treat its effects. It is more likely that preventative advice will be given, perhaps on how to improve your diet and lifestyle; alternatively you may be referred to a nutritionist.

THE HALE APPROACH

Detoxification of the system is best done by complementary approaches unless the condition is life-threatening. For example, poisoning by drugs should be approached via a hospital, although after the dangerous initial toxic levels are reduced complementary treatments can be employed. Generalized detoxification from unhealthy habits and lifestyle is not embraced by orthodox medicine.

The need to clear out and clean up all the systems of the body becomes increasingly pressing in this modern age. No matter how careful we are in choosing organic foods and mineral waters, pollutants are ubiquitous and pervade every aspect of our lives.

The most obvious offenders are polluted water systems, contaminated animal feeds and the pesticides and herbicides used on crops. But the list of possible contaminators is endless: metal poison, organic solvents, aromatic hydrocarbons from vehicle exhaust fumes, never mind tobacco smoke, cleaning products, the contraceptive pill, asbestos and radioactive pollution.

Many of these pollutants are invisible and invasive: we take them in in minute amounts on a daily basis. The effects of drinking cups of tea containing traces of chlorine, aluminium, fluoride and lead from our water pipes may be negligible, you might say, but the cumulative effect of all the pollutants that are silently infiltrating our bodies is enormous. It is a slow but relentless poisoning that can only have a detrimental effect on the way we function.

This situation is compounded by the fact that most of us are lazy about the planning and preparation of our diets. We pay lip service to the nutritional advice of bodies such as the World Health Organization (who recommend at least five pieces of fruit or vegetable every day) and continue to consume over-processed diets rich in fats and simple carbohydrates such as sugar, and low in fruit, vegetables, fibre and complex carbohydrates. The result is that the body's own waste-elimination systems cannot cope with this abuse and we are unable to dispose of waste effectively, so toxicity builds up within us. Statistics document the rise in pollution – and in diet-related illnesses such as allergy, asthma, bronchitis, emphysema, Alzheimer's disease, migraine, hay fever, heart disorders and many others.

Looking back over the centuries, we find that the principle of detox-ification was recommended and practised by most of the world's religions or traditional medical systems to clear the mind and cleanse the body. These ancient principles, which were important to a person's health thousands of years ago, have a particular relevance in today's polluted world. Many symptoms can be alleviated by detoxification.

Moreover, a detox programme can help prevent a recurrence of ill health, as well as supporting other complementary therapies such as homeopathy or osteopathy. Many people's systems are so toxic that treatments take longer to work, so a detox programme can help other therapies to produce faster results.

There are many different methods of detoxification but, with the exception of Buteyko, all those described below will consider and if necessary adjust your nutrition in order to facilitate the detoxification process.

Many detox treatments have a very powerful effect on the body, so it is generally better not to combine too many. Colonic irrigation, lymphatic drainage and the Moor detox treatments can safely be used together. Otherwise, check with your practitioner before undertaking more than one detoxification treatment.

Many detox programmes will help clear the mind and calm the emotions, but it is important to be aware that some patients may need further support from psychology or hypnosis in dealing with any mental or emotional problems.

MOOR THERAPY

The body can't heal itself until it is detoxified,' says one Moor therapist. Moor treatment would involve drinking the pasteurized Moor drink and being given a detoxifying body wrap. The body absorbs what it needs of the hormones, minerals and nutrients contained in the Moor and eliminates the rest through urine and faeces.

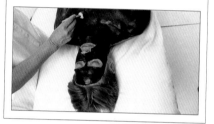

COLONIC HYDROTHERAPY/ LYMPHATIC DRAINAGE

'All the poisons entering our bloodstream cause havoc in our lymphatic system and colon and damage our health,' explains one practitioner of colonic hydro-therapy, lymphatic drainage and nutrition. 'If we look after our body with a detox – think of it as a complete spring cleaning – the whole metabolism will be able to cope much better with the daily demands of stress and toxic substances.'

Colonic hydrotherapy entails the introduction of a gentle infusion of

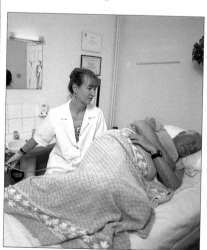

warm, filtered water into the colon to remove the encrusted faecal matter on the colon wall. This allows vital nutrients to be absorbed more easily and makes you feel rejuvenated and healthier. The therapist stresses the importance of starting gently if you have never before done a detox programme. You may be tired or have a headache after the first session; alternatively you may feel euphoric and light-headed.

Lymphatic drainage is an all-over body manipulation and massage of the lymph system that ensures the free flow of lymph fluid and the removal of any blockages. Lymph circulation plays a vital role in the immune system, the elimination of waste and the transportation of nutrients to the cells.

These therapies would normally be complemented by dietary recommendations and exercise advice. Supplements such as anti-oxidant and psyllium husk, alfa detox and the Moor herbal drink would also be endorsed. 'The use of organic herbs further intensifies the process of detoxification,' explains the therapist. 'To complete the session, an implant of friendly bacteria is always given to rebalance the bowel flora.'

Colonic therapy is not suitable for everyone – see page 241 for contraindications.

AYURVEDA

Panchakarma is the Ayurvedic form of detoxification and has been practised in India throughout the ages. It is a way of cleansing and servicing the body which can be used not only to treat certain conditions but also to prevent illness.

The treatment involves four activities: *Nirvha vasthi* (herbal enemas); *vireka* (herbal purgatives); *nasya* (herbal inhalation); and *anuvasana vasthi* (herbal oil enemas). Prior to starting the *panchakarma* treatment, it may be necessary to undergo *snehana karma* (the application of herbal oil either externally, orally or rectally) or *swedana karma* (herbal diaphoretic therapy or steam bath). Depending on the amount of toxins in the body, the treatment could be weekly or once every three months, with the change of seasons.

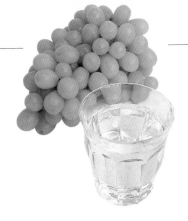

DETOX PROGRAMME

Many of us suffer from an overuse of the liver and the ingestion of toxins. For those who fall into this category, the Hale Clinic detox programme, which is geared towards supporting the liver and clearing the toxins from the system, is an appropriate solution. The clinic's complementary medicine consultant explains, 'This is just an example of a programme, although it is one that can be used by most people with some impunity.'

It comprises a three-day detox diet followed by a seven-day semi-fast diet, as follows:

Three-Day Detox Diet

Day 1: Remember to drink 2l (3½pt) of water in the course of the day, the first ½l (almost 1pt) of which should be before breakfast.
Breakfast: 900g (2lb) grapes (any type), including skins.
Mid-morning: ginger tea, made from two thin slices of fresh root ginger with hot (but not boiling) water.

Lunch: 2 medium-sized apples or pears.
Mid-afternoon: 450g (1lb) grapes.
Supper (at least two hours before bed): 225g (8oz) bran cereal moistened with any fruit juice except orange or apple.

Day 2: Remember to drink 2l (3½pt) water in the course of the day, the first ½l (almost 1pt) of which should be before breakfast.
135kg (3lb) potatoes. These can be divided into any weight for any meal and prepared in any way *but* they must contain the skins and only pepper may be added.

Day 3: 2l (3½pt) water as before.
Breakfast: one whole grapefruit.
Mid-morning: ginger tea.
Lunch: melon – any quantity.
Mid-afternoon: a handful of pumpkin or sunflower seeds (two handfuls if you are hungry).
Supper: a salad of any vegetable content with a fresh lemon juice or balsamic vinegar dressing only. (Remember that tomatoes are a fruit and should not be included.)

Seven Day Semi-Fast Diet

Day 1: Drink freshly squeezed or pressed fruit and/or vegetable juice at approximately four-hourly intervals. Quench your thirst with mineral water or herb tea, and drink at least 2l (3½pt) of fluid. Some suggested juices are apple, orange, grape, pineapple, grapefruit, blackcurrant, mango, cranberry, carrot, beetroot and celery.
Day 2: as for day 1 but add up to 450g (1lb) grapes and three bananas.
Day 3: as for day 2 but add raw and lightly cooked vegetables and any other fruit.
Day 4: as for day 3 but add whole-grain cereals, nuts and seeds.
Day 5: as for day 4 but add fish.
Day 6: as for day 5 but add offal, poultry or game.

Day 7: return to your normal diet as discussed with a nutritionist.

The fast will help to flush the liver but it can be aided by taking one of the following homeopathic remedies: Chelidonium, Berberis or Lycopodium. Ayurvedic herbs may also be useful. 'Milk thistle is popular at the moment. Or there is another compound called LIV-52,' says the practitioner who devised this diet. If people are particularly toxic (if they have been on a binge or have been toxic for a prolonged period of time), he would consider using an intravenous technique. High-dose anti-oxidants, B-complex vitamins and glucuronic acid are very important to help the liver to function well, and, if the liver is working too fast, so producing more cholesterol, an increased dosage of lecithin (1200-1800mg per day in divided doses) is recommended.

On a cautionary note, the practitioner warns, 'Using a detox programme is not a suitable alternative to better living.' He also suggests that if you are under any other medical treatment, you should first consult with your physician before starting a detox programme. It is not suitable for those suffering from diabetes, hypoglycaemia or other serious conditions such as cancer, although there are specific detoxification diets that may be prescribed for cancer patients.

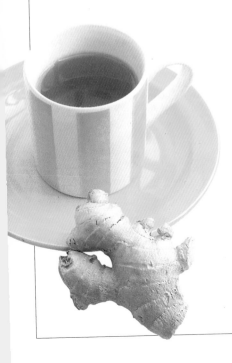

MARMA MASSAGE

·According to traditional Ayurvedic medicine, the digestive tract, liver, kidneys and muscle tissues are major areas where toxins are deposited. Marma deep-tissue massage with special oil together with individual diet advice and herbal teas will help the elimination of toxins and improve the function of the digestive tract. One marma therapist suggests that a single session (45 minutes including consultation and treatment) may be enough for those with low toxicity levels, but six sessions may be necessary if you have a high level of toxins in your system.

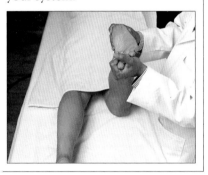

SELF-CARE

Nutrition

Bad eating habits, high alcohol intake and high fat levels in the liver are all components of a toxic body which can be helped by good nutritional advice. A fasting diet will be tailored to an individual's particular requirements. Do not be surprised if you feel terrible on about the third day of a fast. This is a recognized part of the detoxifying process. When fasting, it is recommended that you take Vitamins E and C, zinc and selenium to help eliminate free radical damage, and liver extract, dandelion tea, artichoke juice or milk thistle to improve the action of the liver.

Aromatherapy

Using lymphatic drainage massage and the diuretic/detoxification capacity of certain essential oils such as juniper, rosemary, lemon and patchouli can enhance any dietary detoxification programme.

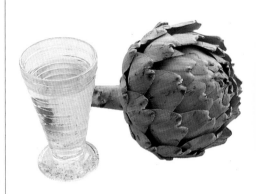

TIPS

• Fasting can be a very beneficial part of a healthy lifestyle, but fasts which last longer than ten days should be supervised.

• Combine fresh fruit and vegetables (i.e. foods with a high water content) to achieve a gently progressing cleanse.

• Colonic irrigation is advisable during a fast to clear the accumulated toxins. A bulking agent and lots of water are also essential.

• Detoxification is a cumulative, on-going process, to be carried out regularly as part of a health programme.

• Skin brushing activates and energizes the body's largest eliminative organ, the skin.

• Worry and fear may increase toxicity in the body – meditation and relaxation can help detoxify the mind and spirit.

SUPPORTIVE TREATMENTS

Buteyko

Buteyko breathing is a very simple yet powerful treatment for many problems and one of its benefits is that it is very effective in detoxifying the body. The techniques can be practised on their own or combined with other detox programmes.

Remedial Yoga

In order to eliminate toxins effectively, the body must have efficient circulation systems. Yoga can be highly beneficial in improving these systems. Good breathing and the effect of pressure and relaxing the muscles during the *asanas* (postures) can improve circulation of the blood and the immune system. Moreover, the endocrine system which secretes hormones into the bloodstream, affecting all organs in the body, can benefit from yoga and this, in turn, leads to more efficient expulsion of toxins. In a nutshell, says one yoga teacher, 'Yoga's basic premise is that you are relieving the body of any minor blockages to the flow of energy. Everybody can do this.'

Peptic Ulcers

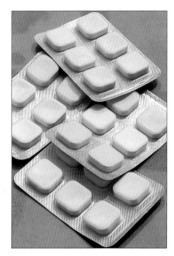

Until quite recently ulcers were thought to be one of the crosses hard-working executives had to bear. They were the mark of a striving go-getter, who strode from power lunch to stock-market take-over bid, pausing only to swallow a packet of antacid tablets. Normally, so the theory went, the stomach doesn't digest itself because a coating of mucus protects it from the hydrochloric acid which, together with an enzyme called pepsin, breaks down the food. But stress and anger can increase the amount of acid in the stomach while aspirin and other drugs can reduce the protective mucus and so the acids begin to eat away at the walls of the stomach or duodenum, creating crater-like sores which can be very swollen and tender. Classic symptoms include burning, intense pain in the mid-upper abdomen and waking in the early morning, often with a sensation of abnormal hunger.

However, in the last few years a radical new explanation for stomach ulcers has made far more effective treatment possible. It now seems certain that about 80 per cent of cases are caused by the action of a spiral-shaped bacterium called Helicobacter pylori which uses its whip-like tail to burrow into the stomach walls.

Most ulcers occur in the duodenum, where the stomach enters the small intestine. They are most common in middle age, though children can get them too. Males are affected twice as often as females, and they tend to run in families.

THE ORTHODOX APPROACH

Before the pylori discovery, treatment consisted of antacids or a newer breed of histamine blockers containing cimetidine. Both sorts relieve the symptoms by reducing the amount of acid the stomach produces, but achieve little in the way of a lasting cure. This approach is still widely used, but some centre claim an 80 per cent success rate with a combination of drugs which eradicate pylori.

Once you have been diagnosed pylori positive with a blood test you are prescribed three drugs in large doses. There's something to keep down the acid such as bismuth subsalicylate (better known as Pept Bismol); a drug such as metronidazole, which is specially effective against bacteria that don't need oxygen; and a common antibiotic such as tetracycline or amoxicillin. The result is that you can end up taking sixteen pills a day. The side effects include temporary grey staining of the teeth, constipation or diarrhoea, and dizziness.

In a few severe cases surgery is necessary. This can range from total removal of the stomach to selective removal or severing of the nerves which stimulate acid secretion in the stomach.

THE HALE APPROACH

Any persistent or severe pain in the abdomen or persisting symptoms of heatburn, reflux or acidity should be brought to the attention of your doctor. Once an accurate diagnosis of an ulcer has been made,

complementary therapies and the Hale approach may be followed, bearing in mind than an ulcer may eat into an artery or perforate the stomach, allowing acid into the abdominal cavity. These are rare but serious complications, and therefore regular review by an orthodox practitioner is advisable.

The Hale Clinic approach to stomach ulcers is to address both the physical and mental causes. A nutritionist/naturopath can advise on adjusting diet and investigating whether any allergies are aggravating the condition. Eliminating allergies will also calm the mind. Alternatively, a patient can practise the Buteyko Method, which will 1) improve the production of gastric juices to promote better digestion and absorption of food; 2) balance the acid/alkaline ratio within the digestive system; and 3) have a calming effect on the mind.

Ayurveda, acupuncture and homeopathy are very effective in the treatment of the mental and physical imbalances which cause stomach ulcers. Various support therapies have an important role in relaxing the mind and improving digestion and absorption of food. Chi Kung and self-hypnosis are self-care tools to be used at home to alleviate symptoms and prevent recurrences.

HOMEOPATHY

Over-acidity is one of the causes of ulcers, and coffee, especially decaffeinated, increases acid production, as does smoking. There are many remedies for various forms of indigestion, which may be related to an ulcer, such as:

• A lot of belching, especially after sweet foods, alternating constipation and diarrhoea, fluttery feeling in stomach, suspected peptic ulcer – Argentum Nitricum.

• Burning sensation in the chest, craving for ice-cold water, which is vomited up as soon as it becomes warm in the stomach, likely peptic ulcer – Lycopodium.

• Burning hunger pangs relieved by food or hot drinks (especially milk), but soon followed by indigestion, person nauseated by sweet things, suspected peptic ulcer – Graphites.

In general ulcers can be helped by eating only small quantities of food at a time. Slippery Elm Food, which can be taken as a drink every two hours, is especially recommended.

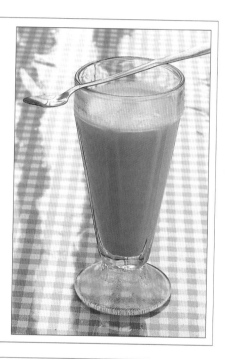

NATUROPATHY/ ALLERGY TREATMENT

The problem with taking antacids is that they disrupt normal digestive processes by lowering the acid in the stomach, which in itself can cause problems, explains a naturopath. They alter the structure and function of the cells that line the digestive tract and can cause kidney problems and a loss of the essential minerals calcium and phosphorus.

The nutritional approach aims at restoring the integrity of the lining of the stomach and duodenum.

Food allergies (see *Allergies*, page 70) are a major cause of ulcers and so patients are tested for allergens – ironically milk, often taken by sufferers, is a prime candidate. A high-fibre diet may help because it slows down the rapid movement of food into the duodenum which often occurs in ulcer patients, but it may itself be allergy-inducing.

There are a number of herbal approaches, the most powerful being liquorice which, rather than reducing acid production, stimulates the body's defence mechanisms against ulceration. It does this by increasing both the number and the effectiveness of the mucus-secreting cells in the lining of the stomach. Raw cabbage juice, 1l (1¾pt) a day, is also very effective.

BUTEYKO

There is a direct link between the levels of carbon dioxide (CO_2) in the body and the production of gastric juices. CO_2 is a key regulatory chemical in the body, where it is in solid, as opposed to gas, form. Buteyko practitioners believe that people with ulcers over-breathe, diluting their supplies of CO_2. The Buteyko technique teaches people to breathe correctly in one-hour classes every day for a week, which corrects the stomach-acid levels.

ACUPUNCTURE

Chinese medicine sees stomach ulcers as arising from an imbalance of yin and yang in the body, and treatment would aim to restore this balance, concentrating on the meridians associated with the stomach and intestines. The therapist would also address the root cause of the problem.

AYURVEDA

According to Ayurvedic principles, stomach ulcers are created more by the mind. When the mind is not in harmony with the body, the stomach functions badly. The person with ulcers is preoccupied and tense and not having meals at the right times - *when* you eat and what type of food is eaten are very important for the digestion. Treatment would involve meditation to help with relaxation and rebalance the mind, encouragement to eat the right foods – not acidic ones – and to eat at the right time. An Ayurvedic physician would also give herbs to cool the digestive tract and detoxification using enemas but not laxatives. Preparations with a cooling effect help to heal ulcers.

SUPPORTIVE TREATMENTS

Healing
This can provide complete relaxation and then reduce the acid in the stomach. It can also clear up associated problems with the liver and gall bladder. Healers recommend sticking to a bland diet.

Shiatsu
This is especially good for ulcers. Massage concentrates on the stomach meridian as well as on those of the kidneys, the liver and the small intestine. According to one practitioner, patients always have a big knot on the upper part of the spine, so their spinal alignment needs to be organized. They should avoid coffee, alcohol or fizzy drinks. The character of people with ulcers is warring and that can be changed with massage to make them more peaceful.

Chi Kung
A few of the many exercises of this system will be right for each individual. Once you have learned them you can concentrate energy and direct it to the stomach area where it will restore the balance.

Moor Therapy
The peat from an ancient Austrian moor is taken as a pasteurized herbal drink to work on the inside of the body. For external use the Moor may be applied to the stomach where the nutrients are absorbed.

Reflexology
Massage will concentrate on the stomach reflex, which covers quite a large area from the inside edge to the middle, just below the ball of both feet. The duodenum reflex is in the same region on the right foot, but covers a much smaller area.

Hypnotherapy
As one hypnotherapist puts it, 'In the language of the body an ulcer is saying, "Something is eating me."' Hypnosis can help people comes to terms with the unresolved issues causing the problem. At the bottom there are usually questions of self-respect and self-confidence. To realize that an ulcer is not just a physical matter can be a great leap for a client. Stress is a major contributory factor in ulcers and stress management techniques are therefore a pre-requisite towards alleviation.

Remedial Yoga
Through body work and breathing practice yoga can help us concentrate on unrelieved tension, anxiety and worry – feelings which affect the flow of acid in the stomach.

SELF-CARE

Indian Medicine
Diet: Eat only steamed food, vegetables or meat. Also eat a mixture of rice and lentils – known as kicherie – every evening.

Gall Stones

It is extraordinary to think that 80 per cent of people with gall stones are walking around completely oblivious to the fact. Gall stones are very common, with thousands of people developing them each year, but only about a fifth of 'sufferers' experience symptoms or complications. Gall stones are the principal disorder of the gall bladder, and the one with which most other such disorders are associated. Women are affected up to four times as often as men, though this figure varies according to age and nationality.

Attempts by the gall bladder to expel the stone(s) can cause severe pain in the upper abdomen (biliary colic) and this pain can radiate into the back, particularly behind the shoulder blades. If a gall stone becomes stuck in the outlet for the gall bladder, the trapped bile may irritate and inflame the gall bladder, which can result in a fever with severe abdominal pain and tenderness under the ribs on the right side.

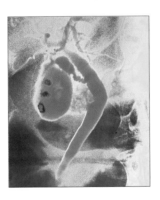

THE ORTHODOX APPROACH

Gall-bladder problems are investigated by physical examination and techniques such as ultrasound scanning, radionuclide scanning or X-ray of the gall bladder after it has been filled with a radio-opaque substance. Blood tests may also be carried out. Small gall stones sometimes disappear without treatment, simply passed out of the body with the faeces. Others can be carried around for years with no adverse effect or pain. However, stones that cause inflammation or pain are removed surgically,
together with the gall bladder. Occasionally, small stones can be dissolved by drugs; some hospitals use sound waves to break them up.

THE HALE APPROACH

Any abdominal pain, especially if it is severe or persistent, must be reviewed by a doctor. Once gall stones have been diagnosed, monitoring by the orthodox profession is essential, since an incorrectly treated blocked bile (gall bladder) duct can be a very serious complication. Complementary ther-
apies may be used in conjunction with orthodox monitoring. Be wary of practitioners who suggest dissolving or shrinking gall stones. Large stones are rarely a problem because they cannot get out of the opening into the gall bladder duct. Once a gall stone is shrunk it may become mobile, cause pain and block the duct.

With the treatment of gall stones it is imperative to ascertain the size of the stone(s) by ultrasound or X-ray. If they are small enough they can be flushed out by a naturopathic or nutritional programme, homeopathy, acupuncture or Ayurveda. For larger stones, a modified treatment would be used to prevent the existing stones increasing in size.

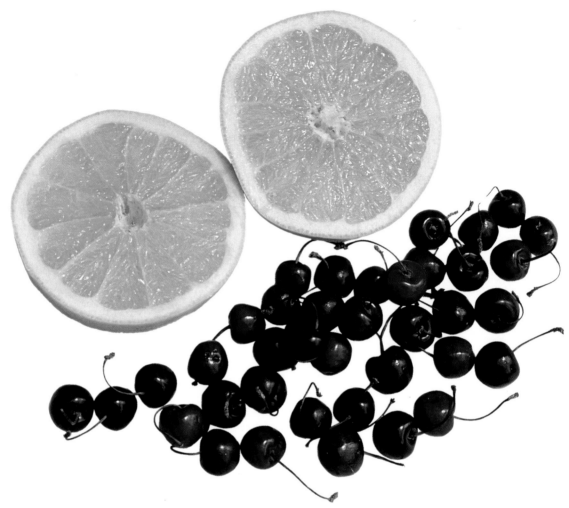

NATUROPATHY

Certain categories of people appear to have a predisposition towards gall stones. These include those who are prone to obesity or bowel congestion and those who eat a fatty, fibre-deficient diet, often with an excess of dairy products. Women who have multiple pregnancies are frequent sufferers from gall-bladder problems, and taking the contraceptive pill can double your chances of developing gall stones.

The first aim of naturopathic treatment is to flush the gall bladder of its stones. However, it is imperative first to ascertain by means of an ultrasound scan that the stones are small enough to be passed. If not, you will experience very considerable pain. Once that is established, a grapefruit diet may be recommended. This comprises:

Stage 1 (3-5 days). A grapefruit mono-diet i.e. grapefruit for all meals and fresh grapefruit juice for drinks.

Stage 2 (minimum one week). Breakfast: grapefruit. Mid-morning: fresh grapefruit, black cherry, carrot, watercress, raw beet or apple juice, parsley or dandelion tea. Lunch: large raw salad with nuts (excluding peanuts) with olive oil plus lemon, honey and garlic salad dressing, or soy-based protein dish with one or two whole wheat crispbreads with vegetarian spread. Mid-afternoon: same as mid-morning. Evening meal: any vegetarian meal, but no dairy products and eggs. Plus any fresh, baked or stewed fruit. Artichoke juice is excellent for the gall bladder generally and is available bottled through health food shops. On its own, it will do much of what is achieved by the diet detailed above. Dandelion tea and wild yam root are also recommended for the treatment of colic.

Alternatively, if the stones are small enough, they can be flushed by taking 300ml (½pt) of raw unrefined olive oil and the juice of two lemons at 8 a.m., repeating at 9 a.m. and 10 a.m., then at 1 p.m., taking two teaspoonfuls of Epsom salts in a glass of warm water

AYURVEDA

According to the principles of traditional Indian medicine, this condition occurs because of a faulty metabolic process. This is governed by the elemental force likened to the bile, *Pitha*, which controls the digestive system and all biochemical processes. Areas to be looked at include the appetite, the efficiency of the digestive enzymes and the quality of the bile in the gall bladder. An excess of fatty and dairy foods is usually responsible. Treatment involves herbal medications and detoxification, plus advice on adjustments to diet and lifestyle.

COLONIC HYDROTHERAPY

A detoxification programme for the liver and colon is important for improved gall bladder function. Colonic irrigation may be helpful in the treatment of gall stones, but only as part of a total cleanse of the gastro-intestinal tract, beginning with a reduction of the amount of fat in the diet.

NUTRITION

A very low-fat diet, excluding all dairy products and animal fats is advised for those suffering from gall stones. Eating plenty of fresh vegetables and whole grains and increasing the intake of polyunsaturated oils such as safflower is also recommended. Also beneficial are fresh lemon juice, and bitter salads such as endive, globe artichoke or chicory.

HEALING

Healing energy is channelled through the healer into the patient as they sit or lie with their eyes closed. This often results in the stones being passed painlessly and unnoticed.

HOMEOPATHY

The most common homeopathic remedy for gall stones is Chelidonium majus. It is very effective in reducing inflammation of the bile duct.

ACUPUNCTURE

After determining the cause of the symptoms by oral and physical examination, the acupuncturist stimulates points on the liver, stomach, bladder, gall bladder, spleen and conception meridians.

SUPPORTIVE TREATMENT

Moor Therapy
This can be extremely beneficial when used in association with other therapies. The medicinal herbs of the Austrian Moor are taken in the form of a pasteurized drink and can help with the elimination of small stones by activating the bile, gall bladder, liver and kidneys.

TIPS

See the advice regarding an ultrasound scan given under *Naturopathy* (opposite) before following these tips.
• Place a hot, wet towel on the gall bladder area for two minutes, then replace with a fresh hot towel. Continue the treatment for ten minutes, changing the towel every two minutes.
• Avoid fried foods.
• Eat papaya for breakfast and take the liver-cleansing tablet Liv-52 twice daily after meals.
• Mix one teaspoon of olive oil with one teaspoon of lemon juice and drink once a day for ten days.

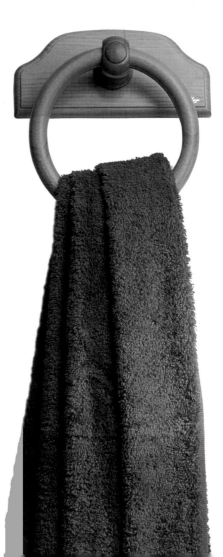

Kidney Stones

The kidneys are responsible for filtering the blood and excreting waste products and excess water in the form of urine. They also control the body's acid/base balance so that when blood and body fluids are too acid or too alkaline, the acidity of the urine is altered to restore the balance.

Kidney stones are quite common, particularly in middle age. They are usually caused by excessive concentrations of various substances, principally calcium; a lack of inhibitors of crystallization in the urine; urine that is too concentrated; or an infection. The calcium and uric acid crystallize into small lumps in the kidneys or the ureters (the tubes that carry urine to the bladder) and are known as stones.

Stones rarely cause pain while in the kidney, but can be agonizing when they become dislodged and start to travel down the urinary tract, or get stuck in it. When this happens, there can be bouts of extreme back pain in the kidney region which sometimes spreads to the abdomen and genitals. Other symptoms include pain on passing urine, and occasionally blood in the urine.

THE ORTHODOX APPROACH

Kidney disorders and urinary symptoms are investigated by urine analysis, blood tests, kidney-imaging techniques such as ultra-sound scanning and X-rays; in some instances a biopsy (taking a small sample of kidney tissue for testing) may be necessary. Ultra-sonic 'shattering' of kidney stones was hailed as a major breakthrough in treatment less than five years ago. Unfortunately, this process has several side effects and may not be as effective as the initial trial suggested. If the stones are causing a blockage in the urinary tract, a variety of other treatments may be called for. Antibiotics are usually prescribed for resulting infections.

THE HALE APPROACH

Diagnosis of a kidney stone will generally require an experienced practitioner or a doctor. Persisting pain in the kidney areas in the back, from the side of the abdomen moving towards the genitals, or in the genitals themsevles should be considered as a kidney problem and initial diagnosis should be made by your doctor. If a kidney stone is diagnosed, then orthodox pain relief is a first-line treatment, but for helping the stone to pass and to prevent a recurrence, complementary therapies are preferred.

If the kidney stone is small enough, complementary medicine can be of great benefit. The Hale Clinic would recommend either homeopathy, Ayurveda, acupuncture or Western herbalism. These can be combined with a naturopathic approach which uses certain foods to dissolve the stone. (The foods used vary with the type of stone.) An Ayurvedic physician will also recommend a specific diet combined with other Ayurvedic treatments.

HERBALISM

A trained herbalist will be able to say whether or not a patient should also see an orthodox doctor. The most effective herbal treatment is an Indian herb called crataeva which is very hard to obtain in the West. A more traditional herb used is pillatory-of-the-wall, which is a general kidney tonic. However, if the kidney stone has passed into the urinary tract, an antispasmodic herb such as khella (used by the ancient Egyptians) is very effective, as is henbane (highly poisonous, so used by trained herbalists in very small quantities). There are also certain substances known as anthroquinones which are thought to be able to bind calcium so that it is not deposited. Aloe is one of these and is used in low doses as a tincture.

AYURVEDA

Medicinal preparations from this traditional Indian therapy help to break down and dissolve existing calcium and phosphate stones in the urinary system. According to Ayurvedic teachings, kidney stones are associated with *Vata* (the basic life force that controls the nervous system) and occur as a result of a fault in the metabolic process. 'Appetite, absorption and distribution systems are restored to normal using Ayurvedic preparations,' explains one Ayurvedic physician. 'Individual lifestyle, diet and the quality of a patient's drinking water would be examined. Ayurvedic medicine is highly effective in the treatment and prevention of renal stones.'

ACUPUNCTURE

The principles of acupuncture are based on the traditional Chinese belief that the body has two opposing yet complementary forces, yin and yang, which make up a balanced whole. Yin is the more conserving, passive force and yang the more positive, thrusting force. Kidney problems are thought to involve a deficiency in the yang element and needles would be inserted to correct this. Acupuncture for kidney problems is given at points on the governor, conception, bladder, large intestine, kidney and spleen meridians. Moxibustion (applying heat locally to regulate, tone and supplement the body's flow of energy) may also be used.

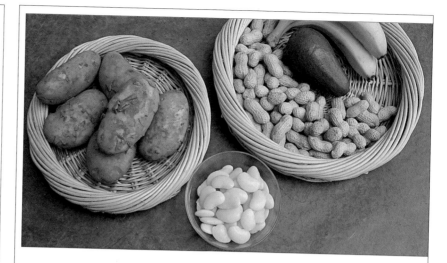

NATUROPATHY

There are several different types of kidney stones and effective treatment requires differentiation between the different types, explains one naturopath. Prevention of a recurrence is also part of the therapeutic aim.

To dissolve the most frequent type of kidney stone, he recommends increasing the intake of fibre, complex carbohydrates and green leafy vegetables and decreasing simple carbohydrates and pureens (proteins made from poultry and yeast). 'You also want a higher ratio of magnesium to calcium, so increase barley, bran, maize, buckwheat, rye, oats, soya, brown rice, sesame seed, potato, lima beans, avocado, banana and peanut.'

Should the kidney stone not be of this type, a naturopath would give specific advice on diet and recommend supplements.

HOMEOPATHY

The most common homeopathic remedies for kidney stones are Pareira brava and Fenecio aureus, although there are others from which to choose and treatment would depend on individual diagnosis.

ENERGY HEALING

Healing energy is channelled through the healer into the patient as he or she relaxes. The healer may see the kidney stones and picture them shrinking. This can result in the stones being passed without any problems.

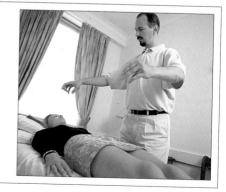

Hiatus Hernia

Hernias are usually associated with 'doing yourself a mischief' by overstraining. However, a hiatus hernia cannot really be said to be caused by anything that you might have done, except perhaps overeating to the point of obesity. Nonetheless, its symptoms are all too real to those affected and can be painful in the extreme.

It is important to understand the anatomy of the chest area before grasping how a hiatus hernia comes about. The stomach lies immediately under the diaphragm, a muscular sheet which separates the chest from the abdomen. The gullet (oesophagus) passes through a small opening in the diaphragm in order to reach the stomach. Normally, the stomach end of the oesophagus and its muscular control ring (sphincter) lie just underneath the diaphragm. When the stomach is distended, pressure pushes upwards against the diaphragm and this closes the sphincter, preventing the stomach contents from passing back up into the gullet.

Sometimes, however, the junction of the gullet and the stomach slips up through the oesophageal opening in the diaphragm and into the chest. This is called a hiatus hernia and the main effect is that the mechanism which prevents regurgitation into the gullet cannot operate properly and so the acidified and highly irritating stomach contents are able to move up into the gullet, damaging the lining and causing a condition called oesophagitis.

Hiatus hernias are most common in middle-aged and elderly women, especially in the obese. They cause severe heartburn (a deep burning pain behind the breast bone) made worse by bending forward, by straining and by lying down. The pain is so intense that it often disturbs sleep and can be mistaken for a heart attack. Other symptoms of hiatus hernia and the associated oesophagitis include acid in the mouth (water brash) and difficulty in swallowing. Sometimes, the condition is complicated by ulceration, bleeding, scarring and narrowing of the gullet. In such cases, anaemia can result from blood loss. Long-term hiatus hernia can cause dangerous changes in the cells lining the oesophagus and some authorities believe this may progress to cancer.

THE ORTHODOX APPROACH

In the first instance, a patient will be advised to lose weight if obesity is part of the problem. More generally, you will be recommended to eat small meals; avoid fatty foods, aspirin and other non-steroidal anti-inflammatory drugs; avoid too much bending from the waist; and sleep with the head of the bed raised. In some cases, H-2 receptor antagonists such as Zantac (cimetidine) or ranitidine are prescribed. If all else fails, surgery may be a last resort.

THE HALE APPROACH

Any persisting or severe discomfort in the throat, chest or upper adbomen – all of which can be caused by a hiatus hernia – should be reviewed by a doctor. Complementary treatment is generally effective and can safely be used, but occasional review by your doctor is recommended if symptoms persist.

With hiatus hernia an immediate adjustment to the patient's dietary habits is essential. We would advise consultation with a naturopath or an Ayurvedic practitioner. Once an improvement is noticeable some of the dietary modifications can be relaxed. However, given that there is a weakness in this area of the body, following a simple diet in the years ahead may be important.

Marma massage (part of the Ayurvedic system) can help a great deal by releasing the pressure on the hiatus hernia. Ayurveda may also use some exercises and medicines. Acupuncture and Shiatsu are very effective, especially when combined with dietary modifications. Homeo-pathy can help relieve the symptoms.

MARMA MASSAGE

According to traditional Indian medicine, the digestive function is controlled by the lower part of the brain which is located at the back of the neck. If the muscles in the neck become weak, it produces pressure in the stomach area and this can result in a hiatus hernia. A marma therapist would use the traditional Indian deep-massage techniques on marma points on the neck to tone up the muscles and relieve the pressure on the hiatus hernia area. Depending on the symptoms – for example, if the patient was producing a lot of gas or acidity – Ayurvedic medicines would be prescribed to complement the massage.

AYURVEDA

Since a hiatus hernia is a mechanical condition, the following Ayurvedic advice should be followed:
• Do not eat raw food.
• Do not eat too much. Reduce the quantity taken at each meal.
• Eat slowly.
• Increase your intake of liquids, but avoid fizzy drinks.
• Do not sleep immediately after a heavy meal.
• Take a walk after meals.
  These principles apply to all hiatus hernia sufferers, but after a consultation Ayurvedic medicines or exercises may also be prescribed to suit the individual case.

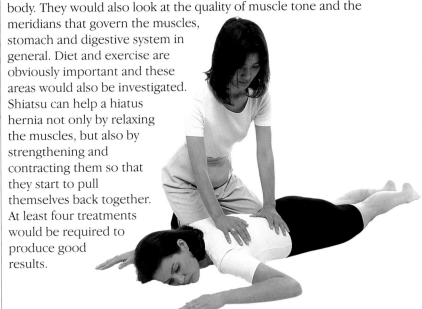

HOMEOPATHY

The philosophy of homeopathy is to treat the whole person by boosting the body's own healing powers. It cannot 'cure' a hiatus hernia, but three or four consultations with a homeopath should result in a marked improvement in symptoms in most cases. Arsenicum or Nux may be used to relieve the discomfort of heartburn, and Bryonia to counteract the acid taste in the mouth. Dietary changes may also be recommended.

SHIATSU

This ancient Japanese pressure-point massage technique has been known to be effective in the treatment of hiatus hernia. Firstly, a consultant would ascertain what was needed from a diagnosis of the meridians and a consideration of all the functional, structural and emotional levels of the body. They would also look at the quality of muscle tone and the meridians that govern the muscles, stomach and digestive system in general. Diet and exercise are obviously important and these areas would also be investigated. Shiatsu can help a hiatus hernia not only by relaxing the muscles, but also by strengthening and contracting them so that they start to pull themselves back together. At least four treatments would be required to produce good results.

ACUPUNCTURE

According to Chinese medicine, a hiatus hernia is caused by energy blockages. These are cleared by inserting needles at points along the liver and stomach meridians. The liver is seen as a yin organ (the passive, gentle aspect) and the stomach as yang (positive, aggressive) – the aim, as always with Chinese medicine, is to achieve a balance between the two.

Menstrual Problems

Most women have experienced some symptoms or discomfort associated with their monthly periods. It may be nothing more serious than feelings of irritation or tiredness a few days before their period which they can easily shrug off. Or it may be much more severe – depression, acute anxiety, food cravings, water retention, abdominal pain or heavy bleeding which can turn the normal menstrual cycle into a misery – for the women concerned and for their families. Most doctors nowadays recognize premenstrual syndrome (PMS) as a collection of symptoms usually experienced in the two weeks before a period. Sore, 'lumpy' breasts, sleep problems, a lack of interest in sex and erratic periods are other symptoms, although some women become much keener on sex just before a period.

The causes of PMS and other menstrual problems are still hotly debated. During this phase of the menstrual cycle levels of the sex hormones progesterone and oestrogen fall, affecting all parts of the body including the brain, which accounts for the wide variety of symptoms reported by women. Hormonal imbalance is certainly a crucial factor, although there is a lively dispute over whether PMS is caused by a deficiency of oestrogen or a problem with the way the body uses progesterone. Poor diet, lack of exercise and stress undoubtedly aggravate the situation and may in some cases turn what might be a mild inconvenience into something much more distressing. There is also evidence that 'oestrogen overload' is something of a modern epidemic caused by a combination of the contraceptive pill, poor diet and stress.

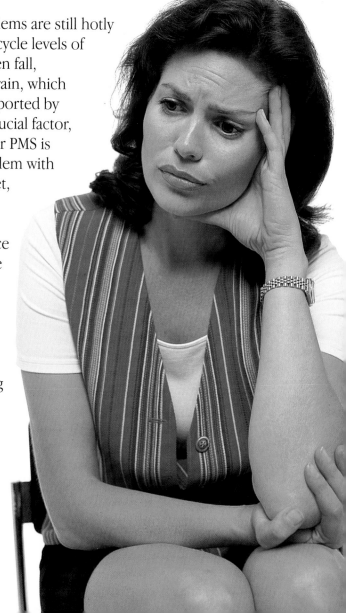

Your symptoms may also be due to something else entirely – a shortage of iron or a thyroid problem, for example – so it is sensible to have a check-up rather than assuming that he problem is related to your monthly cycle.

THE ORTHODOX APPROACH

Vitamin B$_6$ and evening primrose oil are both recommended by doctors: the latter is frequently prescribed for tender breasts, the former for painful periods. For more severe PMS and other menstrual problems the contraceptive pill is often recommended. This suppresses the normal monthly cycle and therefore the symptoms associated with it. The pill can have side effects such as water retention, depression and headaches, but there are many different varieties to try if the first one prescribed does not suit you.

Conventional medicine treats specific symptoms. Diuretics may be prescribed for water retention. Depression may be treated with tranquillizers and antidepressants. Progesterone therapy - natural progesterone in the form of suppositories – is used by many doctors and does not have the side effects associated with taking its synthetic form progestogen, which can actually cause depression. In really severe cases of PMS a hormone known as GnRH, which stops the menstrual cycle completely, may be prescribed, while cases of heavy painful periods might be treated with danazol.

A hysterectomy (removal of the womb and ovaries) may be the drastic solution recommended for women suffering very heavy painful periods and conditions such as endometriosis and fibroids if all else has failed to cure the problem.

THE HALE APPROACH

Complementary medical therapies should be tried for all but the most severe menstrual problems. Orthodox treatment usually revolves around changing the natural hormonal cycle artificially and should be considered only when the alternatives have failed. Persisting or severe bleeding, not responsive within 24 hours to complementary treatment, should be brought to the attention of your doctor or gynaecologist.

Once again, nutrition plays a very important part in alleviating menstrual problems. However, if the symptoms are quite pronounced, treatments such as acupuncture, Ayurveda and aromatherapy, which address the imbalance in the hormonal function will be necessary as well. In cases where patients find it very difficult to change their diet, these treatments are usually sufficient to address the problem. Supportive treatments such as light therapy, reflexology, Shiatsu and hypnotherapy will also have a beneficial effect.

N.B. Amenorrhoea. This means that periods stop completely or occur very infrequently and is a much more serious problem than is generally realized. It shows that the constitution is in a weakened state and not functioning correctly. Amenorrhoea is often aggravated by inadequate nutrition – some vegans and vegetarians, for example, do not make sure that they include all the necessary nutrients in their diet. The Hale Clinic would recommend changes in nutrition. Acupuncture is particularly good at 'jump starting' periods again. (See also *Infertility*, page 180.)

ACUPUNCTURE

Acupuncture treatment is particularly effective for the treatment of heavy or irregular periods. 'In Chinese medicine menstrual problems are seen and treated as an imbalance of the liver function,' says one acupuncturist. 'The liver controls the smooth flow of blood in the body, so energizing that pathway clears the clotting and stagnation and improves the circulation.'

One patient who suffered extremely heavy periods had been told the only solution was a hysterectomy, but after nine months of acupuncture treatment her periods returned to normal. 'It can be a long process,' says the therapist, 'but it has proved a real alternative to surgery for women who have not responded to conventional treatments.'

In Chinese medicine liver imbalance is also believed to be the cause of other symptoms of PMS such as anger, irritability and sugar cravings. These too can be treated successfully by acupuncture.

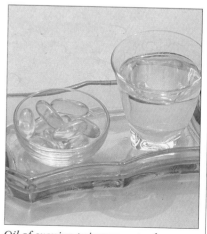

Oil of evening primrose capsules

NUTRITION

Conventional and complementary medicine alike recognize a link between menstrual problems and an inadequate diet too low in important nutrients. 'Dietary factors can have a powerful effect on female hormone chemistry,' says one nutritionist; he believes that many women have found changing their diet far more helpful than hormone treatment in combating period problems and PMS. Shortage of Vitamin B and of essential fatty acids found in seafood, green vegetables and some dairy products, as well as a lack of minerals such as magnesium and zinc are implicated in the physical and psychological symptoms of premenstrual syndrome.

Treatment starts with a nutritional assessment - many busy women do not realize how poor their diet is until they have to compile a list of what they have eaten in the past week or so. A combination of changing your diet and taking supplements can have a significant effect on menstrual problems - but it requires time and commitment. Your diet should be low in salt, caffeine, sugar and animal fats.

There is also a range of herbal remedies that can be prescribed for specific symptoms such as heavy, painful periods, depression and water retention, and for adjusting hormone imbalance. Products containing agnus castus or raspberry leaf may be recommended for heavy periods; burdock for water retention; vervain, lemon balm, St John's wort, ginseng or many others for depression.

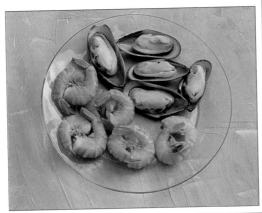

AYURVEDA

PMS and other menstrual problems are defined as an imbalance of *Vata*, one of three *doshas* or forces that control activity in the body. Among other things the *Vata* controls blood circulation and the system of sending messages to the brain.

Ayurvedic therapy aims to calm down the *Vata dosha* by detoxifying the body. This is one of the fundamental therapies of this ancient Indian system. Treatment starts with an assessment of the individual's *prakriti* – their existing state of health – followed by the prescribing of some *panchakarma* herbal treatment. The detoxification may take the form of heat therapy, treatments designed to reduce pressure on the lower part of the body, inhalation, massage with oil or the use of enemas. Monthly sessions over three of four months usually result in significant reduction in symptoms.

HYPNOTHERAPY

No one would suggest that premenstrual syndrome and other menstrual problems were 'all in the mind'. But there is plenty of research to indicate that stress and other psychological factors have a profound effect on the workings of the body, even though the precise mechanisms may not yet be fully understood. Certainly stress aggravates any tendency to PMS, and many of the symptoms – depression, anxiety, food cravings and bad temper – are, of course, quite similar.

One theory is that the body is particularly sensitive to adrenalin in the two weeks before a period, so that any already existing stress symptoms become more acute at this time.

Hypnotherapy treatment helps relieve stress and uncover any psychological concerns that may be exacerbating, or even causing, your problem. It involves a weekly session for some months and combines hypnosis with counselling.

REFLEXOLOGY

'Reflexology provides a deeply relaxing treatment for PMS sufferers,' according to one reflexologist. 'The symptoms of irritation, painful periods and back ache are often stress related and reflexology is also very helpful in relieving pain.' Treatment usually involves around six weekly one-hour sessions. The speed of improvement and length of treatment will depend on the individual and how long they have had the problem. There may be a mild reaction to the first treatment.

HOMEOPATHY

Treatment involves diagnosing 'the maintaining cause' of menstrual symptoms. 'The fundamental problem can be psychological as well as physical,' explains one homeopath, who believes that the stresses of modern life are responsible for a lot of menstrual problems. 'Some women resent having periods, others may suffer because they are in a bad relationship. Coming off the pill after many years can play havoc with the hormonal system and an unhealthy lifestyle will aggravate any problems. Often it is a process of persuading the patient to help herself by making certain changes.'

Apart from a general assessment and advice on the patient's physical and emotional condition, there are specific homeopathic remedies that may be prescribed for menstrual problems. Sepia is one of many remedies that is effective for heavy bleeding, irritability and depression. Pulsatilla may be recommended for premenstrual tension and Folliculinum for regulating periods.

SELF-CARE

Acupressure
Period pain can be relieved by pressing in the centre of the lower abdomen, or a point on the inside of either leg above the ankle.

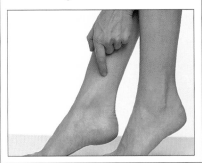

SUPPORTIVE TREATMENTS

Iridology
This diagnostic approach (right) – also known as iris analysis – can help you identify the cause of menstrual distress if there seems to be no reason for it. This should not be used as an alternative to conventional medical diagnosis, however.

Aromatherapy
Massage with essential oils helps rebalance hormones and reduce the effects of stress on them. Hormone-like essential oils such as clary sage, cypress and geranium are particularly recommended for menstrual problems. Aromatherapy massage also eases pain and tension in the lower back and abdomen. Acupressure during the treatment helps to harmonize the internal energies of organs such as the liver, spleen, heart and kidneys, reducing symptoms. A clinical aromatherapist will encourage changes in diet and recommend exercise/meditation for self-care.

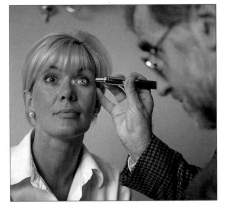

Flower Remedies
Gentle Bach Flower remedies can help relieve PMS. Your therapist will pick a combination to counteract the particular emotions that well up just before your period. Holly may be recommended to counteract 'vexation', while Larch can help those who feel that they are incapable of achieving anything. Other helpful remedies include She Oak (Australian Bush), Japanese Magnolia (Petite Fleur) and Easter Lily (Pacific).

Shiatsu
Concentrating on the spleen, liver and kidney meridians, Shiatsu massage helps adjust hormonal imbalance.

Healing
In cases of heavy, painful or irregular periods healing helps rebalance the hormonal system, reduce stress and control the blood flow.

Light Therapy
This works directly on the pineal gland in the brain to stimulate and balance the hormones. It can be used to treat PMS and to regulate heavy, irregular or scanty periods. You can buy a full-spectrum light box and use it at home to ensure you are getting enough light.

Chi Kung
These exercises rebalance the body energy, reduce stress and tension, and help eliminate toxins from the system. Certain of the exercises support the muscles of the abdominal area, easing symptoms. Other exercises work on balancing the energy of the liver, spleen, kidneys and heart, helping to harmonize the hormones and internal energies, reducing unpleasant symptoms and calming both mind and body.

Cystitis & Thrush

Cystitis is a bladder infection that makes you feel you want to urinate frequently. Each time you do, however, you feel an excruciating burning sensation. You may also get mild fever symptoms such as headaches, a pain in the abdomen and a high temperature.

Cystitis is caused by bacteria, but over-enthusiastic love-making can also cause the urethra to become inflamed, which results in these acutely uncomfortable symptoms. Most women experience cystitis at one time or another, but for some it is a constantly recurring complaint that can have a devastating impact on their lives and relationships.

Thrush is a yeast infection (*Candida albicans*) caused by an imbalance of the organisms in the vagina or gut. The symptoms are a thick, yellowy, 'cottage cheese' discharge and soreness or itching of the genitals. The vulva can become painfully swollen and red. But many women have thrush without suffering any symptoms at all, though their partner may be affected. You may develop thrush when you are run down after an illness, particularly if you have taken antibiotics which kill off the natural bacteria in the gut, allowing the candida to take over. The hormonal changes of the menopause and pregnancy may also trigger vaginal thrush.

THE ORTHODOX APPROACH

Cystitis
Your doctor will take a urine sample to check for infection, which can be treated with a short course of antibiotics. But patients who suffer constantly recurring symptoms without an infection may be advised to seek alternative treatment.

Thrush
Thrush is conventionally treated with vaginal creams and pessaries, and more recently with tablets. Canesten is now available over the counter in Britain as a cream and a pessary – its active ingredient is clotrimazole.

THE HALE APPROACH

Mild urinary tract infections such as frequency of passing urine, stinging or irritation such as burning can be self-treated or treated through a complementary practitioner. Any persistence of the discomfort, severe pain or any suggestion of kidney involvement should be brought to the attention of your doctor immediately. Kidney infections can move very rapidly to destroy the delicate tissues and antibiotics are sometimes required. Complementary therapies can be used in conjunction to protect against the side effects of antibiotics. Persistent urinary tract infections need to be assessed by a urologist.

The use of drugs by the orthodox world has led to resistant strains of the generally unobtrusive yeasts that cause thrush. Complementary therapies promoting the body's immune system rather than directly attacking the yeast are definitely preferable and only the severest of thrush, unresponsive to complementary treatment, should be brought to the attention of a doctor.

For very quick relief, the naturopathic, homeopathic or acupuncture approach can act rapidly to alleviate the symptoms. In the medium term homeopathy, acupuncture, nutritional advice and/ or colonic hydrotherapy should be used to create an environment in which cystitis and thrush are unlikely to recur.

Please note the tips given later in this section.

NATUROPATHY

One of the most successful herbal treatments for vaginal thrush is tea tree (*Melaleuca alternifolia*), an old Aborigine remedy. This has always been known as a powerful natural antibiotic. According to one naturopath, during the Second World War the Australian government exempted leaf cutters from national service so that they could carry on producing tea tree, which was issued to the army as a general disinfectant. Taken in water (under the guidance of your practitioner) and supplemented with the weekly use of tampons soaked in the solution, tea tree has a strong antifungal and antibacterial action. It is available as a lotion, soap, toothpaste and in many other forms for external use as an antiseptic.

Golden seal (*Hydrastis canadensis*) is also used in homeopathic and naturopathic treatments for thrush. Old Romany treatments are particularly successful in treating cystitis. Add a heaped teaspoon of wild cranberry leaves to two cups of water, boil it down to one cup, then drink it.

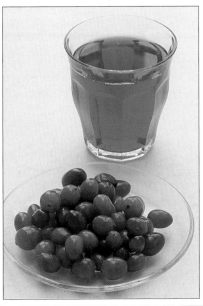

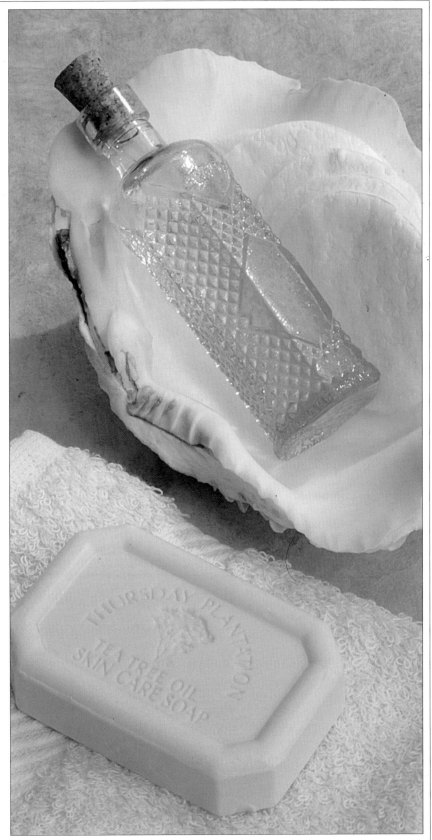

COLONIC HYDROTHERAPY

'Vaginal thrush may be a symptom of candida overgrowth in the bowel,' according to one colonic therapist, who recommends colonic irrigation to help clean out the colon where the candida organism can live. 'We don't force the body in any way,' she says. 'It is a very gentle therapy that encourages the bowel to contract and flush out the waste matter accumulated there.' An implant of acidophilus at the end of each treatment supplements the normal digestive bacteria in the bowel.

Recurrent cystitis may also be linked to an overgrowth of candida and can be helped by colonic hydrotherapy.

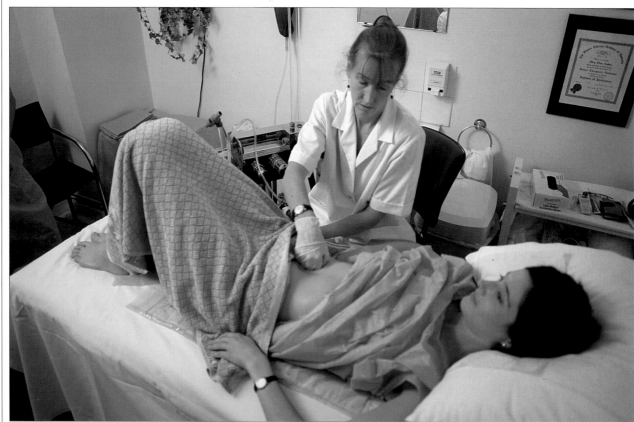

HOMEOPATHY

Homeopathic remedies are very effective for the treatment of both the immediate acute symptoms of cystitis and the underlying problems that cause recurring attacks. It is important to treat the fundamental cause of the problem; reliance on antibiotics can create a vicious circle when the object is to reduce and prevent further repeated attacks.

Antibiotics used regularly to control outbreaks of cystitis, for instance, can result in an overgrowth of candida in the system, since the antibiotic kills the 'good' bacteria in the gut as well as the infection.

Acute attacks can be treated with staphysagria, cantharis or causticum.

Homeopathic treatment starts with a general assessment of the individual's health and includes advice on what food and drink to avoid. The homeopath will try and find out why you are suffering recurring attacks – whether the problem is anatomical (a short urethra), hormonal or psychological, and will prescribe an appropriate constitutional remedy to built up your body's resistance in the future.

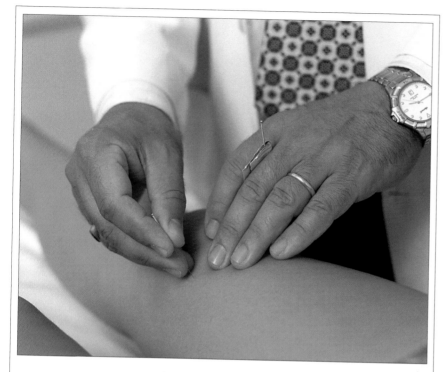

ACUPUNCTURE

In Chinese medicine both cystitis and thrust are commonly diagnosed as a damp heat syndrome. All the lower abdominal organs are prone to damp heat – the heat is in the painful, burning urine that is a feature of cystitis and in the inflammation of the genital area that often accompanies thrush. Acupuncture treatment concentrates on the urine and spleen channels and herbal medicine may also be given. Acute symptoms of cystitis and thrush may subside after one treatment, although more will probably be needed, particularly if the condition has been recurring over a long period.

NUTRITION

According to nutritionists, diet plays an important part in eradicating the root cause of thrush and recurrent cystitis that is linked to candida overgrowth in the bowel. 'If *Candida albicans* has become established it can grow roots (mycelia) that penetrate the intestinal wall and cause a condition known as "leaky gut". Partly digested food can then pass through the gut wall and produce an allergic reaction.' She advises cutting out sugar, which feeds the candida, although you can carry on eating fruit, provided there is no adverse reaction.

Treatment is dependent on the type of candida present, where in the body it is located and the severity of the case. A combination of acidophilus, bifidus, laprylic acid and plant oil complexes is used. This process may take from three to six months, depending on the case.

SUPPORTIVE TREATMENTS

Moor Therapy
Moor herbal drinks and sitz baths soothe inflammation in the urinary tract in cases of cystitis, and help kill off the yeast bacteria that causes thrush.

Shiatsu
Shiatsu massage strengthens the genito-urinary system and helps calm inflammation.

TIPS

Do not take long baths or use soap around the genitals.

Cystitis
Drinking cranberry juice, barley water or a solution of bicarbonate of soda helps relieve symptoms, as does drinking plenty of water. Alcohol and caffeine are aggravants. Citricidal, a grapefruit seed extract, is an effective natural antibiotic to help cope with an attack.

Thrush
The application of plain live yoghurt soothes inflamed genitals. Always wear cotton underwear and trousers made of natural fibres. Avoid tights and very close-fitting trousers.

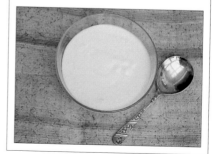

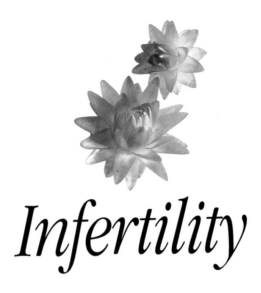

Infertility

Infertility can be difficult to diagnose. So much affects our fertility – our general health, our emotional state, what kind of contraceptive we have been using, when and how often we have sex – that there are a lot of reasons why conception may take longer than expected. Some couples conceive immediately.

Other perfectly healthy couples succeed only after twelve or eighteen months. It is important not to panic if you don't conceive within a few months – stress itself can have an impact on the reproductive system.

Most doctors will be prepared to start a preliminary investigation if you have been trying to conceive for over a year without success. In the case of prospective mothers in their mid-30s or who have a history of miscarriage or pelvic infection, a doctor may want to start investigating sooner or refer you to a specialist fertility unit to see if there is any specific reason for failure to become pregnant. These investigations can take some months and involve both partners from the beginning. Most doctors are well aware that fertility is a sensitive topic. Even so, the process of investigation may seem intrusive, embarrassing and lengthy, and can put a strain on your relationship.

THE ORTHODOX APPROACH

One of the main causes of infertility in women is failure to ovulate properly. This will be investigated only after you have identified your most fertile time and made sure you have had sex during it over a period of months. Ovulation should occur in the middle of your menstrual cycle when the egg is released from the ovary and this is the time you can conceive. Where there are seemingly normal monthly periods ovulation can be checked by using a temperature chart and a basal thermometer. Body temperature falls before ovulation and rises just after as the balance of the hormones change. You can also buy ovulation predictor kits to test your urine for hormonal changes which tell you that ovulation is about to occur. Both these help you pinpoint your most fertile period and you will be urged to make sure you have sex at this point.

If you have been taking the contraceptive pill, however, it may take some months for your cycle and ovulation to return to normal. If you don't have periods at all (amenorrhoea) you will almost certainly not be ovulating. This may be due to underweight, which can suppress hormonal activity, and a healthy diet may be recommended as a first stage to restoring normal periods. But amenorrhoea can also be caused by thyroid problems, drug treatments and stress. Over-exercising can affect hormonal balance – many women athletes have amenhorroea.

If there is a problem with ovulation you may be offered fertility drug treatment, either by pill or injection. Clomiphene or cyclofenil may be taken at a certain point in the month to induce a period to start the menstrual cycle to see if it stimulates the ovaries. Ovulation can be checked by the temperature readings.

Even if your periods appear normal it's possible that hormonal imbalances are preventing ovulation or the successful implantation of a fertilized egg in the womb. Hormone levels can be tested by blood samples taken at certain times in the month to identify which hormones are deficient or overproducing.

If none of this results in ovulation and pregnancy there are other more complex drug treatments that work directly on the ovaries to encourage egg production and hopefully a pregnancy.

Infertility can also result from damage to the fallopian tubes through which the egg travels to the womb. Blockages can be caused by ectopic pregnancy, pelvic inflammatory disease or scars following abdominal surgery. In some cases damage can be corrected with microsurgery which reopens the blocked tubes. But the fallopian tubes are highly sensitive and major damage is unlikely to be successfully reversed by surgery. A laparoscopy (inserting a tube through the abdominal wall under general anaesthetic) will be done to check the state of the reproductive organs. A dye may be passed through the fallopian tubes to check for any blockages. Other investigations will check the state of your uterus and womb – fibroids and ovarian cysts can cause infertility.

Prospective fathers will be offered tests to check sperm counts - in at least a third of all cases the problem is found to be some measure of male infertility. Other tests can be made to determine if there is any problem with sperm production or damage caused to sperm by past illness in

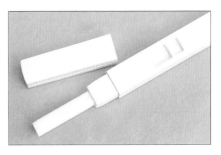

the reproductive organs themselves.

In some cases sperm does not move easily through the cervical mucus to the womb. In other cases antibodies in the cervical fluid kills off the sperm once it gets there. An 'after sex' test may be done in a clinic or hospital on fluid taken from the cervix to see if this is the problem. If so, artificial insemination – introducing a partner's sperm directly into the womb to fertilize the egg – will be recommended.

Conventional medicine has limited help for men with low or abnormal sperm. Hormone and steroid treatment has not yet proved successful. But there may be treatment to clear blockages in the male reproductive system that are preventing the sperm travelling normally through the tubes.

If the problem is found to be the amount or quality of sperm, artificial insemination by donor (AID) can be considered. If there is irreversible damage to the fallopian tubes, assisted conception techniques may be an option. In vitro fertilization (IVF) involves placing fertilized eggs in the womb. In some cases both sperm and egg can be introduced into the fallopian tubes to fertilize naturally.

Investigating infertility is very much a process of elimination and even once they are identified not all fertility problems can be corrected by drugs or surgery. In at least three out of ten cases no convincing medical explanation can be given.

THE HALE APPROACH

If a couple have failed to conceive despite having sexual intercourse at the right time of the month over one year, then initial investigations should take place. These include checking the man's sperm count and the basic hormone levels of the woman. At this time, and before any invasive investigations such as laparoscopies are performed, complementary treatments should commence. If conception has not occurred after six months on naturopathic treatments, then further investigations through orthodox approaches should be considered.

Complementary medicine can be of great assistance in many cases of infertility, though not all – it cannot help with blocked fallopian tubes, for example.

We would address both the mental and the physiological factors behind infertility. As with most illnesses, it is crucial first of all to consider nutrition. Lack of vitamins and minerals, poor digestion and elimination can weaken fertility in both men and women. Organic vegetables are important before conception – research in Denmark showed that organic farmers had twice the sperm count of the average man. Contraceptive devices can also impair some women's absorption of minerals and cause problems with conceiving.

Treatments such as light therapy, Buteyko and Moor will considerably boost the systems of both man and woman, which may be the deciding factor between infertility and conception for some couples.

Acupuncture, homeopathy and Ayurveda are excellent for strengthening the general constitution and particularly helpful in balancing the hormones. Moreover, they can help with the mental/emotional factors which may inhibit conception.

Subconscious fears regarding conception, pregnancy and childbirth can also prevent some couples conceiving. In a study at Queen Charlotte Hospital in London on women who in their conscious minds wanted to conceive and had no medical reason for not doing so, a course of hypnotherapy was shown to uncover and remove subconscious fears about becoming a mother.

For many infertile couples, trying to have a child can put a great strain on their relationship. Counselling and psychotherapy can help them get through this difficult period and derive deeper compassion and understanding from the experience.

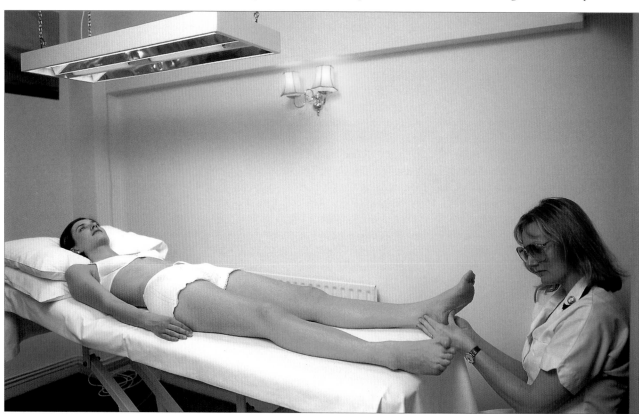

HOMEOPATHY

Constitutional homeopathic treatment and nutritional therapy are recommended; some specific remedies may also be appropriate:

For women:
• Where there is a history of miscarriages – Sabina.
• For irregular periods accompanied by a lack of interest in sex, weepiness and irritability – Sepia.
• Loss of interest in sex accompanied by tender breasts – Conium.

For men:
• Strong libido accompanied by feelings of insecurity – Lycopodium.
• Weak libido, genitals feel heavy – Sepia.

ACUPUNCTURE

Acupuncture has proved successful in treating infertility that is caused by lack of periods, problems with ovulation and hormonal deficiency and is particularly recommended for older prospective mothers. One therapist says, 'I had a recent case where a woman was in early menopause. She had reached the stage where she had no periods and was actually getting hot flushes but was desperate to have a baby. The doctors had refused to let her have IVF. With acupuncture treatment she managed to achieve a pregnancy.'

Acupuncture concentrates on stimulating and toning the kidney function – in Chinese medicine the kidneys and liver are the main organs that control the hormones and menstrual cycle. It can take several months of treatment to regularize periods, which is often the first step to improving hormonal function. Once that is achieved the therapist may organize blood tests to check hormone levels to see whether sufficient progesterone is being produced to create the right environment in the womb for implantation of a fertilized egg.

Acupuncture is also effective in cases of amenorrhoea if periods have stopped completely when a patient has come off the pill or in reaction to some kind of shock or trauma.

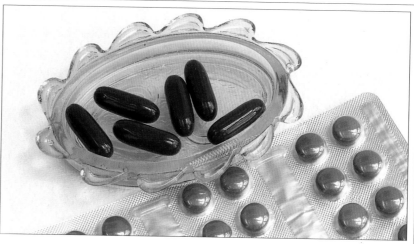

NUTRITION

Nutritional therapy can help both partners increase their fertility by improving overall health, detoxifying the body and identifying any mineral or vitamin deficiencies.

Women who want to get pregnant are warned against the effects of smoking and alcohol on the developing foetus. What is less widely understood is that alcohol and smoking have a direct effect on the amount and quality of sperm produced by the man. Male infertility can be treated with mineral supplements – zinc, for instance, may be prescribed. And high levels of toxic metals such as lead, cadmium, aluminium and mercury which have been shown to affect sperm quality can be identified and reduced by taking Vitamins C and B and other anti-oxidants.

Unexplained infertility in women has often responded to nutritional supplementation, which corrects vitamin and mineral imbalances caused by poor diet, pollution and the contraceptive pill. There may be a shortage of zinc, which affects successful implantation of the fertilized egg in the womb. Other mineral supplements that may be given include chromium, selenium, manganese and magnesium. Essential fatty acids (EFAs) and Vitamin E may also be given to help balance hormones.

Anyone who has been on the pill or used a copper IUD contraceptive or had problems with previous pregnancies should have their mineral status tested before attempting to become pregnant.

Nutritional therapy to address vitamin and mineral imbalances can be particularly effective in achieving a pregnancy where there seems to be no medical explanation for the failure to conceive.

PSYCHOTHERAPY

'There are a huge number of emotional issues involved in fertility, or the lack of it,' says one counsellor. 'That's why couples who have any kind of treatment involving assisted conception are advised to consider counselling, as the procedures can be immensely stressful for both partners. In fact, by law [in Britain] clinics which offer assisted conception have to ensure that counselling is available.'

Counselling – or psychotherapy – can be a great support for couples facing an initial problem with fertility, prolonged and invasive investigations and treatment or – because infertility treatments are not always successful – the realization that they may be permanently childless.

Counselling for individuals or couples creates an environment where the issues of guilt, recrimination and failure, which can be felt by one or both partners with fertility problems, can be openly expressed and dealt with. Many couples find it difficult to talk to each other – they may feel that they have let their partner down or feel resentment towards their partner, for instance. These suppressed emotions may eventually corrode the relationship, although the problem can also bring couples closer together. It

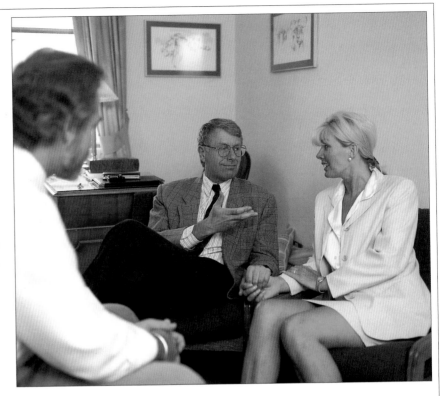

may affect their attitude to the rest of the world around them, their friends and families. The role of the therapist is to help individuals and couples to identify their ambivalences, and then help them work through their emotions so that they can come to terms with their situation. But therapy also aims to help both individuals and couples find ways of helping themselves cope with the inevitable stress and emotional rollercoaster that the problem and its treatments cause.

Finally, in those instances where there is an emotional block causing

fertility problems, such as bad experiences in the past, fears about coping with a pregnancy or childbirth, or worries about the future, counselling, psychotherapy and particularly hypnotherapy may be able to help the client identify such blocks within themselves and then resolve them.

The normal length of a session is just under one hour, with the number of sessions varying both with the nature of the difficulty and with how individual therapists work.

HYPNOTHERAPY

Infertility is said to affect around 17 per cent of potential parents and approximately 28 per cent of those trying to resolve this concern show no apparent medical reason for the problem. For such parents,

conventional medical treatments have proved far less successful than the norm.

Major causes of non-definable medical infertility appear to be acute shock, extreme anxiety or chronic stress. Courses in hypnotherapy and stress management, either on their own or alongside conventional

medical treatment, show positive findings. A recent study of 40 infertile female patients undertaking such courses showed 26 achieving successful full-term pregnancies, with nine of them having also received additional medical treatment such as IVF.

SUPPORTIVE TREATMENTS

Light Therapy

There is a direct link between light and fertility. The pineal gland in the brain which regulates many of our body rhythms is very sensitive to light. Lack of sunlight leads to an imbalance of serotonin, the 'feel good' hormone, and melatonin, the hormone that increases in the dark, helping us sleep. This imbalance can cause depression and lack of energy, and decrease the production of the sex hormones that govern our fertility and our appetite for sex.

Many of us do not actually get enough natural sunlight even in the summer months when permanent wearing of sunglasses out of doors means the pineal gland is not receiving the full benefit of light. Light therapy simulates the effects of bright spring sunshine. Scanning the eyes with light works directly on the pineal gland and has the effect of balancing and stimulating the hormones and increasing fertility in the many cases where there seems to be no particular reason for failing to conceive. It can also help restart periods or a regular cycle if this is the problem.

Light also improves the libido of both partners, which is particularly important if a couple is investigating any possible fertility problems. As a light therapist points out, 'Sunshine makes us happy, more relaxed and much more interested in sex. Couples who have no identifiable or physiological fertility problem have found that light therapy has worked for them.'

The recommendation is a weekly treatment for 8-10 weeks, and possibly installing full-spectrum light in your home.

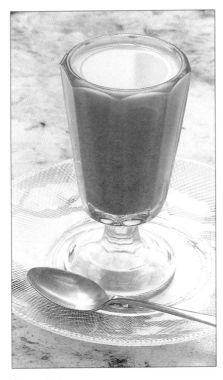

Moor Therapy

Moor herbal treatments, derived from an unique area of moorland in Austria, contain a large number of medicinal herbs, minerals and nutrients. Usually you will be recommended to take the Moor herbal drink and use the Moor bath to help balance your hormones and improve fertility. The Moor also contains anti-inflammatory substances which are believed to be effective in reducing any inflammation in the fallopian tubes.

After consultation with a Moor therapist you can use the baths and herbal drink at home in between visits to your clinic.

Chi Kung

This ancient Chinese system of breathing and movement includes exercises to regulate and balance the flow of energy in the lower abdominal area.

Buteyko

Buteyko training – learning to breathe more shallowly in order to raise the level of carbon dioxide in the lungs – has an invigorating effect on all systems of the body, including the hormonal and reproductive systems. There have been many cases of men and women thought to be infertile proving to be fertile after doing the workshops.

The Buteyko breathing exercises are taught in a series of five one-hour sessions on consecutive days.

Healing

Where there is no physiological reason for the failure to conceive, healing works to relax the patient and make the body more open to fertilization. It can also help to balance the hormones.

SELF-CARE

Nutrition

A poor diet high in sugar leeches minerals from the body. Filtering drinking water will remove lead, excess copper and pesticides. The optimum diet is to vary foods by choosing each day from the four main groups – cereals, dairy products, vegetables and fruits, and proteins, all of which should be organically produced. Fertility can be improved for both partners by a determined effort to eliminate toxins as far as possible.

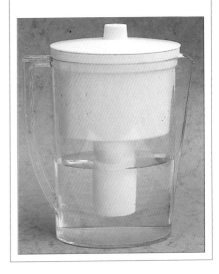

Preconception Care

Preconception care is vitally important and should start at least six months before you try for a baby. Preparation for pregnancy means that both parents can be as healthy as possible when the baby is conceived. This goes a long way towards safeguarding the health of the unborn child, promoting a trouble-free pregnancy and is particularly important where there has been a history of miscarriage, premature birth, birth defects or problems with fertility that seem to have no particular cause. The first few weeks of pregnancy are vital ones for the baby's development and there is plenty of research to indicate that the state of health of parents at the time of conception has far-reaching implications for a child's future development.

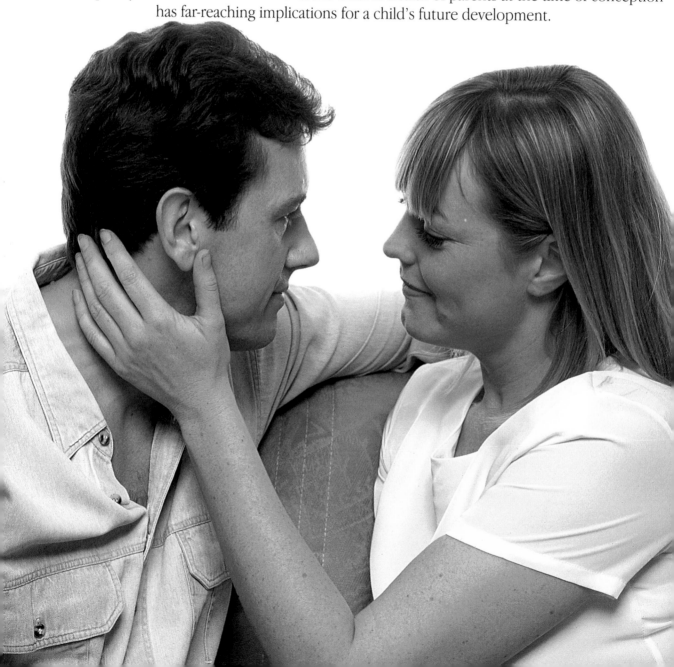

THE ORTHODOX APPROACH

Conventional medicine is only just beginning to take preconception care seriously, largely because of a shortage of resources. It is fair to say that couples planning a family are not as a rule urged to seek medical help before a pregnancy is established, though your doctor will be happy to give you a general check-up and advice if you ask for it, or refer you to a specialist preconception clinic if there is one in your area. From a doctor's point of view it makes sense to check blood-pressure levels before conception so as to establish a 'bench mark' against which changes during pregnancy can be assessed. It is now also accepted that a supplement of folic acid, which reduces the risk of spina bifida, should be taken for several weeks before conception and during the first twelve weeks of pregnancy and that tests for rubella immunity should be done well in advance of any pregnancy as well.

You will also receive advice from your doctor on avoiding infections such as toxoplasmosis from household pets, which are known to damage the foetus in early pregnancy. You should ask your doctor to test for antibodies before you become pregnant and then avoid any contact with cat litter. Since the infection is passed through animal excrement you should wear gloves when gardening and make sure that home-grown root vegetables are properly peeled.

Planning a baby involves giving up any bad habits such as alcohol and smoking well in advance of any pregnancy – and this applies to both partners. While it is widely known that alcohol crosses the placenta and travels through the baby's bloodstream, there is research indicating that alcohol consumption at the time of conception can lead to abnormalities and that it has implications for the health of sperm as well.

Mothers who smoke are more likely to have underweight babies, higher rates of miscarriage and babies with some kind of abnormality. In fathers smoking affects the production and quality of sperm.

If you have been taking the contraceptive pill or using an intra-uterine device (IUD) your doctor will probably advise you to use some other kind of contraceptive for three or four months before you try to conceive. Using the pill lowers the body's level of zinc, manganese and Vitamin A and raises its copper levels. The IUD similarly raises copper levels and lowers the amounts of manganese and selenium. Your monthly cycle may also be irregular when you first come off the pill. Using some other kind of contraceptive helps your system settle down first.

THE HALE APPROACH

The necessary care prior to conception is not a disease process and therefore a doctor's involvement is not required. Complementary practitioners will probably be better versed in nutritional and supplementary care and will be able to offer advice on preparation for pregnancy. A visit to such a practitioner can be contemplated without medical care or concern.

The Hale Clinic sees complementary medicine as fulfilling a very important role in pre-conceptual care – by which we mean both parents being involved in improving their health so that the ovum and sperm produced are of the highest possible quality. A nutritionist will advise on the correct diet, vitamins and minerals, and also try to remove any allergies that may be passed on to the baby.

Monitoring the patients' digestive, eliminative and hormonal systems to ensure optimum function is also important. For example, if the mother is not absorbing her food properly, it will have a direct effect on the development of the embryo and correcting digestive function takes time. The reduction of toxicity in the body is especially important. Research in Denmark has shown that men consuming an 'average' diet of foods containing additives and grown with chemical pesticides have a sperm count 50 per cent lower than that of organic farmers. If the hormones of either partner are not functioning properly, this will effect the ovum or sperm.

Homeopathy combined with nutritional advice will address the above issues by building up the parents' general constitution. Osteopathy can also make a positive contribution to general health, as well as correcting any back problems – particularly important for a woman before she conceives.

Aromatherapy, reflexology, Shiatsu and light therapy are supportive treatments that will further enhance the health of the parents-to-be and their future child.

Nutrition

Nutrition therapy can be very effective in treating chronic conditions like asthma, eczema and migraine that can sometimes be passed on to children. The cause may be a food allergy, a vitamin or mineral deficiency, or a problem with malabsorption, all of which can be treated by eliminating certain foods from the diet or taking supplements. 'It's important to detect and treat allergies well before pregnancy,' says one nutritional therapist. 'It improves general health, and reduces the likelihood of the baby developing an allergic condition if the mother is eating food to which she is allergic during pregnancy or while breast feeding.'

The initial diet may be quite restrictive until the problem is resolved. Then a maintenance diet will be suggested to keep the condition under control.

It is also important to establish adequate levels of essential minerals and vitamins well before pregnancy. Shortage of these can cause problems with conception and premature birth. Use of the pill or an IUD and a poor diet high in sugar or refined carbohydrates can cause deficiencies of zinc, chromium, manganese and magnesium.

Nutritional therapy may involve hair, blood and sweat analyses, followed by a supplement programme.

Ayurveda/Acupuncture

Given its holistic approach, Ayurveda is an excellent therapy for building up the constitution of both parents-to-be. The treatment would be based on the needs of the individual, but might include *panchakarma* (detoxification) and/or herbal massage to relieve stress; it would certainly involve advice on diet and exercise. Acupuncture would be recommended if fertility problems were suspected in either partner (see *Infertility*, page 180). Ayurveda tonics and special preparations may be taken orally during this period to aid conception and prevent miscarriage later.

Osteopathy

'It's a big mistake to see osteopathy just as a way of dealing with bad backs,' says one osteopath. 'It has an important role to play in helping people achieve optimal health, which is vital if you are planning a pregnancy.' The principle of osteopathy is that dysfunction in the structure of the body affects the homeostasis of all the vital organs. 'Stress is a major cause of this dysfunction. Therapy can take pressure off the nervous system to restore balance to the body and improve blood circulation and lymphatic drainage.'

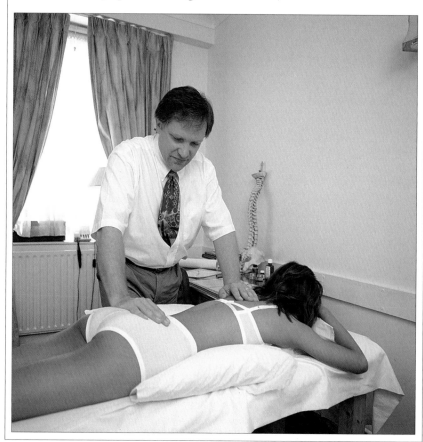

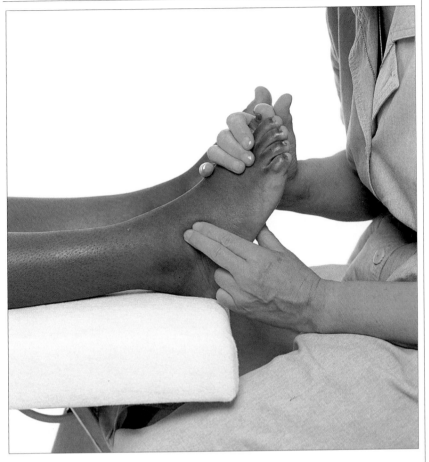

REFLEXOLOGY

'Reflexology is an ideal general therapy for anyone who wants to make a positive effort to reduce the effect of stress on their body,' says one reflexologist. 'It's a very pleasant, relaxing treatment and a very effective way of eliminating toxins, which is important if you are planning to get pregnant.' Anyone who is giving up alcohol or smoking, or who has taken antibiotic or other drug treatment in the past will find that reflexology is a powerful detoxifying therapy.

Reflexology can help balance the hormone levels in the body if you suffer from pre-menstrual syndrome or erratic periods, which may affect your fertility. Four or five fortnightly treatments are recommended.

HOMEOPATHY

A constitutional remedy can improve general levels of health for both partners.

Other chronic conditions may be treated homeopathically, reducing the dependence on drugs for sufferers. Your practitioner will also give you advice on vitamin and mineral supplements and diet.

SUPPORTIVE TREATMENTS

Shiatsu
Shiatsu works to eliminate toxins from the body before conception. This may also help to reduce morning sickness later on.

Aromatherapy
Massage with essential oils can help eliminate toxins from the body. Suitable oils include rosemary, juniper and lemon. Massage and the use of acupressure also help to alleviate stress and its effects on hormone production. Deep relaxation and rebalancing of the body's energies produce a positive environment for conception.

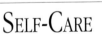

SELF-CARE

The optimum diet is to vary food by choosing each day from the main four food groups – cereals, dairy products, vegetables and fruits, and proteins. As far as possible food should be organically produced. Intake of refined carbohydrates, sugar, tea, coffee and saturated fats should be kept to a minimum.

The effects of stress on the hormonal system may be reduced with the use of aromatherapy oils.

Pregnancy & Childbirth

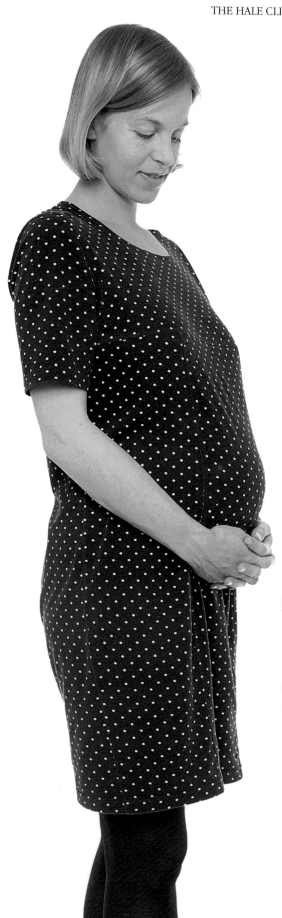

Most women enjoy their pregnancy, although there is no doubt that in the months leading up to childbirth your body goes through huge changes that affect you emotionally and psychologically as well as physically. You may get morning sickness during the first three or four months when the baby's organs are forming – for some women this is the first sign of pregnancy. Hormonal changes can also result in other unwelcome symptoms such as sore breasts, a bloated feeling, dizziness, weepiness or spots in the early weeks. None of these are dangerous either to you or to your baby and most doctors will quite rightly be reluctant to prescribe anything for what is usually a very temporary discomfort.

In the later months of pregnancy it is quite normal to have leg cramps, some sleeplessness and indigestion (heartburn) or constipation. Your increased weight, blood supply and changing shape make a lot of demands on your body. Softening ligaments may cause pain around the pelvis and you will probably experience some back or neck ache. You may have slightly swollen fingers or puffy ankles. You must have plenty of rest and relaxation.

THE ORTHODOX APPROACH

Your doctor will have helpful advice about diet, exercise and posture, and maybe some mild alleviants or self-help tips to recommend. But unless there are reasons for thinking that something is seriously wrong with either mother or baby, medical intervention is kept to the minimum during the months of pregnancy.

Conventional ante-natal care involves regular monitoring, designed to pick up any potential problems. Blood samples, urine samples, blood-pressure readings and a weight check are the main routine tests. In the final stages of pregnancy you will probably be expected to visit the ante-natal clinic once a week. But if you have any severe symptoms you should report them immediately to your doctor. Vaginal bleeding, painful abdominal cramps, vomiting, a high temperature or very noticeable swelling around your feet or ankles can be an early warning of more serious problems such as the toxic condition known as pre-eclampsia.

Preparing for the birth is very important and should begin months beforehand. Most doctors will recommend simple pelvic floor exercises during pregnancy which will help your labour and ensure that these muscles, which support the weight of your pregnancy, return to normal strength afterwards. Antenatal and relaxation classes are highly recommended too.

Nearer the time you will have formed some idea about what kind of birth you want and the options available. Conventional pain-relief possibilities for labour include pethidine injections and an epidural – each method has its advantages and disadvantages. A high-tech delivery will involve monitoring of the baby at the expense of the mother's freedom of movement. Many mothers like the idea of completely natural childbirth. But whatever kind of birth you plan for yourself you must be prepared for the unexpected and not feel disappointed or guilty if things don't go completely according to plan.

THE HALE APPROACH

Pregnancy and childbirth are natural processes and should not need medical intervention. If any problems develop, these must be dealt with initially by your doctor and obstetrician. If treatment or hospitalization is not required, then a variety of complementary therapies are safe and effective.

Nowadays there is a leaning towards home birth, which is fine is your doctor, obstetrician and local midwives are happy. Women have their second or further pregnancices (multi-gravida), having had experience of childbirth, are probably better suited to considering home birth than a first timer (primagravida). Home births should only be considered if a hospital is within five or ten minutes' drive.

Complementary medicine has a great part to play in helping a woman and child through pregnancy, childbirth and post-natal recovery.

During pregnancy, nutritional advice combined with homeopathy and osteopathy will help the baby's development and alleviate the symptoms of back pain and other routine difficulties experienced by expectant mothers. Support therapies such as yoga and aromatherapy are of great assistance at this time.

In the pre-birth stage, acupuncture is very effective in dealing with breach births and in inducing labour. Homeopathic remedies can also be use to encourage birth during a protracted labour. However it is advisable not to combine homeopathy with acupuncture during childbirth.

Aromatherapy can help to prepare the body for birth and some oils can be used to speed up contractions. The mind can play an important part in easing childbirth – mothers-to-be can be taught self-hypnosis techniques to help them relax and thereby considerably reduce pain, as well as speeding up the birth itself.

After the birth there are three people who need support: the mother, the father and the baby. So much emphasis is placed on a woman's health *during* pregnancy that it is often forgotten how much help she needs to recover physically and emotionally from this momentous experience. In India there is a lovely tradition whereby a woman comes to stay with the mother and newborn child for three months. She regularly massages mother and child with special Ayurvedic oils and is there to provide support for them both as they recover from the birth.

Although we do not have this tradition in the West,

complementary medicine can play a similar role. As giving birth can often upset a woman's musculo-skeletal system, it is advisable to have your back checked out even if you are not feeling pain. Acupuncture, Ayurveda, aromatherapy and homeopathy can really help a mother to recover quickly after the birth, and may be particularly helpful in cases of post-natal depression. Homeopathy offers remedies for women who are having trouble producing milk.

Support therapies such as aromatherapy, Shiatsu and Bach flower remedies also help mothers recover mentally and physically. Yoga, T'ai Chi and muscle-toning exercises gently coax the body back into shape after the birth, and later more energetic exercise like running or aerobics is recommended.

One of the most essential treatments for a newborn baby is cranial osteopathy. The cranium is easily distorted during birth, which may affect the child in a number of ways – it may cry a lot, be unable to sleep or suckle, or suffer from colic. Fortunately, there are gentle methods that can return the cranium to the correct position. Ideally a cranial osteopath would be present in the delivery room! One of the cranial osteopaths at the Hale Clinic regularly supports obstetricians, midwives and nurses at a North London hospital. Ayurvedic medicine also has a special herbal oil massage for newborn babies and mothers.

Finally, it is often forgotten that the birth of a child may also bring profound changes into the father's life. He frequently plays a key role in supporting his partner and he too may need support. Self-hypnosis techniques to reduce stress can be very beneficial. Homeopathy, Ayurveda and acupuncture are useful for building up the constitution, particularly after the birth when the father, too, might not be getting enough sleep.

Before, during and after the birth both man and woman will go through a whole range of emotional experiences and it is often very helpful for them (as a couple or individually) to discuss their feelings with a counsellor/psychotherapist. For example, a man may feel rejected because his partner has to give so much attention to the baby. It is always better to tackle these feelings before unnecessary tensions are created within the family.

Unborn and newborn babies respond particularly well to the subtle and gentle approach of healing. It can ease their passage into this world – and help to calm and rebalance the parents during this period of great change.

OSTEOPATHY

'I feel there should be an osteopath at every birth,' says one osteopath, who also practises cranial osteopathy. 'Nothing is quite as stressful as being born. A difficult birth, or even one that appears to be normal, can result in minor neurological faults that lead to childhood complaints like colic, glue ear and behavioural disorders as a child grows up. These can be prevented by gentle cranial osteopathic techniques soon after birth.'

Osteopathic treatment can help mothers before, during and after childbirth. One of the most common complaints of pregnancy and its aftermath is back, neck or shoulder pain brought about by the change in the body's centre of gravity as the baby grows. Hip pain or dysfunction may also occur due to hormonal changes. The effects of incorrect posture and movement during our daily lives are magnified by pregnancy. As well as soft tissue manipulation an osteopath will give you valuable advice on the correct way to sit, stand or move to avoid problems as the pregnancy develops. Treatment is also helpful for after-birth problems such as stress incontinence resulting from the weakening of the pelvic floor, or back pain following an epidural.

A consultation early on in pregnancy is a particularly good idea for anyone with a tendency to back ache. Treatment will take 20-30 minutes, but at the first consultation this will be preceded by a lengthy investigation of your medical history.

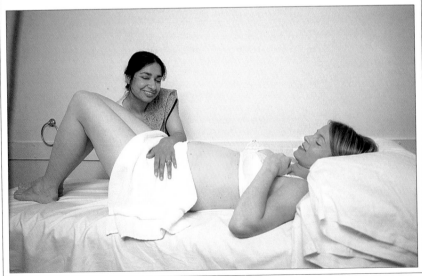

AROMATHERAPY

'Massage using very diluted essential oils can be enormously comforting for mothers in the later stages of pregnancy and in labour as well,' says one aromatherapist, who recommends a monthly treatment. Essential oils are diluted to a third of normal strength in the treatment of pregnant women. The range of oils used is more limited (see page 000 for oils to avoid).

Exhaustion, back or neck ache, oedema, nausea and breathlessness – common complaints in the final months – can be eased with lavender or mandarin, both of which have a calming effect. For puffiness and water retention lemon is gently massaged on the lymphatic drainage points. Ginger or Roman chamomile is also helpful for nausea.

Aromatherapy is a wonderful relaxant, but using oils on the abdomen can also prevent stretch marks after pregnancy and prepare the perineum for birth by softening the tissues, reducing the risk of a tear.

Aromatherapy can be applied during the birth by a partner or midwife. A 1 per cent dilution of clary sage, massaged into the lower back, is believed to speed up contractions. After the birth lavender, calendula and tea tree can be used to help heal any tears.

Herbal teas and dietary changes are often recommended to help alleviate nausea and water retention or to reduce blood pressure.

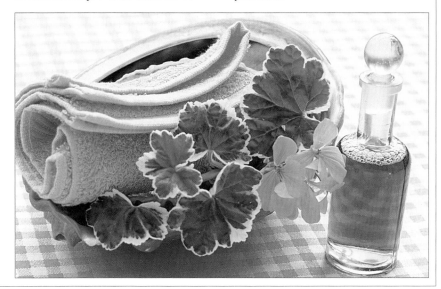

NUTRITION

Eating a wide range of fresh, healthy foods is essential in pregnancy. 'That can be harder than it sounds,' says one nutritional therapist. 'We rely so much on convenience foods and so much of what we eat is sprayed or treated chemically that we have to be very positive about it.'

She advises mothers-to-be to buy organic produce where possible – not just vegetables and grains, but organic dairy produce as well, since the hormones, antibiotics and growth enhancers given to cattle can cross the food chain. Additives such as colourings and preservatives found in convenience food should be avoided if possible,

along with soft cheeses and pâtés because there is still a danger from listeria. There is evidence that too much caffeine (usually taken in the form of coffee) can increase the chances of miscarriage, that alcohol may have a detrimental effect on the developing baby and that smoking may damage its respiratory system. Proper nutrition involves making sure you have sufficient vitamins and minerals, though mothers-to-be are recommended to avoid liver during pregnancy because of the dangers of excess Vitamin A. Folic acid, believed to help prevent spina bifida, is now prescribed to pregnant women, but supplements of zinc, magnesium, Vitamin B_6, essential fatty acids (EFAs) and other trace elements may also be recommended.

A consultation may involve analysis of your diet and mineral status and a follow-up monitoring of changes and improvements.

Good nutrition needs to be continued after the birth, ensuring adequate levels of vitamins and minerals. Zinc is important in preventing post-natal depression.

If breast-feeding, remember that what you eat is passed on to your baby through your breast milk. Keep off alcohol. Keep an eye on your intake of dairy foods, as they may give the baby colic. If the baby suffers from wind, you may be eating too many cruciferous vegetables (cabbages, Brussels sprouts, etc).

It is very important to maintain good health so that you have enough energy to keep up with the demands of the baby!

SELF-HYPNOSIS

Learning the technique of self-hypnosis offers mothers-to-be a method of achieving deep relaxation and effective pain control during labour. 'Much of the work on this method has been undertaken in the United States,' explains one hypnotherapist. 'The potential for promoting the wellbeing of both mother and baby is very exciting for those who believe that childbirth should be a natural and pleasurable experience. Research indicates that not only does it reduce or eliminate the pain of labour, but that the birth can be quicker.'

Self-hypnosis does not in any way interfere with a mother's awareness or capacity to respond to what is going on around her during labour. She remains fully conscious and relaxed, able to respond to instructions and make decisions.

Therapy should start around the thirtieth week of pregnancy. The number of sessions required depends on the individual. Therapy progresses through breathing exercises and relaxation techniques to learning how to concentrate on relaxing particular muscle groups. You will be asked to visualize a favourite place – a warm, sunny beach, for instance, or somewhere that you associate with feelings of pleasure and happiness. The object is to help you reach as relaxed a state as possible during your labour and to reduce feelings of anxiety in the weeks leading up to the birth.

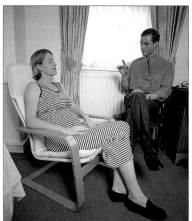

Post-natal depression can also be treated with hypnotic techniques, designed to allow the mother to come to terms with the considerable body changes, both physically and emotionally.

PSYCHOTHERAPY

Having a child completely changes your life - and that of your partner. 'Some of the psychological and emotional problems that mothers or couples may experience after the birth might have been better dealt with in ante-natal counselling, though you can't always predict how you will feel after the birth of a baby,' believes one therapist. 'The dynamics of a relationship change so much during pregnancy and after birth. One of the new parents may have a completely different idea about what life is going to be like on a practical level. It is surprising how little some couples talk about this together. A birth can trigger off submerged feelings about an unhappy childhood, for instance.'

Psychotherapy gives couples, together or separately, the chance to talk through these matters and helps them understand why they feel and act the way they do. Sessions take between one and one and a half hours.

ACUPUNCTURE

Acupuncture is increasingly used to help with breech births. There is absolutely no danger to mother or baby. The treatment involves both acupuncture and moxibustion (warming the needles by burning herbs) applied to a point on the foot in order gently to increase the energy flow. This may be attempted up to three times and is successful in the majority of cases.

Acupuncture is also helpful in late pregnancy to prepare for the actual birth. It can relieve common discomforts like swelling, fatigue and lower back ache. It can also help mothers-to-be who are suffering from high blood pressure. As one acupuncturist says, 'Once-a-week sessions in the weeks before birth relieve tenseness and make the mother feel much more energetic. Acupuncture helps prepare the body for birth, and can also be used instead of drugs to help relieve pain during the birth itself.'

SELF-CARE

Nutrition
Eat plenty of fruit, vegetables and fibre-rich foods and make sure you drink plenty of water to avoid constipation. Prune juice is a natural laxative.

Aromatherapy
Although some essential oils should be avoided in pregnancy there are plenty that you can use – appropriately diluted in the bathor as an inhalation – to help you relax (see under *Aromatherapy*, page 193). You can also get advice on massage techniques your partner can use to help you in labour.

HOMEOPATHY

Fatigue, mood swings, indigestion and other routine discomforts of pregnancy can be helped by the prescription of a constitutional remedy. Morning sickness does not always respond to homeopathic treatment, but there are safe treatments to try. Most women respond particularly well to homeopathic remedies when they are pregnant and homeopaths usually recommend and prescribe a kit to be used during childbirth. Arnica is particularly effective in preventing and treating bruising, Phosphorus can be used to reduce bleeding and Secale can be taken instead of having an injection to help with the expulsion of the placenta. If contractions are sluggish or ineffective, Caulophyllum can be taken. You should have a consultation in early pregnancy and then visit the practitioner as necessary.

Homeopathy can also help with common problems after the birth. Agnus castus is likely to be prescribed in the first instance if you have difficulty breast-feeding, although there are many other remedies that may be useful, depending on the exact cause and nature of the problem. Sepia can help with the listlessness and irritability of post-natal depression.

TIPS

Morning sickness can be helped by eating small, regular amounts of carbohydrate so that your stomach is never empty. Ginger biscuits, sweets or herbal teas also help nausea.

SUPPORTIVE TREATMENTS

Trichology
It is not unusual to suffer some hair loss after birth. This may be caused by hormonal changes, an iron deficiency or simply fatigue. Scalp therapy, combined with nutritional advice, is effective in stopping and reversing the problem.

Healing
Healing can help relax mothers-to-be who are anxious about the birth. It is particularly effective when there have been problems with a previous pregnancy.

Remedial Yoga
This is not recommended during the first three months of pregnancy, but after this time yoga practice, guided by a teacher, can provide a way to keep yourself supple, encourage the free flow of energy and circulation. Also in yogic breathing practice you can learn to relax and control breathing in preparation for labour and delivery.

After the birth yoga is an excellent way for the mother to regain suppleness and tone the internal organs and systems that have been under strain during pregnancy.

Flower Remedies
Bach flowers are entirely safe to use throughout pregnancy and even during childbirth. During early pregnancy they are particularly useful in combating morning sickness. They can also be used to ward off feelings of anxiety and the 'baby blues'. Mustard, for example, is said to be good for 'those who are liable to times of gloom, or even despair', while olive may be recommended for those who are 'so exhausted and weary that they feel they have no more strength to make any effort'.

Pomegranate is useful throughout the whole period of pregnancy – and combined with watermelon good to take during the birth process.

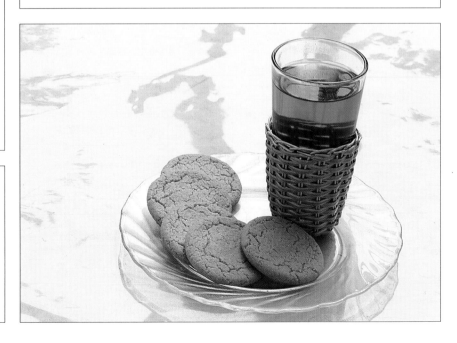

The Menopause

THE ORTHODOX APPROACH

All women experience the menopause, a natural change in the female reproductive system which normally takes place between the ages of 45 and 55. The word menopause specifically means the end of periods, but it is the falling level of the sex hormones oestrogen and progesterone in the body as the ovaries stop working that results in the physical and emotional problems we associate with this phase of women's lives.

Some women experience few or no problems. Others suffer a great deal for several years. The menopause often coincides with the emotional upheaval of children growing up and leaving home, causing women to feel a loss of identity and focus.

Hot flushes and night sweats are two well-known physical symptoms of this temporary hormonal imbalance – working women in particular often say they find hot flushes very embarrassing, though they are not usually obvious to anyone else. Periods may become irregular, heavier or lighter before they stop entirely. Other side effects are general tiredness and depression, irritability, broken sleep and memory lapses and a lack of interest in sex. Vaginal dryness can make sex very uncomfortable and you may be more susceptible to vaginal and urinary infections. Some of these symptoms may occur before periods stop, so it is advisable to have a hormone test once a year from the age of 45 that any appropriate action can be taken.

All these symptoms are temporary and treatable, but the long-term effects of declining hormone levels include a greater risk of osteoporosis and heart disease for some women.

Hormone replacement therapy (HRT) is a comprehensive treatment for the symptoms associated with the menopause, regarded as a deficiency disorder by conventional medicine. HRT replaces some of the hormones that your body is no longer producing with a combination of oestrogen and progestogen or oestrogen alone. It can be taken in the form of pills, as a cream applied to the skin, as a patch or it can be implanted. There are dozens of different preparations now available; some promote a monthly bleed, others do not.

HRT can be taken as soon as symptoms of the menopause, such as hot flushes and vaginal dryness, appear and can, in theory, be taken indefinitely. But HRT, in the UK at least, is controversial and only a relatively small number of women take it for any length of time. Some undoubtedly find it a convenient 'one stop' solution to the problem of hot flushes, night sweats and vaginal dryness. Staunch advocates regard it as an 'elixir of youth', claiming that it improves the appearance of skin and hair and gives a sense of well-being. But many women complain of side effects such as weight gain, hair loss, headaches, tender breasts and water retention. Recent research also indicates an increased risk of breast cancer. On the other hand HRT helps protect against osteoporosis and the post-menopausal risks of heart attacks and strokes.

Anyone who has had breast or womb cancer or fibroids is not advised to take HRT.

Quite apart from HRT there are conventional treatments available for specific problems. Your doctor may prescribe a drug containing clonidine hydrochloride for hot flushes and there are a number of gels and pessaries containing oestrogen to combat vaginal dryness. KY jelly may also help.

THE HALE APPROACH

Menopause is a natural progression, not a disease, and therefore does not require treatment. If the symptoms are unpleasant, complementary therapies should be tried first, with orthodox measures such as HRT used only as a last resort.

Menopause is one of the most important 'passages' a woman has to face in her life. Particularly in the West, it can be a time of great unease, discomfort and uncertainty, or a time to value and respect the past and go forward positively with a body which has adjusted to this new state and with a mental/emotional outlook which is looking forward to experiencing this new cycle in a woman's life.

Many people view the menopause as starting with hot flushes and changes in the pattern or heaviness of periods. They are not always aware of the pre-menopausal state which starts about five years before the onset of the 'real thing'.

As most menopause starts around the age of 50, the average time for pre-menopause is 45. At this time you could start having mood swings and other symptoms without realizing that you are in a pre-menopausal state. The Hale Clinic would advise women from about 45 onwards to have yearly hormonal tests to ascertain whether hormonal changes have

already started. If this is the case, the treatments used for the 'menopause proper' will also be of great assistance during the pre-menopausal years.

In addition, good nutrition, exercise and massage to promote good circulation and reduce stress levels can help prepare the body and mind so that 'the passage' becomes much easier.

The closest complementary treatment to HRT would be a combination of herbal remedies which contain phytoestrols, which mimic the role of oestrogen, thereby preventing the menopausal symptoms (although periods will stop eventually).

Trichology and Oxypeel treatments can help any external effects on the hair and skin caused by the menopause.

Osteoporosis screening is also recommended to assess bone density; advice on future courses of action would be given on the basis of the results.

Finally, because the menopause can be such an important time of change in a woman's life, the Hale Clinic would highly recommend counselling or psychotherapy to assist a woman in integrating this new cycle into her life, and from there approaching the future with an awareness of the many opportunities it can bring.

NATUROPATHY

Herbalists have for centuries used certain plants to treat menopausal symptoms. Now we know that several of them contain phytoestrols, which stimulate hormone levels, acting as a mild, safe form of HRT. A naturopath explains: 'Phytoestrols are compounds that have a molecular structure similar to that of oestrogen and have effects comparable to, but weaker than oestrogen. This offers the benefits of conventional HRT without the well-known attendant risks.'

Celery, fennel, ginseng and alfalfa are among the many plants and herbs that contain these compounds. Extract of rhubarb root and hops are also particularly rich sources. These active oestrogen-like alternatives can easily and safely be taken by most women and are effective in treating

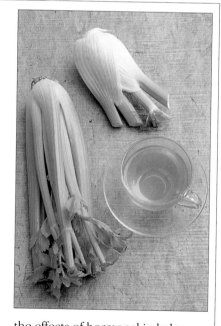

the effects of hormonal imbalance.

Herbal mixtures of black cohosh, blue cohosh, dandelion, *dong quai* and agnus castus may be prescribed for hot flushes and night sweats. These work primarily on the liver, which controls the release of hormones in the body.

ACUPUNCTURE

The changes of the menopause affect the functions of the liver and kidneys which regulate the hormonal balance in the body. 'In Chinese medicine the kidney is "water" and the liver is "fire" or "wood",' explains one acupuncturist. 'When these get out of balance the water function becomes sluggish and the heat, the liver function, is too dominant, resulting in the irritability, anxiety, hot flushes, water retention and other symptoms of hormonal imbalance women experience at menopause.' Acupuncture aims to rebalance the body by stimulating the kidney function, increasing the energy flowing through this pathway. It may be used in conjunction with Chinese herbs, which will be prescribed for use at home. Treatment with acupuncture takes about half an hour and 7 to 10 fortnightly sessions are recommended to get the full benefits.

PSYCHOTHERAPY

The hormonal changes of the menopause are frequently associated with a number of psychological problems such as depression, loss of confidence and self-esteem or feelings of acute self-doubt and eating problems. Psychotherapists believe that hormonal changes are part of the cause of these problems, but many are due at least in part of the stage of life. Women may be particularly vulnerable when their children leave home, an event which often coincides with the menopause. 'Often you find that they are faced with feelings, problems and insecurities they had many years ago that were effectively submerged while they were bringing up a family but now come to the surface again,' explains one psychotherapist.

Talking to a psychotherapist should help you understand your reactions and feelings through examining your past; you can then start challenging your behaviour. Developing new attitudes and becoming more conscious of the way you react to stressful situations can help overcome many of the emotional difficulties associated with the menopause.

HOMEOPATHY

Homeopathic treatment for the menopause aims to help your body adapt to change. Change is inevitable, but it needn't be disruptive. Advice should be sought as soon as periods become irregular so that the effect of the inevitable hormonal changes – hot flushes, irritability and sleep disturbance – are managed and contained. Treatment starts with an assessment of the individual's overall health and personality and may include a blood test to check hormonal levels.

Sepia, belladonna and agnus castus are among the natural remedies prescribed to combat menopausal symptoms. Calc. carb., gelsemium and graphites may be prescribed for hot flushes. There are also treatments to counteract the side effects of HRT and to help women who want to stop taking it without suffering the return of menopausal symptoms.

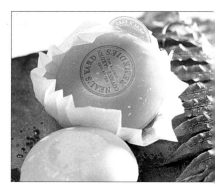

NUTRITION

Menopausal problems can be exacerbated by poor eating habits developed over a long period. Re-establishing a healthy diet with a wide range of fresh foods is of prime importance. Leafy greens, soya products and broccoli should play a major part in your diet; intake of red meat and caffeine should be reduced. In general, guard against having too much protein in your diet, since this is believed to rob the body of calcium and other essential nutrients.

'There may be vitamin and mineral deficiencies in the diet and a good multi-vitamin programme designed for the individual will include supplements of selenium, Vitamin E and Vitamin C,' is the view of one nutritionist, who also believes that many of the psychological problems experienced at menopause may be due to poor nutrition.

Examining not just what you eat but the way you eat is crucial. Taking smaller meals throughout the day rather than leaving long gaps between meals maintains blood sugar levels and helps fend off nervousness and low energy.

An initial consultation with a nutritionist will take about an hour and your therapist will work out a diet and supplement plan for you to follow at home.

LIGHT THERAPY

Light plays a vital role in our physical and mental well-being and it is now widely appreciated that the lack of it can lead to depression and low energy. 'Every living thing responds to light,' explains a light therapist. 'Light regulates the hormones in the body and so can be used to counteract many of the problems associated with menopause.'

Light therapy involves exposure to full-spectrum light equivalent to what you would experience on a 'bright spring day in the northern hemisphere'. Sessions last about an hour and the effects can be instant. Light absorbed through the eyes works on the pineal gland in the brain, stimulating production of serotonin, the 'feel good' hormone, and improving the circulation. It is an effective treatment for the sleep disorders, depression, irritability and panic attacks experienced during menopause.

Light therapy can also be used on the skin. The dilation of the blood vessels helps hot flushes and the treatment stimulates the body's lubrication to counteract vaginal dryness.

MOOR THERAPY

A Moor bath or body wrap is particularly recommended as a treatment for water retention and hot flushes. The nutrients are easily absorbed through the skin and they improve the circulation and lymphatic flow.

This relaxing treatment also improves the feel and texture of the skin itself, which may become drier during the menopause The body wrap is particularly effective if there are problems with cellulite around the hips and thighs.

SELF-CARE/TIPS

• Spicy foods, hot drinks and alcohol can all trigger hot flushes.
• A Vitamin E capsule inserted into the vagina each day is effective treatment for dryness.
• Avoid powerfully scented soaps or vaginal sprays: these may irritate the vaginal area, which is often more sensitive at menopause.
• Weight-bearing exercise such as brisk walking will build up bone density and improve circulation, which is of benefit during pre-menopause and menopause.

SUPPORTIVE THERAPIES

Osteoporosis Screening: This is a simple test for measuring bone density. It can identify early signs of bone loss, establish a 'base' for future reference and suggest strategies for building up bone density.

Remedial Yoga: Learning to relax and keep the body supple are important in restoring and maintaining an equable and confident approach to life.

Healing: Feelings of fatigue and lethargy can be helped by healing, which works to put energy back into the body.

Hypnosis: Hypnosis can reassure and empower the unconscious mind to intervene, balance and harmonize the body's natural rhythms.

Chi Kung: Exercises can help counteract specific symptoms of hormone imbalance and make you feel more in control.

Trichology: There are a number of scalp therapies and treatments for hair loss due to hormonal changes. These aim to improve circulation and stimulate follicular cell activity.

Oxypeel: Treatment with plant extracts can help remove brown marks on the skin caused by hormonal changes and can also reduce the problems of dryness of the skin which many women experience as they get older.

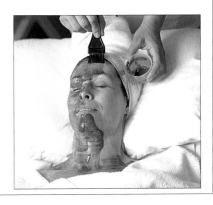

Osteoporosis

THE ORTHODOX APPROACH

As more people live longer osteoporosis or 'brittle bone disease' has become a major health concern. It affects far more women than men, though either sex can suffer the progressive loss of bone density that leads to fractures of the wrists, spine or hips. Bone is not a static tissue – it is constantly being broken down (a process known as resorption) and rebuilt throughout our lives. If less bone is being made than is disappearing it becomes porous and easily broken.

Known as 'the silent epidemic', osteoporosis often makes its presence known only when a sufferer incurs a surprise fracture after a minor fall. Visible symptoms are loss of height and the development of a stoop or 'dowager's hump' as the skeleton weakens and shrinks.

Up to one in four women are believed to be at risk of osteoporosis, which is thought to be closely linked to the fall in hormone levels during the menopause; this interferes with the absorption of calcium and slows down the formation of new bone.

Particularly at risk are those who have had an early menopause or who have had their ovaries removed. Smoking, habitual dieting, prolonged absence of periods and treatment with corticosteroid drugs are also risk factors. Heredity also plays an important part. Increasing number of young men now suffer from osteoporosis, which indicates that diet and lifestyle may be important factors in the cause of this disease.

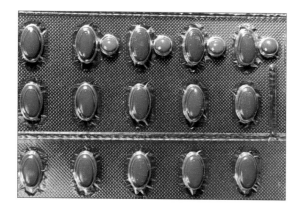

Hormone Replacement Therapy (HRT) is the prime treatment prescribed for women at risk of osteoporosis or already showing some bone loss. HRT replaces the oestrogen that declines at the time of the menopause. There is known to be a link between low levels of oestrogen and the development of osteoporosis; research shows that women who take HRT are at less risk of bone fractures. However it is accepted that HRT has to be taken for at least five to seven years, maybe longer, to be effective against osteoporosis and many women are uneasy about that.

The decision whether or not to take HRT is a very personal one. Research shows that HRT may be linked to increased cases of breast cancer, but that it also reduces the risk of heart attacks and strokes. Many women experience side effects when taking HRT -weight gain, water retention and depression are typical. But there is now a wide range of different HRT products available and some will suit you better than others. Treatment with testosterone, the male sex hormone, can be helpful in treating men with osteoporosis. Women who do not want to take HRT may be prescribed other bone-strengthening drugs. The pharmaceutical companies are currently investing substantial sums of money in the development and marketing of new remedies. Calcitonin is a hormone included in a number of prescription drugs that helps conserve bone mass by slowing down the resorption process. Established osteoporosis can be treated with bisphosphonates.

THE HALE APPROACH

Unless your doctor or hospital specialist is prescribing HRT for a serious medical problem, it would be best to have complementary treatment from a knowledgeable therapist who specializes in this area. Complementary treatments can be very effective and this, combined with the fact that 50 per cent of women who start HRT stop it within the first year, suggests that avoiding HRT is a possible and safe route. If you are already taking HRT, complementary therapies can be very beneficial, but withdrawal from HRT should be done under the care of a complementary therapist who knows the subject, or through your doctor.

With osteoporosis or suspected osteoporosis the first course of action is to take a screening test. This is a quick, painless scan of the heel bone, giving a patient an accurate measurement of current bone density and a likely prognosis. Treatment and corrective action may then be advised. It is a good idea to have an osteoporosis screening in your early 20s so that preventative action may be taken if a potential weakness is identified.

The right nutrition plays a vital role in preventing osteoporosis. Eating calcium-rich foods, as well as making sure your digestion is working properly to ensure absorption of this bone-building mineral, is imperative. If you do not spend much time in sunlight, Vitamin D supplements are important to help with the absorption of calcium. Research done by US doctors has shown that natural progesterone (from Mexican yams) increases bone density by 40 per cent in women suffering from osteoporosis, as well as playing a preventative role by building the bone density of women whose tests indicated their bone density was less than it should be.

Acupuncture can be of great assistance bothin the treatment of osteoporosis. Finally, weight-bearing exercise such as running or walking is of vital importance in building up bone density. By taking some of the advice given here, men and women can look forward to enjoying the positive aspects of aging without the fear of being incapacitated by brittle bones.

LIGHT THERAPY

Sunlight is known to be essential for the production of Vitamin D, which enables calcium to be absorbed and used for bone formation. But many of us do not get enough sunlight in our daily lives, which means that taking calcium supplements may not be sufficient to prevent bone loss. Exposing the skin to full-spectrum light corrects any Vitamin D deficiency and enables the body to utilize calcium more effectively.

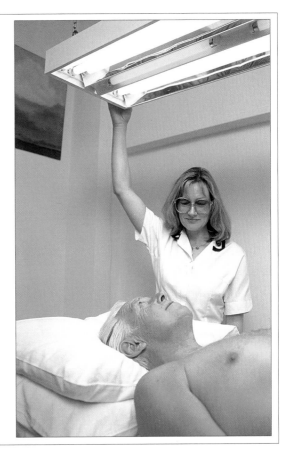

NATUROPATHY

Most of us consume enough calcium through eating the proper food and by taking supplements if necessary. The problem is that much of it is not properly absorbed and put into bone. This may, according to one naturopath, be due to inadequate levels of Vitamin D_3, which is synthesized into calcitriol, which in turn regulates calcium absorption through the gut lining and stimulates bone production. Vitamin D_3 is actually a hormone, formed by the action of sunlight on a substance in the skin. Taken as a supplement it increases the amount of dietary calcium absorbed into the bloodstream, stops most of the magnesium and calcium we consume being lost in our urine and ensures that more calcium enters the bone.

OSTEOPOROSIS SCREENING

Ultra-sound screening tells you whether your bone-mineral density and structure are low, average or high for your age, providing a 'benchmark' for future monitoring. It is a simple test, painless and non-invasive, carried out on the heel, where the metabolic activity of the skeleton is highest.

'The heel is on the same axis as the hip joint,' explains one practitioner, 'and the hip joint is a major concern in osteoporosis.' The screening takes no more than 30 minutes and you receive an immediate reading and interpretation, plus advice on diet and exercise. Osteoporosis screening provides an important 'early warning' of bone loss, which may otherwise remain undetected until you break a limb. It enables you to make any lifestyle changes to prevent future problems. 'I would like to see more people, men and women, being screened in their 20s and 30s,' says the same practitioner. 'Most people who have screening are women in their 40s concerned about the menopause. But bone loss can start long before then.' People who are at risk of osteoporosis, or who have lower than average bone density, are advised to have a screening once a year. Screening is also a good idea if you have had a serious illness or prolonged drug treatment, both of which can result in a loss of bone density.

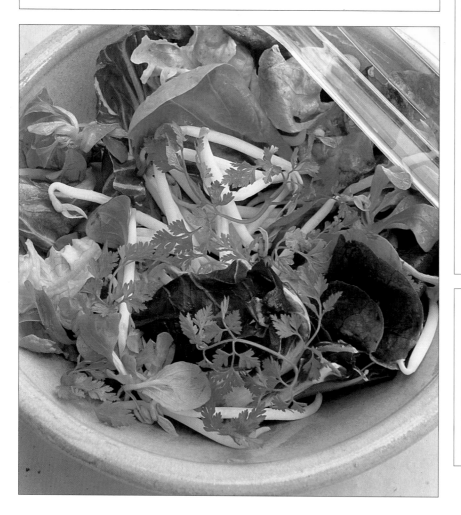

NUTRITION

Eating a wide range of nutritious food and cutting down on alcohol, smoking and caffeine, all of which leech calcium from the body, is the sensible approach to preventing osteoporosis. But it is also important to check that your digestive system is functioning properly. One nutritionist points out that our levels of stomach acid can fall as we get older, or as the result of stress, resulting in poor absorption of the nutrients contained in what we eat. A simple test will establish whether or not the body is digesting and utilizing food properly, and if necessary supplements will be recommended.

Dairy products are by no means the best source of calcium – there is a school of thought that suggests too high an intake of these foods may interfere with the process of putting calcium into bone. Better to increase your intake of green vegetables, nuts and seeds, tofu and oily fish, all of which contain large amounts of calcium and essential fatty acids. Excessive meat eating should be checked, as this stresses the kidneys, which lose calcium as a result.

SUPPORTIVE TREATMENT

Acupuncture
Acupuncture treatment can be used very effectively for pain relief in established cases of osteoporosis.

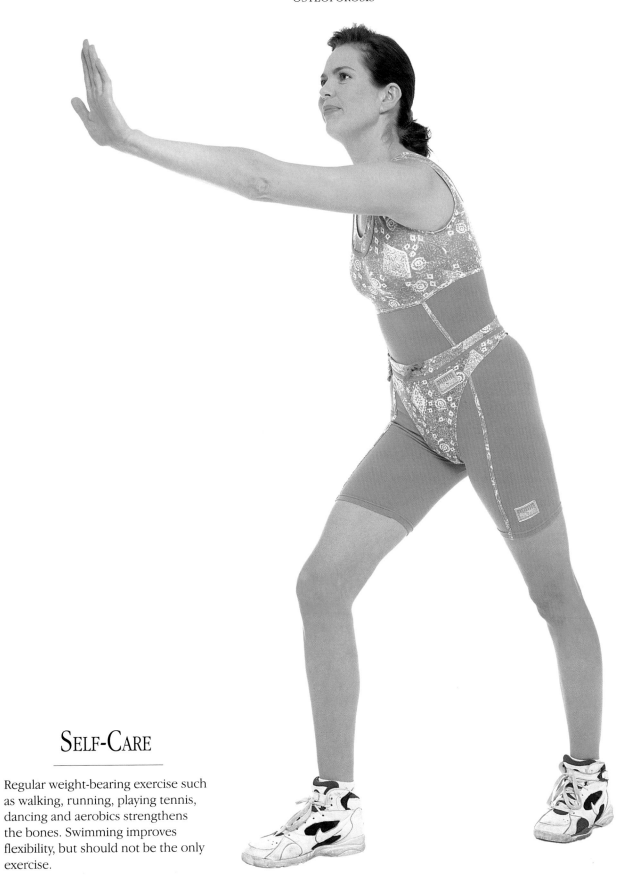

SELF-CARE

Regular weight-bearing exercise such
as walking, running, playing tennis,
dancing and aerobics strengthens
the bones. Swimming improves
flexibility, but should not be the only
exercise.

Impotence

There are a number of medical conditions that make it physically difficult or impossible for a man to have an erection. These include injury or surgery to the spinal cord, certain chronic illness such as diabetes, some nervous disorders and a number of different drugs – tranquillizers, diuretics, antidepressants, barbiturates, drugs for high blood pressure and stomach ulcers. Of course, there's also one more cause none of us can escape – old age. By the age of 65 the average angle of an erection has declined from 120 to 75 degrees.

However, there is something of a debate in the medical profession as to whether most cases of impotence are due to such physical causes or whether they have a psychological origin because, while erections are certainly the result of a reflex, there is nothing automatic about them.

They can be helped by trust, relaxation and fantasy and they can become a problem because of guilt, sexual taboos and fears of inadequacy when there are no physical problems at all. In fact the psychological reasons for being unable to make love can be all too mundane – job worries, money problems, depression and fatigue all have a habit of getting into bed with us. Some experts claim that 90 per cent of cases are due to the mind, though others put the effect of physical causes much higher.

THE ORTHODOX APPROACH

When it comes to treatment there is a sharp division between the strict medical view and the ideas of the caring, therapeutic professions. The most commonly recommended treatment for psychological impotence is that developed over 30 years ago by Masters and Johnson. Couples are encouraged to slow down, relax, and practise touching and mutual stroking, but to delay penetration for anything up to a week while they follow a series of increasingly imaginative sexual exercises.

Doctors and hospitals, on the other hand, rather ignore the mental element and tend to rely on injections of papavarin, a drug that will guarantee erections but won't deal with any underlying emotional issues. Other more radical treatments include surgically implanting a pump that can be activated when needed.

THE HALE APPROACH

Problems with erection should first be analysed by a urologist or specialist in sexual medicine. Try complementary treatments before you proceed with the orthodox options.

Impotence can often be caused by an interplay of physical and mental factors, so it is advisable to choose a programme or a combination of treatments which addresses both these aspects.

Homeopathy, acupuncture and Ayurveda will treat both the physical and mental sides of the problem and can be combined with supportive treatments such as light therapy, aromatherapy and healing. Chi Kung and yoga can be used as self-care tools to strengthen the body and calm the mind.

Hypnosis and psychotherapy focus more on the mental aspects of impotence and can be particularly helpful in treating the more deep-seated psychological problems associated with this problem.

ACUPUNCTURE

According to acupuncturists, impotence is generally caused by damage to kidney yin or yang energy resulting from repeated seminal emission or excessive sexual activity. It may also be due to an imbalance in the heart and spleen energy, resulting from emotional factors such as fright or worry; stagnation of liver energy; or the presence of damp and heat, causing relaxation of tendons and muscles. Impotence may also result from other diseases such as hepatitis or prostatitis. These primary diseases should be treated first.

Although impotence is characterized by failure to achieve erection, or by weak erection, there may be other symptoms: if the kidney yang is deficient, there may be weakness of the lower back and knees, dizziness, blurred vision and the need to urinate frequently; if the heart and spleen are involved there will be palpitation and insomnia. Full consideration of the patient's symptoms, including examination of the pulse and tongue, will determine the exact cause and the most suitable programme of treatment, directed towards relieving the cause of the problem. Treatment may include body and ear acupuncture, moxibustion (the use of hot needles) if appropriate, change of diet and exercise to strengthen the kidneys and improve energy flow. Acupuncture gives satisfactory results in the treatment of impotence, especially when it is combined with lifestyle advice to help prevent a recurrence. During the period of treatment sexual activity must be avoided.

HOMEOPATHY

The very specific nature of homeopathic remedies means that it regards impotence as coming from a number of different causes which need different remedies. For instance, there are cases where the problem stems from a fear of sex, which may derive from worries about AIDS or a strict upbringing where sex was frowned upon. These cases may respond to the following remedies:

• For a man who is torn between an intense desire for sex and a fear of sexual failure plus a general insecurity – Lycopodium.
• For phobias and irrational fears about catching something – Pulsatilla.
• When there are difficulties caused by grief or disappointment in a previous relationship – Ignatia.

In cases where there is a specific problem with getting an erection the following remedies are advised:

• A surge of desire followed by the anticipation of failure and the penis cold and small – Lycopodium.
• Erection does not last, a great surge of sexual feeling after long abstinence, legs feel cold and cramped – Conium.

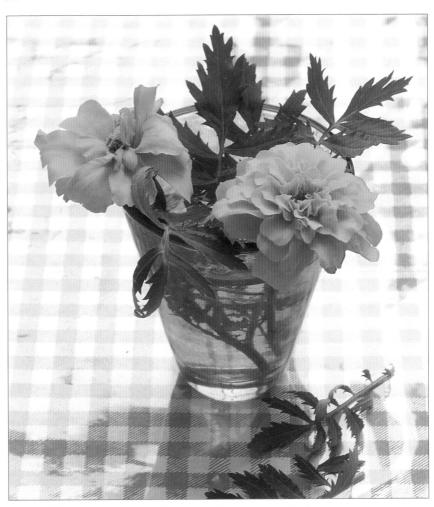

Marigold flower essence is said to be good for hormonal imbalance

HYPNOTHERAPY

'This is a question of confidence, of relaxation and how you relate to your partner,' explains one hypnotherapist. 'If you are consistently failing to make love it may be that there are some unacknowledged feelings about her – perhaps you are angry or threatened – and hypnosis can help to let them out.'

Alternatively a cycle of anxiety can be set up. A man is tired or worried, can't perform – as is quite natural – but feels 'less of a man' because of it. He becomes anxious about making love and so the next time his worry causes him to fail again. Here hypnotherapy can help the person to relax.

Some men feel threatened if their partners are more successful then they are. The way out is to bring the complex emotions involved to the surface.

PSYCHOTHERAPY

In dealing with sexual problems such as impotence, the primary goal of therapy is to create or restore mutual sexual comfort and satisfaction. This is achieved through emphasizing mutual pleasure, closeness and the enhancement of one's own and one's partner's satisfaction. Placing an emphasis on performance is often counter-productive, creating more anxiety and ultimately contributing to the problem. Therapy therefore focuses on non-performance goals, but the establishment of a more pleasurable and non-demanding sexual process will often have a pleasant side effect, more effective sexual performance.

The therapist needs to earn the trust of both partners, not taking sides and being careful to allow for the discussion of difficult and sensitive subjects in a non-threatening environment. Religious and cultural beliefs need to be taken into consideration, as well as more general matters pertaining to lifestyle and family life.

There are several approaches to therapy in this area, falling under the general heading of cognitive-behavioural therapy. One common method is what is referred to as 'sensate focus' exercises, which involve encouraging a couple to approach intimate physical and emotional involvement with each other in a series of safe but gradually more intense stages. This 'homework' allows people to engage in sexually related exercises and the on-going therapy sessions review progress, identify positive changes, and help the couple express and resolve any anxieties or problems.

Education is a fundamental part of the process, and providing information may be the most important aspect of sex therapy.

Giving consideration to the environment and circumstances in which the sexual relationship exists is also essential, as is challenging negative beliefs or attitudes and reducing thoughts which interfere with sexual satisfaction. Communication problems are often encountered in sex therapy, and indeed often present as more specific issues around sexual matters. The therapist identifies these and helps the couple work towards more effective, non-threatening styles of communication, which in turn contribute to the development of a mutually satisfying sexual relationship.

Psychological therapy with impotence is therefore a complex process comprising several different facets, all of which need to be considered if the couple is to achieve the kind of sexual relationship they desire.

SELF-CARE

Flower Remedies
Marigold (Petite Fleur) is said to be good for hormone imbalance and sexually related problems, and so is banana (African Essences AK).

SUPPORTIVE TREATMENTS

Healing

'The important thing here,' according to one healer, 'is completely to de-stress the patient. After a treatment they may sleep especially well because there was a lot of tension there that has now been released. Then healing energy can make them feel good about themselves again and help with circulation, which is useful with problems of impotence.'

Ayurveda

According to Ayurvedic principles, impotence is created by the mind and by physical disability, possibly because of unhappiness or depression. Treatment involves herbs to improve potency and a total detoxification using enemas, laxatives, steam baths and oil massage to tone up the whole body. But probably the best treatment is for the person to have the right partner.

Chi Kung

These gentle exercises can direct *chi* (intrinsic) energy to the affected area. There are many hundreds of exercises and your teacher will guide you as to which are most appropriate. Chi Kung exercises rebalance the *chi* (intrinsic) energy, improving control of muscles and nerves. Once mastered, these are ideal for self-care at home and form a useful support to other forms of complementary treatment.

Light Therapy

Light therapy relaxes the patient, reducing stress levels and significantly improving circulation. In this way, it helps break the cycle of stress–impotence–increased stress.

Aromatherapy

Stress, poor diet, inability to relax and low kidney energy can all be factors in causing impotence. Clinical aromatherapy massage helps rebalance the body's energies and induce relaxation, boost circulation of the blood and *chi* energy, improving self-esteem. Oils such as jasmine, cedarwood, sandalwood, rosewood and juniper help to overcome these difficulties. Use of the oils at home between clinical sessions is essential.

Remedial Yoga

Yoga encourages a healthy energy flow in the body, decreasing any blockages that may be present. Blockages can disturb the flow of hormones, influenced by the functioning of the glands. Through body, mind and breath yoga teaches us how to rebalance, stimulate and relax any tensions that may be the cause of blockages.

Buteyko

No person who breathes correctly (shallow breathing) suffers from impotence, unless they have a specific physical problem.

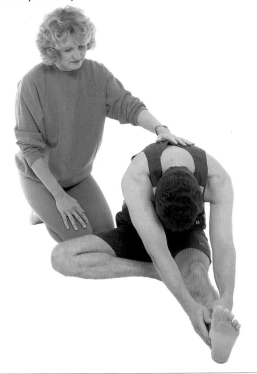
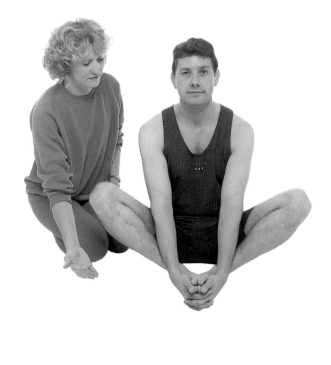

Prostate Problems

Something like 60 per cent of men over the age of 45 have an enlarged prostate gland and a significant proportion will go on to develop cancer there. In fact cancer of the prostate is the second most common cause of death in males and the rate is increasing – up 66 per cent in Britain between 1979 and 1990.

Often, however, the cancer develops slowly, without symptoms, and it is discovered only at a post mortem. Detection is tricky because of where the prostate is located. It is a bulb-shaped gland that goes round the urethra just where it leaves the bladder, so when it swells up urination becomes a problem. In fact, the first symptoms include finding it hard to urinate, wanting to urinate often, a burning sensation when you do, or blood in the urine. But cases often aren't spotted until quite late because the basic method of diagnosing an enlarged prostate is by rectal examination and many men prefer to avoid that. For cancers there is now an prostate-specific antigen test.

The prostate's job is to add acids, trace elements and enzymes to seminal fluid at the moment of ejaculation; these activate the sperm and give semen its distinctive smell. For reasons we don't understand the prostate tends to enlarge and stiffen with age, but it is probably connected with changing levels of various hormones. About a third of cases clear up of their own accord, but an enlarged prostate can cause related infection in the bladder and the kidneys.

In cancer cases doctors are increasingly recognizing a connection with high-fat diets. Cancer of the prostate is rare in Japan and China, for instance, where low-fat diets containing lots of vegetables and fish are the norm.

THE ORTHODOX APPROACH

The favoured treatment is surgery, whether to remove the excess tissue from an enlarged prostate or to cut out a cancerous one. Entry is either via the abdomen, up the urethra or in from behind the scrotum. The drawback to surgery is that it can cause impotence – you may have a problem either with achieving an erection or with ejaculating – and you may become more or less incontinent. On the other hand, an enlarged prostate can cut off the flow of urine altogether.

In contrast to the prevailing attitude in America, where they tend to operate at the first sign of cancer, in Britain many physicians leave it alone if it hasn't spread, and give radiotherapy if it has. Another approach to prostate cancer that has spread is to combat it with doses of feminizing oestrogen, with or without castration.

A new approach for cancer cases is cryotherapy, which involves injecting liquid nitrogen into the prostate via a metal probe.

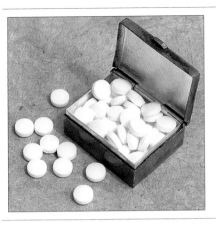

HOMEOPATHY

Specific remedies include:
• Difficult or painful urination with spasms of the bladder – Sabal.
• For a senile person who urinates frequently at night, complains of pressure on his rectum and has a smarting sensation at the neck of the bladder – Ferrum pic.
• When there is a frequent urge to urinate but this produces only a slow stream and the person is thin, underweight and prematurely impotent – Baryta.
• For someone who has a frequent and urgent desire to pass urine – Thuja.
• For impotence because erection is lost on penetration or a lack of desire for sex or pain during intercourse – Argentum nit.

THE HALE APPROACH

Any symptoms of prostatism should first be checked out by your doctor. If cancer is diagnosed, then referral to a cancer specialist and assessment of the severity of the problem is essential. If orthodox treatment offers a high percentage chance of success, then complementary treatments should be used alongside. If the orthodox treatment is unlikely to be effective, then one must ask the question, 'Might the treatment be worse than the cure?' In that case alternative therapies can be used without their orthodox counterpart.

The constitutional treatments of homeopathy, acupuncture and Ayurveda can be of great assistance with prostate problems. Following a specific nutritional programme and having osteopathic treatment will also strengthen the body's ability to fight this illlness.

Supportive treatments such as reflexology and healing can also be helpful, with Chi Kung giving the patient a self-care tool to use at home to increase resistance to prostate problems.

OSTEOPATHY

Benign prostate hypertrophy (BPH) is a common condition which may benefit from osteopathic manipulative therapy. Prostate disorders relate to dysfunction of other parts of the body such as the lumbar spine and sacroiliac joint, as well as pelvic congestion. The aim of the osteopathic treatment is to decrease the pelvic congestion and correct the spinal and/or cranial dysfunction through muscle release, manipulation, stimulation of neuro-lymphatic reflexes and visceral manipulation. These techniques help improve the lymph and blood drainage of the area as well as increasing the circulation and nerve outflow to the prostate.

NUTRITION/ALLERGY TREATMENT

Changes in the level of several hormones are involved with prostate enlargement, but the key one is a version of testosterone, known as dihydrotestosterone (DHT). Reducing levels of DHT reduces the size of the prostate. DHT levels go up with alcohol (especially beer) consumption and with stress, and come down with zinc and Vitamin B_6. Zinc also cuts down the rate at which testosterone is converted to DHT.

Conditions favouring an increase in DHT include exposure to pesticides and other drugs found in the environment such as dioxin and biphenyls. Therefore a diet of natural whole foods is advised. Also recommended are various supplements – calcium, magnesium, bio-flavonoids and carotenes – which can help the body deal with the presence of toxic chemicals. The herbs saw palmetto and ginseng both inhibit the production of DHT.

Supplements of essential fatty acids (linseed or oil of evening primrose) should also produce improvement, as may adding amino acids to the diet.

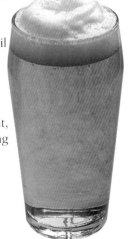

AYURVEDA

According to Ayurvedic principles, prostate problems are due to too much stimulus in the lower part of the body, which usually means too much sexual activity or toxic chemical matter passing with the urine, although having a high level of acid in the blood from excess alcohol can also play a part. Treatment involves the use of Ayurvedic enemas and laxatives, a steam bath and some herbal preparations to cool down the urinary system. Herbs might also be given to reduce the appetite and bring about balance of the *doshas* (the three main energy forces in the body).

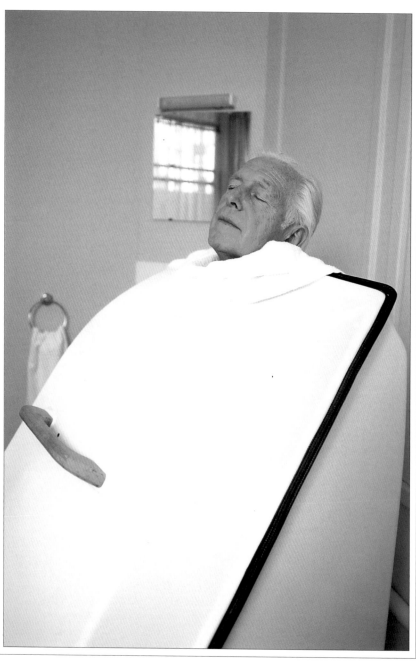

ACUPUNCTURE

According to Chinese medicine, the pattern of disharmony and its contributing factors which lead to prostate problems are as follows:

• Accumulation of damp and heat resulting from excess consumption c spicy, greasy food and alcohol, or fro liver and kidney imbalance.
• Retention of cold damp resulting from too much raw and cold food, or exposure to cold, wet weather over a period of time.
• Weakness of the kidneys due to ageing, too much sex or heavy physical work.
• Liver energy stagnation due to emotional factors, lack of exercise, to much sitting, repression of sexual energy, chronic constipation or local trauma.
• Stagnation of the blood due to sedentary occupations.

In Chinese medicine it is believed tha deficiencies in the kidney, especially i kidney yin, in senility cause the prostate carcinoma. Investigation by Western medical methods is sometimes necessary, so a patient could benefit from a combination of Western and Chinese treatment. Chronic prostatitis is often resistant t antibiotics. For benign prostate cance the side effects and consequences of surgery need to be weighed up. Whei orthodox medical treatment is being held off in order to watch for developments, acupuncture and Chinese herbal treatment may improve the symptoms and significantly reduce the need for surgery or other invasive treatment.

Chinese medicine requires a holisti approach. Patients should take advice on diet and lifestyle and make necessary changes. Acupuncture treatment will follow a flexible plan tailored to the needs of the individua patient.

SELF-CARE

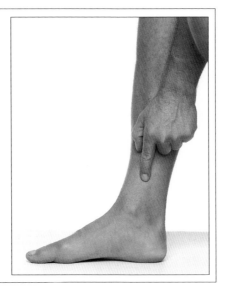

Indian Medicine
Pressure points: there is a point called kidney 3 two to three fingers above the ankle bone on both sides of the leg. Press that for one minute on both legs three times a day.

Yoga postures: sit in a chair position and breathe deeply 20 times.

Diet: drink three glasses of water as soon as you wake up in the morning.

SUPPORTIVE TREATMENTS

Healing
This can help to keep the problem to a minimum. The healer channels healing energy from an outside force to encourage the body to heal itself.

Chi Kung
A practitioner will guide you to which of the many hundreds of Chi Kung exercises are appropriate. These exercises can direct energy to the affected area, relaxing and balancing the body and mind. Once mastered they are easy to practise at home and form a useful support to other complementary therapies.

Reflexology
Massage will concentrate on the prostate reflex, which is on the inside of the ankle, halfway from the ankle bone to the back corner of the heel.

Hypnotherapy
Very often the symptoms of an enlarged prostate can be helped by visualization exercises which concentrate on generating a feeling of comfort. The condition is made worse by stress and tension and hypnotherapy can help with that too.

Gout

Contrary to popular belief, this painful affliction is rarely caused by too much of the good life. True, an excess of red wine can be a contributory factor, but overeating and overindulgence generally are not causes of gout. In fact, it is a disorder of the body chemistry whereby too much uric acid and its compounds (urates) accumulate in the blood. This results in acid and urate crystals collecting in one or more of the joints, causing extreme pain, swelling and redness. The joint at the base of the big toe is particularly prone to gout and repeated attacks can damage the bones of the joints.

Urate crystals can also collect in the kidneys, leading to kidney stones (see page 168), kidney failure and high blood pressure (see page 128). They can also collect in the skin where they form hard lumps – the ears, fingers and toes are all common sites.

THE ORTHODOX APPROACH

Diagnosis is made by a blood test. It is known that excess red wine and some medicines, such as diuretics (which encourage urine excretion) increase the risk of contracting gout, so these factors could be indicative.

Anti-inflammatory drugs are usually prescribed to relieve pain and inflammation. A sufferer would also be advised to avoid excess alcohol and medicines that raise the blood urate level in order to prevent further attacks. Drugs that increase urate excretion may also be prescribed. Some prescription drugs reduce urate production and therefore the risk of subsequent attacks. However, they have to be taken every day for some years.

THE HALE APPROACH

Diagnosis, as mentioned above, is made by a blood test which generally requires a doctor's opinion. Once the diagnosis is established, complementary treatments are safe and effective. Orthodox drugs may be required initially and you should notify your complementary specialist of everything you are taking or being given.

Nutrition plays a vital role in the treatment of gout – and in the prevention of a recurrence – so nutritional/naturopathic or Ayurvedic advice on a suitable diet is highly recommended. Colonic irrigation would complement a nutritional programme, while homeopathy has some remedies which are particularly effective in the treatment of gout.

HOMEOPATHY

Although homeopathic treatment is very individualistic, taking into account such factors as a patient's emotional and psychological state, their diet, etc., in general terms one of the most common remedies for gout is colchicum. Dietary advice is also given if necessary.

AYURVEDA

According to Ayurveda, gout is known as *Vatarakta*, meaning toxicity in the blood causing toxic deposits or inflammation commonly in the joints of the toes or fingers. In the treatment an understanding of the *dosha* state (the patient's general 'type') is important, as is looking into diet and lifestyle.

Specific oral preparations are available, but a detoxification programme using *panchakarma* (revitalizing) methods is the most important aspect of controlling gout successfully. In general dietary terms, avoid any acidic foods, fat, 'cooling' foods, meat and meat products, and eat plenty of fish, vegetables and fruit.

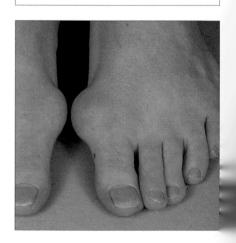

COLONIC HYDROTHERAPY

According to one colonic therapist who is also a nutritionist, gout is a form of arthritis. If the body is not eliminating efficiently, it will obviously retain waste. The body protects its most vital organs and so it dumps its waste at points that are not as important, depositing uric acid in the joints. In general terms, if you can improve elimination through the bowel, it will help the other organs of elimination. The nature of toxins is to be acidic. Poor bowel elimination stresses the lymphatic system (our second major waste-disposal system). In the light of this, one colonic hydrotherapist believes that the fluid retention of gout is the body's way of protecting itself, increasing alkaline levels in an overly acidic system.

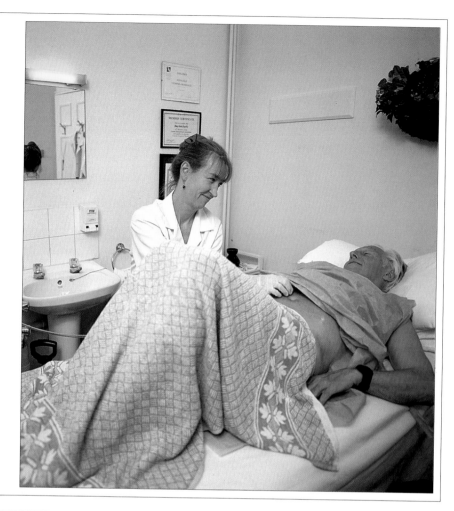

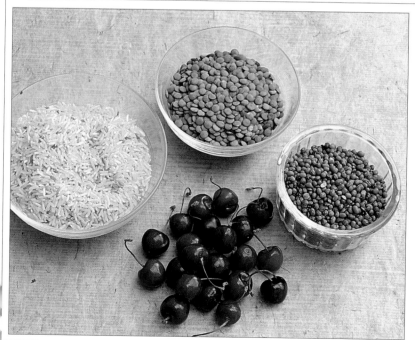

SELF-CARE

Nutrition

A nutritionist will put together a specially tailored, low-protein, rehydration diet which is strongly recommended for gout. You are likely to be recommended to concentrate on alkaline foods to counter excess uric acid production; suitable foods include vegetables, brown rice, pulses, millet and lots of water. 'Cherries are very good for gout,' says one nutritionist. 'As are aloe vera and the essential fatty acids.' Foods to avoid include spinach and rhubarb, and you should cut out altogether red meat, alcohol, tea, coffee and dairy products, all of which are acidic.

Feet Problems

The feet are possibly the most maltreated and maligned part of the body. We cram our feet into tight, unyielding shoes, we stand or stomp around for hours at a time and, in the case of women, often in high heels, and proclaim at the end of it all that 'we hate our feet, they're really ugly' or that 'our feet are killing us'.

These unsung heroes of the body in fact perform two vital functions, namely to support the weight of the body and to act as a lever to propel the body forwards. The foot is an extremely intricate and delicate structure, yet despite the abuse it often suffers, it stands up pretty well under the strain. Naturally, some people (especially sportsmen and women) do suffer injuries to the foot, particularly fractures of the metatarsals and phalanges (the bones of the toes). Deformities of the foot are also reasonably common and include talipes (club foot), flat feet, claw foot and bunions (thickened, fluid-filled pads over the joint at the base of the big toe). Skin disorders are also common on the feet. Principally, these are conditions such as corns (small areas of thickened skin), often caused by tight-fitting shoes; plantar warts (verrucas) on the sole (see page 219); and athlete's foot, a fungal infection which affects mainly the skin between the toes, causing it to become itchy, sore and cracked.

An in-growing toenail is an affliction peculiar to the foot and, although it is the butt of many jokes, it can be an agonizing condition. It most commonly affects the big toes, causing painful inflammation of the surrounding tissues. Another painful condition which features heavily in comic material is gout, a fairly common form of arthritis which often affects the joints of the foot (see page 212).

Flat feet tend to occur in small children and the elderly whose ligaments are generally slack. Virtually anyone who can bend their fingers right back or who is 'double-jointed' will flatten out the arches of the feet when standing. If the feet ache, arch supports can be worn in shoes, but otherwise no treatment is necessary.

The winter months can spell misery for those with sensitive skin or poor circulation, as it is during these cold periods that chilblains make an appearance. These reddish-blue swellings on the toes and fingers occur when blood vessels shrink so much that the skin's supply of blood and oxygen is severely reduced. Chilblains can itch and burn furiously, but scratching them can only make them worse (see also *Circulation Problems*, page 120).

214

THE ORTHODOX APPROACH

Doctors rely on powerful chemical preparations to clear up many of the common foot problems. In the case of athlete's foot, chemists keep a selection of proprietary foot powders and creams which can be bought over the counter without prescription. If the infection is minor, doctors usually prescribe a cream containing econazole nitrate or sulconazole nitrate and, if this does not work, tablets containing griseofulvin. For in-growing toenails, antibiotics would be prescribed if infection were present. In severe cases, part of the base of the nail would be removed so that the nail was narrower and therefore less likely to grow into the skin.

Chilblain sufferers would be advised to keep the feet from getting chilled, and, if they experienced poor circulation, to take regular exercise to stimulate the blood flow. Doctors may also prescribe creams to soothe the burning and itching.

Standard treatment for skin conditions such as verrucas and corns would be similar to the methods used by chiropodists, while severe bunions may eventually need an operation to cure them.

THE HALE APPROACH

Complementary treatments following the Hale Approach are fine for all feet problems, and an orthodox angle need only be sought if treatments are not beneficial.

In nearly all cases of bunions and corns we would recommend a chiropodist, who would treat the affected area of the foot. But, again in nearly all cases, we would also suggest other treatments which may treat another part of the body in order to relieve foot pain. In certain cases a manipulation therapy such as osteopathy or soft-tissue massage such as the GDS Techniques may be indicated. These treatments, like the Alexander Technique, also address the patient's posture, which will often have a beneficial effect on the feet. In certain cases reflexology is also very effective for the relief of foot pain.

Paradoxically, when biomechanics are used to help a recurring foot pain, this often has a beneficial effect on the rest of the musculo-skeletal system.

Finally, never underestimate the importance of good shoes!

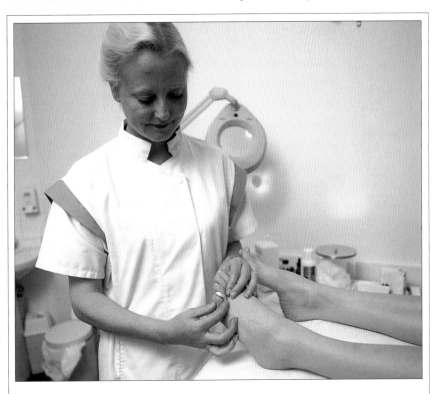

CHIROPODY

Often a corn is a problem that recurs because it forms on an area of the foot that takes excessive pressure. Hard corns are pared away with a scalpel and the core removed (nucleation). Sometimes the area is softened in advance by treating it with a salicylic preparation.

Vascular corns (where blood vessels are involved) can be very painful. These are treated by a combination of chemical applications, the scalpel and padding. Soft corns between the toes are generally approached by scalpel treatment and pads. These are sometimes caused by footwear, but also occasionally by anatomical irregularities, which may be helped by silicone orthotics. For a bunion a chiropodist would provide padding and deal with the accompanying side effects of the bunion, such as corns.

A specialization within the field of chiropody is biomechanics. If you are plagued by a recurrent foot problem, then the biomechanic study of your foot (where a cast will be taken and your walk filmed and analysed) can help identify the error. Tailor-made appliances that fit neatly into the shoe may be recommended to correct the root cause of the problem.

OSTEOPATHY

The body's framework of bones, joints, muscles and ligaments is used by the osteopath to diagnose and treat problems. After taking a medical history, the osteopath will carry out a detailed physical examination of the joints and tissues of the feet as well as analysing the patient's gait to assess what might be causing either the foot problem or problems

elsewhere in the musculo-skeletal system. A treatment session, which usually lasts about 30 minutes, may include soft-tissue manipulation techniques – soft, gentle, repetitive movement of joints and rapid guiding of the joints through their normal range of movements (producing the characteristic clicking that most people associate with osteopathy). Where relevant, there will be advice on posture and specific exercise and relaxation techniques.

GDS TECHNIQUES

GDS Techniques offer a holistic approach that treats the whole body. With any feet problems, a GDS Techniques practitioner will firstly identify the dysfunction by analysing the patient's posture and movement. They then concentrate on improving this with movement and exercises that include isometric techniques, gentle stretching, postures and soft-tissue massage. In GDS Techniques, it is important to consider the body as a whole unit. The treatment does not focus only on the pain, which is not often the root of the problem, but may be a reaction to something that has built up over a long period.

To give one example, a flat foot (where the arches have collapsed) is often the result of an imbalance in the muscles controlling the inside and outside of the foot.

This may be due to hip problems or to an excessive shortness of the muscles which run along the outside of the lower limbs from the hips down to the feet. In this case, GDS Techniques would work to loosen the hip or the muscles along the leg and would educate the patient to maintain optimal foot position in relation to the correct posture of legs, pelvis and trunk.

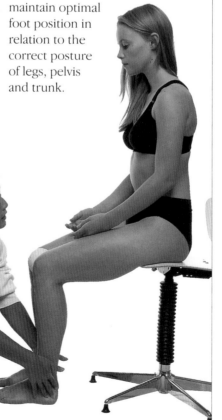

ACUPUNCTURE

One acupuncturist blames feet problems – indeed all health problems – on the external cold of the British climate and on internal cold, caused by eating or drinking cold foods or sitting on cold floors. Internal cold may also be the result of an operation trauma or prolonged stress. The effect of this internal and external cold is to cause cramps that block the flow of blood to the feet, eventually causing pain, hardness, weakness and lumps on the feet. Any previous accidents also increase blockages. Acupuncture is used to treat the kidney, liver and spleen, warming and strengthening the body. Acupressure is used on the specific blockages in the feet and legs, freeing the flow of blood.

CHIROPRACTIC

Foot pain may often result in spinal and postural problems, and chiropractic manipulation may bring relief to sufferers whose foot problem has a mechanical origin. At the first consultation, a chiropractor will take your medical history and details of the current problem, give you a full examination, inclduing looking at your overall posture, gait and the kind of shoes you wear. If he or she then decides that chiropractic treatment may help, it usually begins on the same visit. The treatment uses various manual techniques concentrating on adjustments to the foot, spine and pelvis. These are not painful and, once the cause of the problem has been corrected, the foot and spinal pains should clear up.

ALEXANDER TECHNIQUE

An imbalance in the body's movements and posture has a direct effect on the feet. An Alexander teacher will be able to pick up these problems by watching you walk and conducting a physical examination. He or she will then correct the imbalance by showing you correct postures and how to use your muscles with minimum effort and maximum efficiency.

Lessons last about 45 minutes and a course of 30 is usual, after which time your foot problems should be solved and you should know enough about the Alexander Technique to be able to continue its teachings on your own.

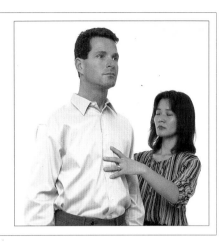

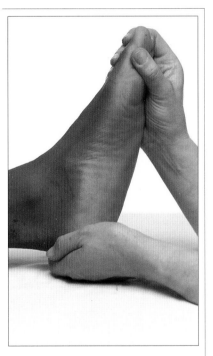

REFLEXOLOGY

A therapist will begin by giving a full reflexology treatment and then concentrate on specific areas relating to the adrenal glands, spine, solar plexus and corresponding zone-related areas on the hand. As one reflexologist explains, 'Reflexology treats areas that, on the surface, appear to have no relation to the affected area but, because it works on energy zones, you will pick up points that relate to that zone.'

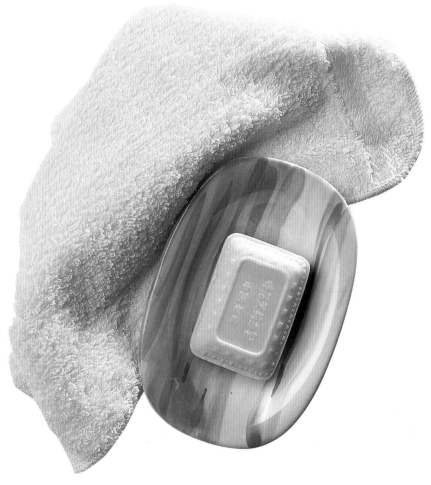

SUPPORTIVE TREATMENTS

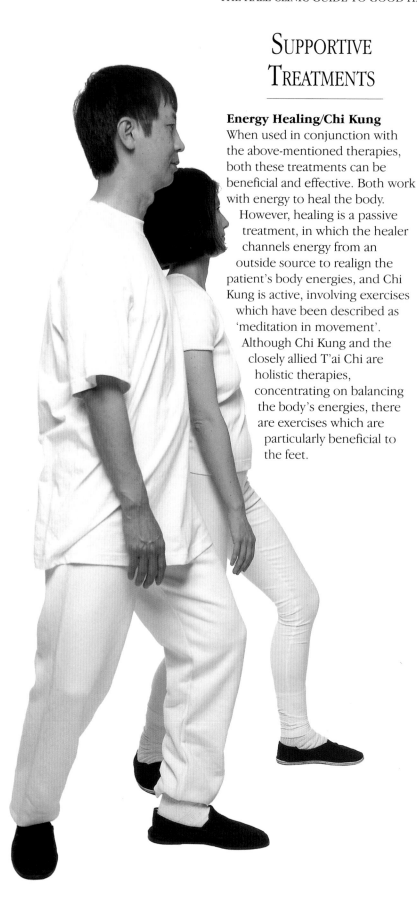

Energy Healing/Chi Kung

When used in conjunction with the above-mentioned therapies, both these treatments can be beneficial and effective. Both work with energy to heal the body.

However, healing is a passive treatment, in which the healer channels energy from an outside source to realign the patient's body energies, and Chi Kung is active, involving exercises which have been described as 'meditation in movement'.

Although Chi Kung and the closely allied T'ai Chi are holistic therapies, concentrating on balancing the body's energies, there are exercises which are particularly beneficial to the feet.

SOME TIPS ON SHOES

Children

• Always go to a reputable shoe shop where the foot is measured.

• Choose leather shoes wherever possible.

• Do not always wear training shoes.

• Avoid second-hand shoes, especially if they are well worn.

• Socks are as important as shoes – make sure they have good toes and heels, and are neither too big nor too small.

Women

• Vary the height of the heel on high-heeled shoes, and wear flat shoes sometimes to prevent the calf muscles from shortening.

• 'Fashion' shoes are OK for an evening out but not for regular daily wear. Try not to wear high heels on a regular basis.

• When choosing shoes for extended wear, make sure they have ample room for your toes.

Men

• Wear sandals rather than shoes occasionally to give your feet an airing.

Herbal foot creams such as Weleda Foot Balm and Moor Life Foot Bath can bring relief from some foot problems.

Warts & Verrucas

Regrettably, warts are not the sole preserve of fairy-tale witches and goblins. In fact, they are an extremely common skin condition that can affect anyone at any age. They are contagious but completely harmless, growing on the skin or mucous membranes such as the nostrils. A wart affects only the top layers of skin (it has no roots, seeds or branches) and so, in theory, it should be possible to remove it with no more than a little discomfort.

Caused by the human papilloma virus HPV (of which there are 70 different types, although not all are associated with warts), there are at least 30 different types of warts which can affect various parts of the body, principally the hands, face, neck and genitals. Common warts, which are particularly prevalent in young children, are firm, sharply defined and usually round, although some are irregular in shape. They range in hue from flesh-coloured to brown, and can be anything up to 6mm (Gin) in diameter, often with a rough surface. Common warts usually appear on parts of the body that are prone to injury, such as the hands, face, knees and scalp.

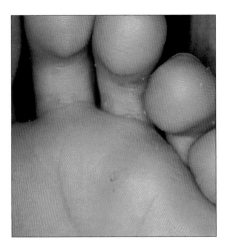

Also common on the wrists, backs of hands and the face are flat warts, so named because they are flat-topped. They can be itchy but you should try to resist the temptation to scratch, since it is scratching that causes the virus to spread, leading to the appearance of more warts.

As you get older, you may discover small, finger-like growths, sometimes dark in colour, growing on your face, neck or arms. These are completely harmless and are known as digitate or filiform warts.

The bane of the public swimming pool and communal changing rooms, plantar warts, commonly called verrucas, are simply flat warts which occur on the soles of the feet. They don't look like the flat warts you might find elsewhere on the body because they have become flattened by the pressure exerted on them. In fact, this prevents them from growing outwards and forces them inwards, which can make them more painful. They appear hard and horny to the touch. Verrucas sometimes occur singly, sometimes in clusters.

In spite of being classified as a sexually transmitted disease, genital warts are part of the same harmless family of growths. They are transmitted by sexual contact and can appear anything up to 18 months after infection, emerging as extensive, pink, cauliflower-like areas on the genitals. Since there have been links with genital warts and cases of cervical cancer, women affected by genital warts should be particularly careful about keeping up-to-date with smear tests.

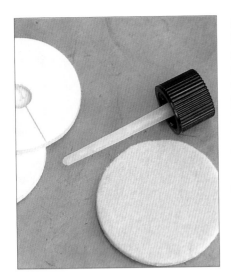

THE ORTHODOX APPROACH

In about 50 per cent of cases warts disappear of their own accord within 6-12 months. If they persist, common, flat and plantar warts can be treated by applying a chemical liquid or special plaster. Several treatments may be needed before the wart disappears and, like the proverbial bad penny, they sometimes return. Warts are also commonly treated by cryosurgery. (Liquid nitrogen is used to freeze the wart solid. As it thaws, a blister forms, lifting the wart off.) They can also be cut out using electro-cautery, curettage or laser treatment and, specifically for plantar warts, salicylic acid plasters may be used. Surgery or applications of podophyllin are usually the options for removing genital warts.

THE HALE APPROACH

External warts in areas that are not liable to be disfiguring can be treated by complementary therapies effectively and with safety. **Internal warts such as bowel polyps or cervical warts must be dealt with by an orthodox practitioner. Genital warts should also be monitored by a doctor or hospital specialist. For these latter cases surgical treatment may be required and complementary therapy before, during and after the operation is highly recommended.**

The obvious external treatment for warts and verrucas is chiropody. However, if a patient wants to approach the problem internally and get at the root cause, then homeopathy or acupuncture can be very effective, with hypnotherapy, Bach flowers and aromatherapy as support treatments.

CHIROPODY

Not all verrucas are the same, varying from single growths to clusters of warts through to mosaic types of verrucas which can be quite large. As such, the choice of treatment a chiropodist might apply will vary according to the individual patient and to the type of verruca they present.

Cryosurgery is perhaps best suited to new growths, whereas chemical treatment (solutions of salicylic acid in varying strengths, monochloro-acetic acid – sometimes used in its crystal form and rubbed on the area – or trichlorocetic acid) is more widely used. Chemical treatment does not actually destroy the verruca; rather it changes the condition of the surrounding skin so that the virus can no longer survive there. However, strong chemical treatment does not suit everyone – anyone who suffers from diabetes or poor circulation is advised against it.

Many people report that their verrucas clear up after a beach holiday, where the combined effects of salt water and sand are of great benefit. Other home treatments occasionally recommended by chiropodists include bathing the feet nightly in a saturated solution of vinegar and salt; or applying garlic paste every few days, then rubbing the area with a pumice stone and reapplying the garlic paste. Unfortunately, verrucas have a habit of apparently clearing up completely and then, when you think it's safe to go back in the water, reappearing having lain dormant for some time. So be vigilant.

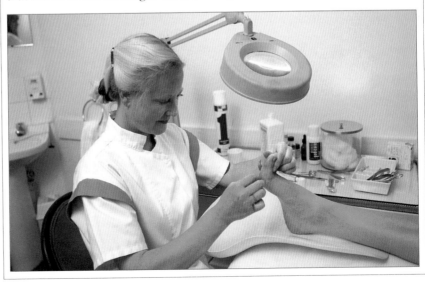

HOMEOPATHY

The homeopathic approach aims to treat the whole person and the underlying causes of a problem rather than its physical manifestation. Warts are caused by a viral infection, HPV, and so this, and any other reasons for disharmony or imbalance in the body, are matched to corresponding remedies that will enhance the body's ability to fight the HPV itself. The most commonly used remedy is Thuja occidentalis, which has a deep-acting effect and can be applied locally as a tincture or cerate, or taken internally.

ACUPUNCTURE

In traditional Chinese medicine the skin is related to the lungs and the spleen, so treatment is given both at points surrounding the wart(s) and at points on the governor, spleen and stomach meridians, as these points are believed to be anti-inflammatory and to stimulate the immune system.

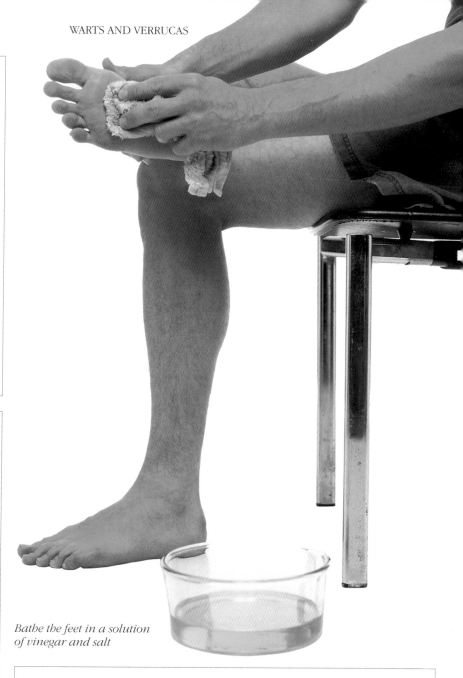

Bathe the feet in a solution of vinegar and salt

SUPPORTIVE TREATMENT

Hypnotherapy
While in a hypnotic state the sufferer is given suggestions that the warts are gradually losing their food supply, fading away and eventually dropping off.

SELF-CARE

Flower Remedies
'Pansy (Pegasus FES) is great for warts,' says one flower therapist. 'They just drop off and disappear.' Spinefex (Australian Bush) and K9 (Andreas Korte, African Essence) are also good for warts.

Aromatherapy
Onion and garlic oils can be highly effective, but are often taken in capsule form because of their strong aroma. However, raw, chopped onion or garlic applied regularly as an overnight compress has also been successful in removing warts. For persistent warts, a combination of garlic, lemon oil, *Thymus linalol* and *Origanum compactum* may be applied directly to the wart twice a day with an earbud.

Acupuncture/Acupressure

One of the best known and respected of complementary therapies, acupuncture is a part of a comprehensive system of traditional Chinese medicine that dates back thousands of years. Most people know treatment involves having fine needles inserted in parts of the body. But the philosophy behind acupuncture is fascinating and completely different from Western medical thinking. The *chi* or energy flow through the body is believed to be the main determinant of our physical and mental wellbeing. It flows through 12 main invisible channels known as meridians. Too much or too little activity in one or more of these is believed to be the cause of illness. The needles are inserted at various points to reduce or increase the energy flow, remove blockages, tone and restore balance in the system. This releases the body's own healing mechanisms.

Acupressure is based on the same fundamental concept, but the points will be pressed by the therapist's fingers, often in two or three different places at the same time. Acupressurists believe that the energy flow can be monitored and directed by the fingers.

Achieving balance and harmony are in fact the fundamental objectives of a complex and sophisticated system that

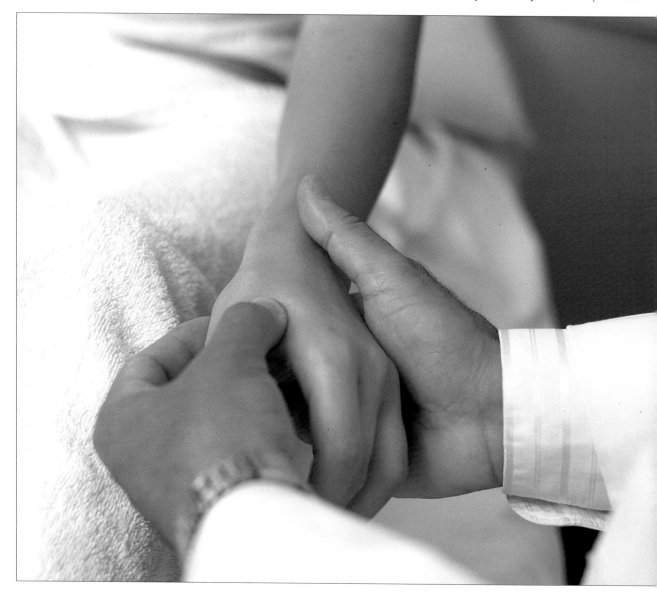

recognizes the close interaction of mind and body. Our moods as well as our health are regulated by two opposing forces – yin, a dense, passive force and the yang, the active force. The five basic elements of Chinese thought - fire, water, earth, matter and wood – also play a vital role in our wellbeing. The heart, for instance, is a fire organ, the kidney is water and the liver and gall bladder relate to wood. If these functions get out of balance illness results.

Symptoms will often be described as 'hot', 'cold', 'damp', etc., in various combinations. A practitioner will point out that people with heart and blood pressure problems typically have red faces – a sign that the 'fire' is not functioning as it should.

Conditions Treated

In theory virtually any complaint can be treated with acupuncture because, according to Chinese medicine, all illness is caused by some kind of imbalance. In practice Western acupuncturists usually find themselves dealing with a range of problems, often long-standing, that conventional medicine has failed to tackle successfully because it is treating only the symptoms. Recurrent back pain, neck pain, headaches and migraines respond extremely well to acupuncture treatment. The therapist will be searching for the fundamental cause of the problem – which is why six patients with stomach ulcers, for instance, may find themselves being treated in six different ways.

Acupuncture has a very high success rate with stress-related problems such as painful periods, skin complaints, digestive problems and high blood pressure, and sufferers may well find treatment recommended by their doctors.

Conditions such as arthritis may be treated with moxibustion, where the needles are warmed by burning herbs. Specific problems such as sports injuries, where increasing the local circulation promotes healing, can also

be treated. In addition acupuncture is increasingly employed as a pain reliever during labour.

Acupressure is a very effective treatment for stress disorders. The therapy is more general than acupuncture, though specific problems such as back ache, PMS and migraine respond well.

Infants and Children

Children may be frightened of the idea of having needles stuck in them, which could reduce the benefits of the treatment. But acupressure is an effective alternative.

How to Choose a Practitioner

The Council for Acupuncture is the ultimate governing body for registered UK acupuncturists. It provides a list of trained, accredited practitioners on request. Contact the Council for Acupuncture, 179 Gloucester Place, London NW1 6DX, tel 0181 964 0222.

There are five recognized acupuncture organizations in the UK. Their members must have a minimum of two years' training, which includes study of anatomy and physiology. A registered acupuncturist will have one of the following set of letters after his or her name: MBAAR, FBAAR, MIROM, MRTCM, MTAS or CSAS.

The British Medical Acupuncture Society, Newton House, Newton Lane, Lower Whitley, Warrington, Cheshire WA4 4JA, tel 01925 730 727 has a list of medical doctors who have trained in acupuncture.

An acupressurist's training lasts two and a half years. The Shen Tao Foundation, Middle Piccadilly Natural Healing Centre, Sherborne, Dorset DT9 5LW, tel 01963 23468 keeps a list of qualified practitioners.

Insurance Recognition

Most private medical insurance schemes will pay for treatment if you are referred by a doctor or consultant. Some may insist you go to an acupuncturist who is also medically qualified.

What to Expect at a Consultation

Treatment is preceded by a very careful, detailed questioning about every aspect of your health and life. You will be asked some very personal questions. Your tastes, physical appearance, colouring and personality are all crucial aspects of the diagnosis. Your tongue will be inspected for colour, shape and condition. The therapist will also feel the six pulses on your wrists. These relate to the 12 main organs in the body and tell the therapist which are strong and which are weak.

Most people just don't feel the insertion of the very fine acupuncture needles. Your therapist will probably use only a few at the first session, and only for 6-10 minutes initially, building up to 20 or 25 minutes in later sessions. But it would be misleading to say you don't feel anything at all. Acupuncture is a very powerful therapy. You may have an itchy, tingling sensation or feel quite uncomfortable, though it is rare to feel any actual pain.

The majority of acupressure points used are below the knee and elbow, although points on the middle line of the body, back and front, may also be used depending on the precise complaint. The needles may be manipulated by the therapist or left still, depending on whether the energy flow needs to be stimulated or calmed. Six to ten fortnightly session may be recommended.

Contraindications

Anyone who is nervous of needles will obviously have a problem with acupuncture. Some acupuncturists will not treat pregnant women. Infected joints should not be treated with acupuncture. Anyone subject to fits or convulsions should not have this treatment.

Compatibility with Other Therapies

Acupuncture works well in combination with Chinese herbal medicine since it is part of the same medical system. Homeopathy and the massage therapies are also particularly compatible with acupuncture.

Ayurveda

In India a sophisticated and all-encompassing system of medicine flourished long before the Ancient Greeks or the Chinese developed their own healing philosophies. Sanskrit texts indicate that Ayurveda was scientifically well evolved by 1500BC.

According to the principles of Ayurveda, marma points on the body govern our muscular, skeletal and nervous systems. The seven *chakras* – the major centres of spiritual power in the body – form its main energy centres. The mind has considerable influence on the body, and in common with other great systems of medicine the concept of balancing the energies or life forces to achieve harmony of mind and body is central to the Ayurvedic philosophy.

Each living thing in the Ayurvedic universe contains five different elements, which in the human body combine into three distinct kinds of energy forces or *doshas*. *Vata* is air, governing our nervous and circulation systems, *Kapha* governs our cells and structure, and *Pitta*, which represents heat, governs our metabolism. In a perfect state these would all be in balance. In practice we each tend to have one or two dominating *doshas* and this predetermines our *prakriti* – how we look, think and move and what kind of person we are – our very being, in fact. In Ayurvedic thinking illness is caused by an imbalance of the *doshas* brought about by poor diet, the environment, our mental state and previous life, all of which represent a certain kind of energy.

Each individual has a unique *dosha* combination. Certain foods may be beneficial for one person but not for another if they upset the energy balance. *Vata* dominance, for instance, makes people more nervous – they need things to calm them down. *Kapha* types tend to have a slow metabolism, be lethargic and inclined to overweight. Knowing what is right for you is an important part of preventative medicine which is very much at the heart of Ayurvedic thinking.

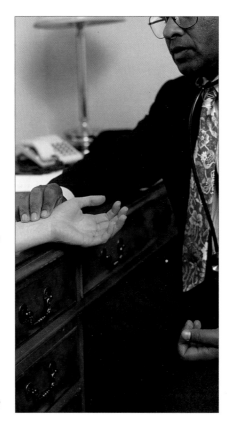

Conditions Treated

Any illness and disorder can be treated with Ayurvedic therapy, except conditions that require surgery. Allergy-based disorders such as asthma, hay fever, migraines and eczema, and such complaints as ME and arthritis might be treated with a detoxification programme (known as *panchakarma*), herbal medicine and yoga exercises. Stroke patients respond well to massage of the body's marma points with herbal oils. Impotence and prostate problems have also been successfully treated. Ayurvedic aphrodisiacs stimulate the blood circulation and neurological systems.

Diet is certain to be a central feature of all treatment – foods are regarded as medicine and the basis of a healthy lifestyle. As well as successful treatment of chronic disorders that conventional medicine has failed to cure, Ayurveda is an effective way of promoting a healthy lifestyle and thus preventing disease.

Infants and Children

Ayurveda is suitable for children.

Insurance Recognition

No.

How to Choose a Practitioner

Ayurvedic practitioners study for six years in India and Sri Lanka and should have a recognized degree. But there are few graduates practising in the UK. Contact the Ayurvedic Medical Association (founder – Dr Shantha Godagama) at the Hale Clinic, 7 Park Crescent, London W1N 3HE, tel 0171 631 0156, for a list of qualified practitioners.

What to Expect at a Consultation

Diagnosis takes the form of very close observation to determine your *dosha* or energy type, together with examination of your Ayurvedic pulses. Your tongue and the colour of your skin and eyes may also be inspected.

At your first consultation the practitioner will want to know everything about you – absolutely everything, including your toilet habits. Then a regime will be worked out for you. Once a treatment is prescribed you should have a consultation every three or four weeks until the condition clears up. There are a wide variety of treatments including herbal preparations, massage, therapeutic steam baths and exercise techniques. You will also be given advice on diet.

Contraindications

None.

Compatibility with Other Therapies

Ayurveda is compatible with most other therapies, but yoga exercise is part of its healing regime.

Reflexology

Reflexology is an ancient therapy, probably eastern in origin, involving the gentle manipulation of the feet or hands to stimulate the body's own healing and balancing processes. The underlying principle is similar to that of acupuncture in that each pressure point on the sole or sides of the foot is directly related to a particular function or part of the body, though the actual meridians or zones of the body are described differently in reflexology. All the organs and systems of the body have their corresponding reflex points'.

Reflexologists believe that applying pressure to a specific point on the foot energizes the corresponding zone or function of the body, getting rid of toxins and enabling the body to heal itself. Reflexology also improves blood circulation and reduces stress, and in some cases practitioners can identify a previously unsuspected problem in its early stages.

Conditions Treated

Reflexologists treat a very wide variety of conditions. Menstrual problems, endocrine problems, allergies, arthritis, high blood pressure, back and neck pain and stress-related problems have all responded to treatment and there is currently medical interest in its use for pain management for the chronically ill. Reflexology is also used to treat irritable bowel syndrome and other digestive problems, ear complaints, sinus problems, migraines, recurring headaches and some skin complaints. It has been claimed that having reflexology during pregnancy can significantly reduce the length of labour.

Infants and Children

Size of feet is an obvious limitation, so children can only be treated from the age of one or two. Reflexology has been successful in treating childhood problems such as hyperactivity and 'glue ear'.

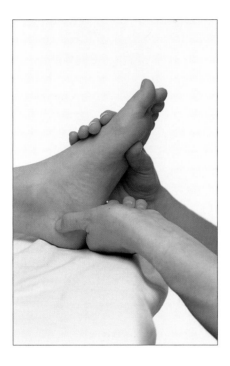

How to Choose a Practitioner

At the moment anyone can describe themselves as a reflexologist. To make matters more difficult there are over a dozen reflexology organizations in the UK, but no central governing body. Trained reflexologists will have one of the following sets of letter after their name – IFR, MIFR, MBRA, MBFR or AOR – depending on which professional body they belong to. The two largest, who will give you a list of trained therapists in your area, are the Association of Reflexologists, 27 Old Gloucester Street, London WClN 3XX, tel 0990 673320, and the International Federation of Reflexologists, 78 Edridge Road, Croydon, Surrey CR0 1EF, tel 0181 667 9458.

Insurance Recognition

Some private health schemes may be persuaded to cover the cost of treatment if it is recommended by your doctor or consultant. You may be able to get reflexology treatment on the National Health for conditions such as migraine and pre-menstrual syndrome.

What to Expect at a Consultation

The first consultation will involve treatment of the whole body, not just the specific ailment, since the therapist is concerned to investigate the fundamental cause of the symptoms. Most people find the treatment quite relaxing. The therapist exerts a firm pressure with the thumb on each reflex point, working from toe to ankle. The massage is not at all uncomfortable, though there may be a pricking pain from time to time as a particularly sensitive area is worked on. There may be a slight reaction to treatment the following day – mild flu-like symptoms, for instance, or a slight skin rash. It is also possible that the actual complaint might feel a little worse for a couple of days. You may want to urinate more frequently and you may feel quite tired. These side effects indicate that the body is beginning to detoxify and heal itself and they should subside fairly quickly. Weekly sessions for six weeks are recommended.

Contraindications

Anyone who has had recent replacement surgery for the knees or hips should not have reflexology therapy until completely healed. Some therapists will not treat anyone who has had a thrombosis, osteoporosis, a heart condition or epilepsy or who is suffering from an acute infection or fever. Women who are having a 'risky' pregnancy should not have reflexology, and therapists may also be concerned about treating anyone suffering from diabetes, particularly if they are injecting.

Compatibility with Other Therapies

Reflexology is not incompatible with any other therapy, and works particularly well with acupuncture, osteopathy and light therapy.

Massage

Massage is one of the most ancient forms of therapy. At its most basic it is an instinctive method of soothing pain. Physiologically increasing the circulation to a sprained limb by massage helps its healing. Gentle massage can be used to help people relax. More vigorous techniques can be used to stimulate the workings of the various systems of the body in a very precise way. Massage can also be used to help the body 'relearn' movement and posture and counteract the effects of stress in everyday life, which causes many of us to stand, walk and sit in ways that cause long-term problems for our musculo-skeletal system. Massage with essential oils acts directly on the bloodstream. Massage, it is now acknowledged, can help pain management through releasing endorphins and help comfort those in emotional or psychological distress. The skin is an organ in its own right. Massage can release toxins from the system, disperse the lactic acid in muscles that causes shoulder pain and move energy in the body.

In Asian medicine, various forms of massage developed as highly skilled techniques philosophically integrated with the central focus on maintaining energy and circulation flows round the body and maintaining balance. Nowadays there is a rich if confusing range of massage techniques available to tone up the system, deal with specific aches and pains and treat the more generalized problems of stress.

Marma massage is part of the Indian Ayurvedic system of medicine, dating back thousands of years. The principle is that the human body, like any other machine, needs servicing if it is to function properly. There are 107 marma points on the body where flesh, veins, arteries, bones, joints and tendons meet up. An injury to these points, it is believed, can result in permanent damage. Massage of the marma points,

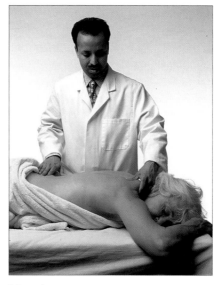

Marma massage

which relate to the internal organs and body systems, improves the circulation in the particular area of the neuro-muscular system and tones up the surrounding muscles.

BodyHarmonics combines traditional Chinese, Indonesian and Thai techniques. *Tuina* (which means 'push and squeeze') massage is part of the system of Chinese medicine involving pressure on the acupuncture points on the body, soft-tissue massage and joint manipulation. Indonesian traditional massage is done with aromatic oils and works on the circulation and lymphatic system. Thai massage involves yoga-like stretches for improving flexibility.

Hellerwork is an intense direct massage which is particularly effective for dealing with problems caused by poor posture. The theory is that our body movements become distorted from poor habits or from physical or psychological trauma. The object of Heller's massage is to reveal the integrity of the structure of the body. Hellerwork, which is essentially a series of classes, concentrates on manipulating the fascia, the connective

tissues that are the 'wrapping' for the muscles and link them with the bones and the rest of the body. It emerged as an offshoot of the work of a US scientist, Dr Ida Rolf, the developer of rolfing, a body-work technique designed to restore the body's proper balance. One of her pupils, Joseph Heller, incorporated a psychological element into the therapy in the belief that individual experiences and emotions had a powerful influence on the way we moved our bodies. To produce permanent change, he believed, you had to change the emotional 'holding pattern' as well as the fascia.

Lymphatic therapy is a very gentle massage to stimulate the lymph system, which controls the elimination of toxins and waste matter from the body. The lymph plays a vital role in the immune system and the supply of nutrients to the cells. The circulation of the lymph system is three times greater than that of the blood. Our skin is the body's largest elimination organ and we have some 660 lymph nodes, many of them in the throat and neck, that filter out toxic wastes and store antibodies which are released into the lymph system when the body is under threat.

Lymphatic therapy, or manual lymphatic drainage (MLD), was developed in the 1930s by a Dr Vodder, who treated many patients from the UK who had gone to the South of France to recover from chronic colds. He discovered that characteristically they all had swollen lymph nodes in the neck, and that when he massaged these the colds vanished and the patients' health improved. The theory is that if the lymph system is loaded with toxins the body becomes acidic and catarrhal, increasing our vulnerability to disease. MLD helps the free flow of lymph fluid and frees blockages.

Conditions Treated
Marma massage improves co-ordination

by stimulating communication between the muscles, the nerves and the brain. Stroke and multiple sclerosis victims find it particularly beneficial because it helps the brain 'relearn' how to control and co-ordinate the muscles and nerves after illness or injury. Unspecified aches and pains, general lack of energy and nervousness can also be helped by marma massage, which is regarded by Ayurvedic practitioners as an important preventative therapy.

Body harmonics is particularly good for musculo-skeletal problems – neck and shoulder pain, lower back pain, sciatica and repetitive strain injury. *Tuina* Chinese massage works on the energy meridians and acupoints on the body to release the blockages that cause chronic pain.

Hellerwork does not treat particular problems, but back, neck and shoulder pains caused by poor posture respond well to what is essentially an educative therapy that works on the psyche as well as the body. Anyone who feels that stress and occupational pressure may have distorted their movements and balance can be helped by Hellerwork, which aims to change the way you move and hold yourself.

Lymphatic therapy is a direct treatment for water retention (lymphoedema), puffy ankles and legs, sinus problems and cellulite. MLD is an important part of any general detoxification programme.

Infants and Children
Massage therapies can safely be used on children of any age.

How to Choose a Practitioner
Anyone can call themselves a massage therapist. The International Therapy Examinations Council (ITEC) diploma is a recognized qualification. Contact the Institute for Complementary Medicine, PO Box 194, London SE16 1QZ for a list of ITEC practitioners. The Clare Maxwell-Hudson School of Massage , PO Box 457, London NW2 4BR has lists of trained therapists, including MLD therapists. The International Association of Ayurveda, PO Box 3043, Barnet, Herts EN4 0QZ has a list of recognized Ayurvedic practitioners in the UK.

There are very few Hellerwork practitioners in the UK. Lists of therapists who have trained with Hellerwork institutions in the USA and New Zealand are available from Roger Golten at the Hale Clinic, 7 Park Crescent, London W1N 3HE, tel 0171 631 0156.

What to Expect at a Consultation
A marma therapist will check muscles and nerve reflexes and the acidic levels of the tongue before treatment. A balance of 60 per cent alkaline and 40 per cent acid food is believed to be desirable for optimum health, so you may be given advice on diet as well as other treatments. Massage takes between one and one and a half hours and is quite vigorous. Two to six sessions are recommended. Stroke sufferers will benefit from regular weekly massage over a period of three to six months.

A number of different techniques are used in BodyHarmonics. *Tuina* therapy involves a rolling pressure on the body's acupoints and joint manipulation. Indonesian traditional massage is done with aromatic oils. If you have particular problems with neck and shoulder pain, some of the massage may be given while you are sitting on a chair. The session ends with a series of yoga-like stretches

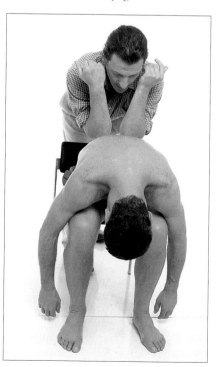

Hellerwork

on the floor to improve flexibility and relax both mind and body. A massage every week or two weeks is recommended.

Hellerwork consists of 11 standard sessions which systematically work on all the different parts of the body in turn. Although Hellerwork does not address particular symptoms, the therapist will observe the way you move and hold yourself before treatment – some even take 'before and after' photographs to identify problems and changes in posture. You lie on a table and the therapist exerts deep pressure through very slow 'leaning' movements while talking to you about how your beliefs, opinions, feelings, thoughts and attitudes affect your body. Hellerwork therapists believe that it is important for you to understand and work through the feelings that influence the way you hold your body so that it will not revert back to its habitual movement after treatment.

Lymphatic drainage is a very gentle, all-over body massage – a pumping motion against the lymph flow to free any kind of blockage. An MLD session may end with an aromatherapy massage. The therapist will also advise on diet and exercise to counteract any sluggishness of the lymph, reduce the intake of toxins and improve the body's capacity to eliminate them naturally. For chronic conditions such as sinus problems a weekly session may be recommended until the condition improves.

Contraindications
Hellerwork therapy is not recommended for anyone with bone or joint diseases such as arthritis or osteoporosis. Lymphatic drainage is not suitable for anyone with cancer.

Compatibility with Other Therapies
Marma massage is an integral part of Ayurvedic therapy and *tuina* is part of traditional Chinese Medicine. Hellerwork is thought to be particularly beneficial in conjunction with psychotherapy since it involves changing the ideas and emotions that are limiting or blocking physical movement. Lymphatic drainage may be combined with colonic hydrotherapy for a detoxification programme.

Shiatsu

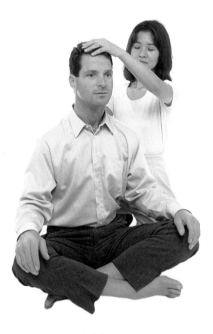

The principles of Shiatsu have much in common with those of acupuncture; in fact Shiatsu is often described as acupuncture without the needles. Both originate from traditional Chinese medicine, which believes that energy flows through the meridians of the body and that illness or dysfunction are the result of blockage, overactivity or underactivity in these pathways, which can be accessed by acupoints at various places on the body.

The word *shiatsu* means 'finger massage' in Japanese and part of the therapy is the application of gentle pressure to the acupoints along the meridians. Shiatsu in its present form was revived in Japan in the early 20th century as a serious health-promoting therapy combining massage, acupressure and body stretching, and incorporating elements of Western anatomy and physiology.

It is a much more personal and less clinical therapy than acupuncture. Therapists aim to 'feel' the energy flows in the body, using not just their fingers but their own arms and legs as well to adjust the flow in the meridian. The aim is to 'move' the energy from where it is accumulating to weaker areas, stimulating the blood circulation and the lymph system.

Shiatsu therapy also has an important psychological element, since it seeks to put the individual in touch with the body's own healing processes.

Conditions Treated

All stress-related conditions respond particularly well to Shiatsu therapy. Back pain, shoulder tension, headaches, migraine, asthma and some skin conditions can be treated successfully. The Shiatsu therapist, however, will be treating the fundamental cause of the problem rather than local symptoms. Irritable bowel syndrome and other digestive problems respond well. With skin problems the object may be to improve the blood circulation.

Infants and Children

Therapists will not treat babies or toddlers, but children over the age of five may benefit from Shiatsu.

How to Choose a Practitioner

The Shiatsu Society, 31 Pullman Lane, Godalming, Surrey GU7 1XY, tel 01483 860771, has a register of members who have obtained a diploma at a recognized school and have satisfied the society's own assessment panel.

Insurance Recognition

Some private health insurers may pay for treatment if it is recommended by a consultant.

What to Expect at a Consultation

Hara diagnosis is one of the most important parts of the consultation. Shiatsu therapists regard the *hara*, the abdominal area of the body, as a 'map' which can give them a guide to the energetic state of the person and the relative weakness or strength of its major systems. The diagnosis takes about five minutes. The practitioner kneels beside the person with the palm of one hand on the abdomen, the other hand feeling with the tips of the fingers. This process tells the therapist which meridians should be worked on.

Before the *hara* diagnosis the therapist will question you about your medical history, look at your tongue, observe your posture and take your pulses. In traditional Chinese medicine the 12 pulses on the wrist are an important part of the diagnosis. The therapist will obviously enquire about your particular complaint, but he or she will be mainly concerned with identifying those parts of the body where the quality of the energy needs to be changed.

Treatment should not be painful. The level of pressure is adjusted to the individual. You lie on the floor, normally on a futon, fully clothed, while the therapist works on the relevant meridians or parts of them. To start with, the therapist may well stretch parts of your body, using leaning movements. As well as massaging the acupressure points the therapist will work along the whole of the meridian, since the object is to shift the energy to a part of the body that needs it.

Most people feel very relaxed after a Shiatsu session. During the two or three days after treatment you may get a slight reaction like a headache - part of the process of eliminating wastes from the system. After ten days you should feel the full benefits. Sessions take between an hour and an hour and a half, and a course of six treatments, one every two weeks, is recommended.

Contraindications

Anyone with osteoporosis or who has painful joints as a result of conditions such as rheumatoid arthritis should not have Shiatsu.

Compatibility with Other Therapies

Shiatsu is closely linked to traditional Chinese medicine, which embraces herbal medicine as well as acupuncture. It may also work well with psychotherapy.

Chiropractic

Chiropractic is a manipulative therapy developed at the end of the 19th century by Daniel David Palmer, who believed that if a vertebra is displaced, it may press against nerves, the channels of communication in the body, and so cause an imbalance, resulting in disease. The name comes from the Greek *cheiro*, meaning hand, and *praktos*, meaning to use. The early chiropractors believed that symptoms stemmed from disorders in the nervous system and that most problems occurred because of misalignment of one or more of the spinal vertebrae This was hypothesized to result in irritation or pressure on a nerve as it left the spinal cord to supply an organ. Thus it wa s believed that pain or dysfunction of an organ could have its cause elsewhere.

Chiropractic treatment is aimed at restoring normal function to stiff and irritated joints and their supportive structure, especially those related to the spine and pelvis. Treatment is carried out by means of precise adjustments. The emphasis is on alleviating existing problems and promoting long-term preventative health care. Thus, depending on individual circumstances, treatment may also include exercises, ergonomic and nutritional advice, and counselling.

Conditions Treated

Chiropractic treatment can relax muscles in spasm, and thus restore or improve normal movement when the problem is associated with, for example, lower back or neck pain. A lack of mobility in the spinal joints places considerable stress on the intervertebral discs and may lead to early wear and tear. For sciatica, adjustments are usually made to the lower spine and pelvis. Pregnant women often suffer from lower back problems due to the strain on the back caused by the enlarging abdomen; chiropractic can help and has no harmful side effects for mother or baby. It can also ease back problems caused by a difficult birth.

Chiropractic is recognized as a safe and effective method of treating back

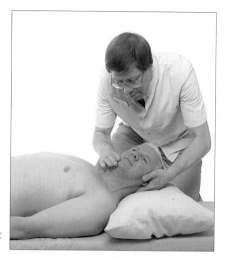

problems. One study funded by the Medical Research Council has added weight to this, finding that chiropractic treatment was more effective than hospital outpatient therapies for those with chronic or severe back pain.

Other commonly seen conditions which may respond well to chiropractic treatment include shoulder and arm pain, pins and needles, hip, knee and foot problems (sports injuries), tension headaches, migraine, menstrual pain, asthma and non-organic abdominal symptoms such as constipation.

Insurance Recognition

Most private health schemes will pay for chiropractic treatment, but some require referral from a general practitioner or consultant.

Infants and Children

Age is not a barrier to chiropractic treatment: the gentle treatment of young children or babies, for example after a traumatic birth, may be beneficial and prevent functional problems in later life.

How to Choose a Practitioner

Your chiropractor should have one of the following qualifications: DC, B. App Sc (Chiro), BSc (Chiropractic). To become a chiropractor students follow a five-year full-time course, resulting in a BSc degree

from the Anglo-European College of Chiropractic, Bournemouth. Those with an existing BSc degree in an appropriate subject can follow a three-year full-time course to obtain an MSc (Chiropractic) from De Montfort University, Leicester.

Only after another year's post-graduate course at an established clinic may they apply for membership of the British Chiropractic Association, which can be contacted at 29 Whitley Street, Reading, Berkshire RG2 0EG, tel 01734 757557. It maintains a register of all qualified chiropractors in membership, which is limited to graduates of recognized chiropractic colleges in Britain and abroad.

What to Expect at a Consultation

The chiropractor will want to know about your medical history and lifestyle. He or she will examine you, feeling for areas of muscular spasm and tenderness. He or she will also examine your joints to establish whether any are not working as efficiently as they might be. X-rays may also be.taken.

A course of treatment usually lasts some weeks and the chiropractor may then recommend a maintenance session every few months to prevent problems recurring.

Contraindications

After careful preliminary examination and the taking of a medical history, the chiropractor may consider that manipulation would be unsuitable – for some forms of arthritis, for example – or that conventional medical advice is needed instead.

Compatibility with Other Therapies

Chiropractic can safely be used in conjunction with other treatments, which may facilitate the body's self-healing processes. Depending on the nature of the problem and the patient's lifestyle, these adjunctive therapies may include for example acupuncture, herbal medicine or yoga.

Osteopathy

Osteopaths believe that our bones and muscles are not just a framework for the body and its vital organs. In fact our musculo-skeletal system has a profound influence on the workings of those organs and on our general health. The mechanics of the body can be distorted by bad posture, injury and stress, leading to pain and strain, which can in turn affect functions like breathing and digestion. Equally, internal problems can lead to muscular pain as our body structure tries to compensate - frequent menstrual pain, for instance, can result in neck and shoulder strain.

Osteopathy was developed in the late 19th century by an American doctor, Andrew Taylor Still. His theory was that if you could adjust the structure, by massage and manipulation, then the body would heal itself.

Cranial osteopathy is a more recently developed branch of the therapy concerned with the gentle manipulation of the 28 movable bones that make up the skull. Cranial osteopaths believe that imbalance in the rhythms or pulse in the cranium – sometimes caused by a difficult birth or an accident, for instance – can result in problems such as colic, migraine or even behavioural disorders.

Conditions Treated
Osteopathy is a prime therapy for back, neck and shoulder pains and for sports injuries, which will be treated by a combination of massage, manipulation, stretching and sometimes what is known as the 'high velocity thrust' – a rather dramatic technique used to free up a joint. Osteopathy can also help enormously if you are suffering from 'occupational' problems – caused by spending your working day at a computer, for instance. Therapy aims to get to the fundamental cause of the problem and will include advice on posture and sitting positions.

But osteopathy involves far more than joint and muscle manipulation.

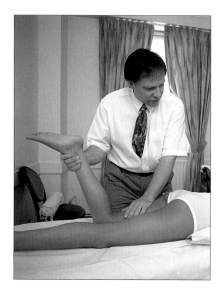

Conditions such as premenstrual tension, asthma and migraine also respond well to therapy since they may be exacerbated, or even caused, by structural dysfunction.

Mothers-to-be will find osteopathy particularly helpful in treating and preventing back ache. After-birth problems such as stress incontinence can also be helped.

Cranial osteopathy also treats back ache and musculo-skeletal problems, working with the muscles and joints. In addition it is used to treat head injuries, 'glue ear' and sinus problems. It can be particularly helpful in treating babies for colic or constant crying, and older children with behaviour difficulties.

Infants and Children
Even newborn babies can be treated by a cranial osteopath. Quite small children can benefit from osteopathy.

How to Choose a Practitioner
Osteopaths are now regulated by law in Britain, as are doctors and dentists. However, until all the measures of the 1993 Osteopaths Act come into force anyone can claim to be a practitioner.

Osteopaths should be members of one of four professional bodies, the largest of which, the General Council and Register of Osteopaths, will become the umbrella organization when the Act is in force. Lists of its registered members are available from 56 London Street, Reading, Berkshire RGl 4SQ, tel 0l734 576 585. Registered osteopaths should have had a four-year training leading to a Diploma of Osteopathy (DO) or a BSc (OST).

Insurance Recognition
Most private health insurance will pay for treatment by a registered osteopath on the recommendation of your doctor or consultant.

What to Expect at a Consultation
The osteopath will want very full details of your complaint and your past medical history, your work and your lifestyle. He or she will look carefully at the way you move and your posture when sitting, standing, etc. Your reflexes, muscles and spine will be examined. The therapist may want you to have an X-ray or a blood test before deciding whether or not treatment can help you, and will also decide if cranial osteopathy will help.

Treatment, which will probably be a combination of massage and manipulation, is not usually painful but it may sometimes feel a little uncomfortable. It will take about half an hour. You may be given advice on posture and exercise. Expect to have at least three or four weekly treatments before you feel the benefits.

Contraindications
Osteopathy is not recommended for anyone with pathological problems of the bone or joint, such as cancer, nor to treat a fracture. However it can treat the weakness that results from a fracture.

Compatibility with Other Therapies
Osteopathy can be used alongside all other treatments, but can be very effective when used with naturopathy and other detoxifying programmes.

Alexander Technique

Every day we make hundreds of movements. Routine movements such as answering a phone, picking up a child, opening a window, working at a desk, getting up from a chair are rarely thought about in terms of the movement itself. Our focus is usually on what we are trying to do, rather than how our body is doing it. It is hardly surprising, then, that over time and under pressure we develop bad habits which, repeated again and again, distort and undermine the balance and functioning of the body.

The Alexander Technique is a process of re-education in movement aimed at making us more aware of how we use our bodies in daily life. Most doctors and physiotherapists endorse the technique as a very practical approach to dealing with back, neck and shoulder pain caused by poor posture and inappropriate muscle movements. Practitioners believe the technique can help breathing problems, headaches and stress-related disorders as well.

The technique was developed in the late 19th century by Frederick Matthias Alexander, an Australian actor who began to lose his voice during performances. He observed that he had a habit of pulling his head backwards and downwards before he delivered his lines. This habitual movement, he discovered, compressed the spine, chest and ribs. By focusing on lengthening his neck muscles Alexander regained his voice control. He then went on to explore how rethinking and relearning movements could help numerous other problems and make us generally more alert, healthy and poised.

Conditions Treated

The Alexander Technique is regarded as a prime programme for promoting good posture. Stiff necks, shoulder tension, back aches and headaches caused by stress and constant misuse of muscles respond particularly well to the technique, which encourages a forward and upward movement of the head,

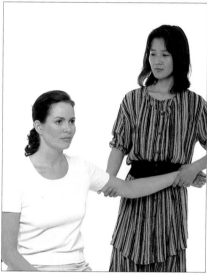

changing the pattern of reflexes and therefore the way we move, sit and stand. Shoulder pain, for instance, may be caused by holding our chin too far forward, or it may be related to pushing the pelvis forward. Both these habits should be corrected as the general technique is understood and learned. Conditions such as asthma, hyperventilation and other breathing difficulties can also be helped.

Infants and Children

The Alexander Technique is not a passive therapy. A child should be old enough to understand what is being taught. It is therefore unlikely that Alexander will be appropriate for anyone under the age of about 12.

How to Choose a Practitioner

Teachers of the Alexander Technique should have completed a three-year full-time course recognized by the Society of Teachers of the Alexander Technique. Details of qualified practitioners in your area are available from the society at 20 London House, 266 Fulham Road, London SW10 9EL, tel 0171 351 0828.

Insurance Recognition

Most private medical schemes will cover the cost of lessons if you have been referred by your doctor or consultant.

What to Expect at a Consultation

The Alexander Technique does not seek to 'cure' complaints. The teacher will be interested in your specific aches and pains, but much more interested in how you stand, sit and move. You may be asked to sit or lie down while the teacher gently manipulates your body. This will indicate problem areas where there is tension in the muscles. The teacher will be able to feel your responses to certain movements which will indicate any habitual misuse of muscles. Through this manipulation the teacher will try and demonstrate the possibilities of change and focus attention on the actual process of movement, encouraging you to 'feel' how your body is working and to think of the movements you are making.

The teacher will give instructions to help you become more aware of your own subconscious reflex pattern and teach you to project simple messages from the brain to the body that will help you alter it. The idea is that these changes can be carried through in daily life. Lessons, which are one to one, take up to 45 minutes. At the beginning it is a good idea to have two lessons a week, but teachers believe that most of us need between 20 and 30 lessons to get the Technique working successfully.

Contraindications

None.

Compatibility with Other Therapies

Lessons can be taken alongside any other therapies but are particularly compatible with yoga.

Naturopathy

Naturopathy is often described as the Western equivalent of traditional Chinese medicine or Ayurveda - a distinct and total philosophy of life and health that addresses the individual rather than just his or her symptoms. The principles of naturopathy were established in ancient Greece by Hippocrates, the patriarch of conventional medicine, who taught that the body had the power to heal itself and that illness was a reaction to disharmony and imbalance. The cause could be physical or psychological and emotional. But health could be regained provided nothing interfered with the natural process of healing and recovery. Disease is defined as a crisis of this natural process, so the object of naturopathy is to help the body restore its natural balance rather than to deal with the symptoms. Naturopaths regard drug treatments, which may suppress symptoms, as counter-productive and likely to cause worse problems in the future. A fever or diarrhoea is a sign that the body is fighting and shaking off an infection or an intrusion.

Modern naturopathy holds true to the original principles, seeking to treat and avert disease by bolstering the body's defence system, primarily through a healthy diet and sensible lifestyle. Many naturopaths, however, have incorporated other techniques such as osteopathy, homeopathy and herbalism into their treatments, all of which are based on the idea of restoring the body's homeostatic balance and energy.

The naturopathic way can appear positively spartan since treatment largely involves changing the diet and making a commitment to exercise; yet fasting and hydrotherapy are also important features of this therapy. Naturopaths believe that the individual must take responsibility for his or her own health; they see themselves as teachers as much as healers.

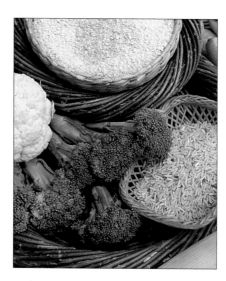

Conditions Treated

Skin disorders, asthma, rheumatoid arthritis, allergies, hormonal and digestive problems respond particularly well to the naturopathic approach, even where other therapies and conventional medicine have failed.

Infants and Children

Anyone can benefit from naturopathy.

How to Choose a Practitioner

Anyone can call themselves a naturopath. But qualified UK practitioners will have completed a four-year full-time course at the British College of Naturopathy, or a post-graduate course run by the British Naturopathic and Osteopathic Association; they will have the letters ND or MRN after their name. The General Council and Register of Naturopaths is the governing body for qualified naturopaths and has a list of registered members. Its address is Goswell House, 2 Goswell Road, Street, Somerset BA16 0JG, tel 01458 840072.

Insurance Recognition

No.

What to Expect at a Consultation

The practitioner will want to know everything about you - your work, relationships and eating habits as well as your medical history and actual complaint. Standard medical techniques, including X-rays, blood tests and urine tests, are also used in diagnosis, and some naturopaths make an iris analysis.

Once a diagnosis is made you will be advised on diet, exercise and any other treatment. If a food allergy is suspected you may have to stop eating whatever is thought to be causing the allergy for a time. Naturopaths regard a healthy – and preferably raw food – diet as the best form of medicine, but some will use acupuncture and herbal or homeopathic remedies to stimulate the body's vital force, though not to suppress symptoms. If you have joint problems such as rheumatoid arthritis you will be advised to reduce your intake of protein. Many naturopaths are also osteopaths, so massage and manipulation may be a part of your treatment, along with poultices and water treatment for inflamed joints.

You will need to have follow-up sessions to check progress at least once a fortnight, depending on the complaint and treatment. The longer you have had the complaint the longer treatment is likely to take. You will be warned to expect a 'healing crisis' – the return of symptoms from time to time as the body's energy is restored.

Contraindications

If you are being treated by a doctor you should check if fasting is appropriate. Naturopaths are not allowed to treat conditions such as cancer, TB, venereal diseases or diabetes, but people with those diseases can have naturopathic therapy, under medical supervision, to improve their overall health.

Compatibility with Other Therapies

Acupuncture, chiropractic, osteopathy, herbal therapy and homeopathy are based on similar principles to naturopathy and work well with it.

Nutritional Therapy/ Allergy Treatment

Nutritional therapy, the use of food and supplements to cure and prevent disease, is an increasingly scientific and highly complex field that conventional medicine is only beginning to take seriously. There has been a great deal of research, for instance, into why heart disease is less common in Japan and the Mediterranean countries than in the United States or the UK, and a diet high in vegetables and low in saturated fats seems to be a significant part of the answer. Research has also demonstrated that junk-food diets are associated with anti-social behaviour and that the disposition of young offenders, for instance, can be dramatically improved by better food and supplements.

It is hardly surprising, then, that a very wide range of everyday ailments – asthma, irritable bowel syndrome, migraines, mood swings and skin disorders, to name but a few – can be successfully treated with nutritional therapy when conventional medicine has failed. And increasing numbers of us seem to have an allergic reaction to certain foods, though we may not realize that this can be the cause of any number of chronic ailments.

Conditions Treated

Many minor chronic conditions such as migraine, hay fever and irritable bowel syndrome can be successfully treated by excluding certain foods from the diet. Wheat and dairy products are often found to be the cause of these – and of skin conditions like eczema, which may also result from an unsuspected food allergy. Inflammatory diseases such as osteoarthritis may be helped by eliminating animal fats. Food allergy can also be the cause of fluid retention and weight gain.

Food intolerances may also be linked to poor digestive function or a 'leaky gut', which has allowed undigested food

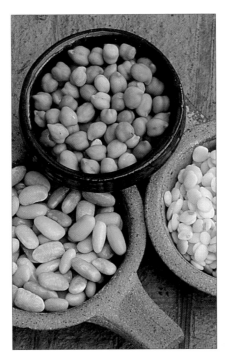

particles into the bloodstream. A nutritional programme will include herbs and nutrients to improve the absorption of food, as well as supplements to correct the balance of intestinal flora.

Problems such as fatigue, ME, headaches and fluid retention may also be due to toxic overload and may be treated by diet and supplements designed to detoxify the system and improve liver, gall-bladder and bowel function.

Pre-menstrual syndrome (PMS) is often treated with a combination of diet (eliminating sugar, for instance) and vitamin supplements.

Infants and Children

There is no reason why young children should not have nutritional therapy.

How to Choose a Practitioner

Anyone can claim to be a nutritional therapist. The Society for the Promotion of Nutritional Therapy has a register of members who have completed a recognized training. Write to the society at PO Box 47, Heathfield, East Sussex TN21 8ZX, tel 01435 867007.

What to Expect at a Consultation

Expect to fill in a large, detailed questionnaire. This gives the therapist your medical history, a guide to your symptoms and some idea of your diet and lifestyle. The initial interview may take about half an hour to an hour and the therapist will try and pinpoint any dietary deficiencies, allergies or digestive problems. There are a number of tests that might be used – blood tests, stool samples or hair mineral analysis, for instance. But some therapists prefer to rely on their own observation – looking carefully at the condition of your nails, for instance – when making a diagnosis.

Treatment programmes consist of nutritional education, a short-term diet and a course of supplements which may include vitamins, minerals, herbs or evening primrose oil. The therapist will probably want to contact your doctor, too.

The number and frequency of follow-up consultations will vary according to individual needs. You may be advised to come once a month or even once a fortnight for several months; or two or three consultations followed by a check-up after six months may be sufficient.

Contraindications

Anyone receiving conventional drug treatment should consult their doctor before having nutritional therapy.

Compatibility with Other Therapies

Many nutritional therapists are also osteopaths, homeopaths, acupuncturists or trained in another holistic therapy.

Herbalism

Herbalism is certainly the oldest form of medicine, developed by the most primitive societies, many of whose traditional plant-based remedies have now been demonstrated by modern science to have healing and therapeutic properties. Many drugs are based on the active elements of plants – digoxin, used in the treatment of heart disease, is the synthesized version of digitalis (foxglove), for instance. But the principle of herbalism is completely different from the pharmaceutical approach. Herbalists believe that the true therapeutic value of plants and herbs, which have a complicated biochemical structure, lies not just in the isolation of active ingredients, but in providing a natural balance that promotes healing. A plant may contain substances which modify the side effects of the main active ingredients, making it easier and safer to use.

Each culture has its herbal tradition, but Chinese herbal medicine is now proving to be very popular in the West, particularly for the treatment of skin problems. Traditional Chinese medicine works with about 10,000 different herbs, often used in conjunction with acupuncture.

In the UK, unlike in China, orthodox medicine attempted to suppress herbalism from around the 15th century. The traditions of Western herbalism survived among the colonists and refugees who emigrated to the New World and adopted Native American herbal medicine.

Conditions Treated

In Chinese medicine skin problems such as acne, eczema and psoriasis are seen as a 'damp heat' symptom. Herbs will be prescribed to help cool down the blood and correct the function of the spleen, which is regarded as responsible for the movement of fluids around the body. While Chinese herbs are increasingly popular for treatment of skin diseases, practitioners can treat all physical

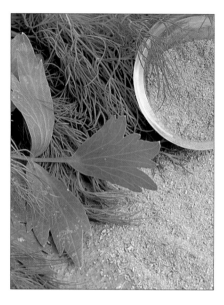

conditions that don't require surgery or manipulation, and psychological problems such as depression as well. Pre-menstrual syndrome (PMS) and menopausal problems may be treated by a combination of herbs and acupuncture. Often acupuncture will help relieve immediate symptoms, while the longer-term herbal treatment will restore the balance of the body.

Western medical herbalists treat a wide range of complaints, including menstrual disorders, breathing problems, irritable bowel syndrome (IBS), candida and arthritis.

Although herbalism is generally understood to be a 'gentle' therapy, herbs can have a direct and powerful effect on the internal organs and systems.

Infants and Children

Anyone of any age can take herbal medicine.

How to Choose a Practitioner

Herbalists have a four-year training and should have the letters NIMH or FNIMH after their name; this shows that they are a Fellow or Member of the National Institute of Medical Herbalists. The

NIMH has a list of registered practitioners available from 56 Longbrook Street, Exeter EX4 6AH, tel 01392 426022.

Insurance Recognition

Private medical insurance does not usually cover the cost of this therapy.

What to Expect at a Consultation

In Chinese medicine diagnosis will be made from looking at your tongue, taking the pulses in the wrists and observing your general appearance. Western herbalists use several standard medical tests when making a diagnosis.

Herbal treatments may be prescribed in the form of a tincture, an alcohol-based liquid, a cream or compress or a dried herb powder used to make up a tea that is drunk several times a day as prescribed. A herbalist may prescribe something to help acute symptoms, but long-term treatment will involve changes in diet and lifestyle as well. The initial consultation will take about an hour and follow-up sessions are recommended every couple of weeks.

Contraindications

Several plants and herbs that stimulate hormones should be avoided during pregnancy. Anyone with liver disease such as hepatitis or high blood pressure should consult their doctor before taking Chinese herbs.

Compatibility with Other Therapies

Chinese herbs are often most effective in conjunction with acupuncture. Herbal therapy is particularly compatible with osteopathy, chiropractic and naturopathy.

Light Therapy

All living things respond to light. It is as important to us as food, air and water. When the sun comes out we all feel happier. But the idea that light has a serious therapeutic role is a novel one to most of us, although doctors and other practitioners have been using light therapy successfully since the beginning of the century to treat a variety of skin disorders. Before then several innovative physicians had discovered that sunlight could help cure patients of numerous diseases.

Pollution, long office hours and fears about ageing the skin mean that many of us simply don't get enough natural light even in the summer. Seasonal Affective Disorder (SAD), a depression that many people suffer during the winter months, is believed to be directly linked to a shortage of sunlight. But light therapy – exposing the skin and eyes to full-spectrum light – is now used to treat this and a wide range of other problems too.

Light has a direct effect on the workings of the body and on our moods. It stimulates the pineal gland in the brain to produce serotonin (the 'feel good' hormone) and balance the amount of melatonin (the 'hibernating' hormone manufactured in the dark). Melatonin controls our sleep patterns but an excess can lead to depression and tiredness. Sufficient light is needed to keep these hormones in balance. Light therapy simulates the effect of the natural light of 'a bright spring day in the northern hemisphere'.

Conditions Treated

Light therapy is used to treat a range of problems associated with hormonal imbalance. Women suffering menopausal symptoms such as hot flushes, or menstrual problems such as pre-menstrual syndrome or period pains, have found it very beneficial. The effect on some of these problems can be very quick. Light therapy advocates believe that it has a stimulating effect on the sex hormones. Problems such as

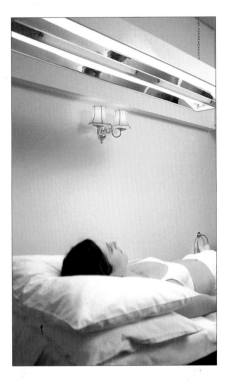

infertility and loss of libido have also responded to light therapy.

The body needs light in order to manufacture Vitamin D_3, which is essential for maintaining healthy bones and skin. Debilitating diseases such as osteoporosis may be due in part to poor digestive function, which leads to calcium being lost from the body instead of forming bone. In these cases light therapy may be particularly appropriate for older people or for those who have suffered a serious illness, althogh osteoporosis is increasingly affecting younger people too.

Light therapy is also used to improve blood circulation, boost the immune system and treat skin disorders such as acne, eczema and psoriasis.

People with dark skins can benefit greatly from light therapy, as they absorb less light that those with pale skins.

Infants and Children

There is no problem about children having light therapy.

How to Choose a Practitioner

As yet there is no recognized qualification for light therapy practitioners training in the UK, although a Light Therapy Association is being established. This will have a central register of therapists. At the moment you should look for a therapist qualified in another area who offers light therapy as well, or send a stamped addressed envelope to the SAD Association, Box 989, London SW7 2PZ.

Insurance Recognition

Some private insurance schemes will refund the cost of treatment for SAD.

What to Expect at a Consultation

Consultation will begin with a check on your overall health and discussion of your symptoms. Then you will lie on a couch facing an overhanging light for around 45 minutes. The light may scan only the eyes if you are being treated for hormonal problems or depression – light on the eyes works directly on the pineal gland in the brain.

You take some or all of your clothes off if you are being treated for skin problems or Vitamin D_3 deficiency. The therapy is entirely safe and there is absolutely no danger of sunburn or eye damage as the harmful rays are screened out. For acute symptoms a once-a-week therapy session is recommended until the problem is under control – response to light therapy can be very fast. Then you may be advised to have a 'boost' every few months.

Contraindications

If you are having frequent light therapy sessions you should not take Vitamin D tablets at the same time.

Compatibility with Other Therapies

Light therapy can be used with other therapies and treatments. It is particularly effective combined with reflexology in the same session.

Homeopathy

Homeopathy is a system of treatment founded by a German doctor, Samuel Hahnemann, in the early 19th century. Hahnemann found that giving his patients tiny doses of substances that would cause the symptoms of their illness in a perfectly healthy patient could in fact cure them. The founding principle of his system, then, is to treat like with like – similar to the medical theory underlying vaccination or immunization. This method of treatment is said to stimulate the body's own healing processes to cure the particular ailment or overpower the bacteria, rather than treating the symptoms themselves, which may merely suppress the problem temporarily. By introducing a remedy that mimics the symptoms, homeopathy builds the body's resistance. Homeopaths regard symptoms as the result of the body's attempt to stay healthy, rather than the real problem.

There are several thousand homeopathic remedies, many of them produced from herbs or plants, though conventional drugs can also be prescribed homeopathically, in very small amounts. Another homeopathic principle is that all remedies, given as tablets or medicine are prescribed in minute, dilute amounts. (The designation 6c, 30c, etc. after the name of a remedy refers to the amount of dilution.) Homeopaths believe that the more dilute the concentration, the more powerful and effective it is. Remedies are prepared by a process known as succussion (shaking), which releases the energy from the remedy.

Many conventionally trained doctors also practise homeopathy and there are several National Health Service homeopathic hospitals in the UK.

Conditions Treated

In principle any disorder can be treated homeopathically. Constantly recurring but non life-threatening problems such as menstrual disorders, allergies,

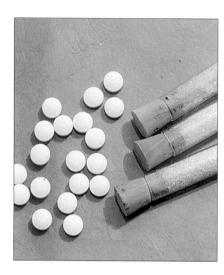

asthma, migraine, eczema, cystitis, constipation and IBS, that conventional medicine finds hard to treat successfully and permanently, are particularly responsive to homeopathy.

Infants and Children

Homeopathic remedies are safe even for young children and a homeopath will prescribe remedies for babies suffering from problems such as colic.

How to Choose a Practitioner

Members of the Society of Homeopaths have the initials RSHom or FSHom after their name. They will have had a four-year part-time or two-year full-time training at a recognized institution and one year's supervised clinical experience. You can get a list of registered homeopaths from the Society of Homeopaths, 2 Artizan Road, Northampton NN1 4HU, tel 01604 21400.

A list of members of the UK Homeopathic Medical Association (MHMA) can be obtained from 6 Livingstone Road, Gravesend, Kent, DA12 5DZ, tel 01474 560336.

Doctors who have taken a postgraduate training in homeopathy have MFHom or FFHom after their name. A list of medically qualified

homeopathic practitioners is available from the British Homeopathic Association, 27a Devonshire Street, London W1N 1RJ, tel 0171 935 2163.

Insurance Recognition

Your doctor may be able to refer you for homeopathic treatment through the National Health Service; if he is a fundholder he can refer you to a private homeopath. Most private insurance schemes will refund the cost of homeopathic treatment if you are referred by a doctor.

What to Expect at a Consultation

An initial consultation may take one to two hours. The therapist will want to know a great deal about you – your general health, diet and medical history, relationships, moods, what you perceive as your strengths and weaknesses, as well as your particular complaint. The therapist will want to prescribe a remedy that 'matches' you. As well as these *constitutional* remedies designed to treat long-standing conditions he or she will also prescribe something for any immediate *acute* symptoms.

Some people are concerned that homeopaths use substances like digitalis (derived from foxgloves), arsenic and belladonna, all known to be potentially poisonous. But because of their dilution the remedies are completely safe. You should visit your homeopath as you do your doctor – to check how the remedies are working and when you feel you need help.

Contraindications

Homeopathy is not recommended for surgical emergencies.

Compatibility with Other Therapies

Homeopathy is compatible with other therapies, although some homeopaths do not like you to have aromatherapy while you are being treated because some essential oils can interfere with the remedies.

Buteyko

Most of us assume that deep breathing is healthy because it increases our oxygen intake. But because the air around us contains a much smaller proportion of carbon dioxide (CO_2) than our own bodies and because CO_2 is essential for the body's uptake of oxygen, over-breathing results in a deficit and reduces the level of oxygen in our blood circulation and tissues, affecting the function of every system in our body. So the more we breathe the less oxygen we actually manage to send round our bodies.

The Buteyko Mehod aims to retrain breathing patterns to ensure optimal oxygenation of the body and its tissues and is a direct therapy for the treatment of asthma and other breathing disorders. The technique was developed by a Russian medical scientist, Dr Konstantin Buteyko, some 40 years ago when, as a young intern working in a hospital for terminally ill patients, he observed that an increase in breathing was an indicator of approaching death. He realized that he could predict the time of death by monitoring patients' breathing patterns and that deepening breathing was associated with a very wide range of diseases and chronic conditions.

From studies of hundreds of patients, Buteyko developed the theory that much ill health was the result of the body's defence mechanisms trying to compensate for a lack of carbon dioxide. Observing that patients with hypertension, cardiac problems, allergies, piles and breathing disorders all breathed more than normal, and concluded that deep breathing was not just a symptom but a cause of their ailments. The technique he developed as a result of his observations is a series of exercises designed to restore breathing patterns to a normal level by retraining the body's involuntary respiratory centre.

Conditions Treated

With asthma sufferers the object is to change the breathing pattern to reduce

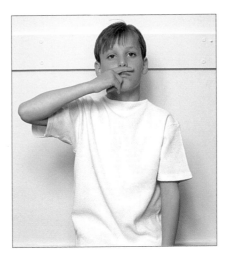

or eliminate spasms and enable the patient to be less dependent on medication. Conditions such as hyperventilation and angina also respond to the reconditioning of the respiratory function through breathing-retention exercises.

With eczema, diabetes, hay fever and other allergies the treatment aims to reduce the oversensitivity to outside stimuli which is believed to be one long-term result of over-breathing. High blood pressure and heart conditions are also said to benefit from the Buteyko Method, which has had success in helping people stop snoring as well. Normalizing breathing stimulates the metabolism, so it can also help people who want to lose weight.

Infants and Children

Children who suffer from asthma and/or eczema and who are old enough to understand what is being taught can benefit from Buteyko. Indeed, children who do not have a lifetime of bad habits to unlearn may achieve results very quickly.

Insurance Recognition

No.

How to Choose a Practitioner

Qualified Buteyko practitioners have a five-year training. Details of UK practitioners are available from the International Association of Buteyko Practitioners, 12 Harley Street, London W1N 1AA, tel 094111 5484.

What to Expect at a Consultation

Buteyko can only help people who are breathing more than the normal rate. This is established by a simple control pause test to see how long you can comfortably hold your breath. If you are over-breathing you can have one-to-one therapy or join a workshop in order to learn the technique. Continuity is important and you are expected to practise between classes. The most effective way of learning is one one-hour session a day for five consecutive days. You will be taught how breathing relates to physiological function and the rationale of Buteyko will be explained. You will then learn a number of breath-retention exercises to help establish a new pattern of shallow breathing. This can be quite difficult for asthmatics and people with breathing disorders.

You will also be advised to eat less and temporarily to exclude animal protein from your diet since over-consumption of meat and dairy products in particular is thought to increase breathing levels.

A bona fide qualified Buteyko practitioner offers a money-back guarantee of substantial improvement for every patient he or she has agreed to treat, no matter what the complaint.

Contraindications

Buteyko is not suitable for anyone suffering from an infectious disease in acute form.

Compatibility with Other Therapies

Buteyko is compatible with all other therapies, but may work particularly well with meditation and yoga, since both these promote shallow breathing. It does not interfere with any other treatment you may be having for asthma or allergies.

Psychotherapy & Counselling

Essentially psychotherapists believe that our past experiences can distort our perceptions of the present. This can affect our feelings about ourselves, our relationships and the way we react to events and other people. The object of psychotherapy is to help us explore the reasons why we think, feel or behave in a certain way in order for us to change these patterns.

The psychotherapist will guide this self-exploration, but will not tell you what to think or how to behave. Through understanding why you react the way you do, you can start responding in a different, more rational way. Because so much communication is involved it is important that you have good rapport with the therapist.

Counselling is a more short-termform of psychotherapy, which will usually deal with very specific problems and crises – the aftermath of bereavement or job loss, for instance, or some other kind of difficulty.

Conditions Treated

Depression, phobias, anxiety and eating disorders can all be treated successfully with psychotherapy and counselling. Problems such as obesity, impotence, menstrual and menopausal stress may also have a psychological root which therapy can help resolve. Major life changes like bereavement and divorce may require supportive counselling and therapy on a shorter-term basis.

Infants and Children

There are specialized child and family psychotherapists who believe that any child over the age of about 12 can benefit from psychotherapy, but this is a controversial issue. Children with behavioural problems are often referred to educational psychologists, who are trained to deal with children who – for whatever reason – are experiencing difficulties in learning at school or in their behaviour.

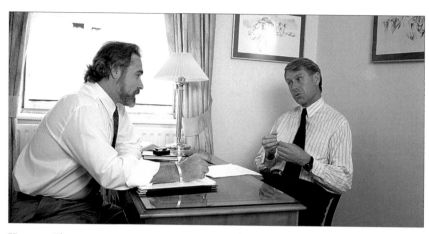

How to Choose a Practitioner

Anyone can call themselves a psychotherapist or a counsellor. However, recognized practitioners often have a background in health or social work and a relevant training in addition to their original professional qualification.

The United Kingdom Council for Psychotherapy, Regents College, Inner Circle, Regents Park, London NW1 4NS, tel 0171 487 7554, has a list of registered therapists. The Register of Chartered Clinical Psychologists, British Psychological Society, St Andrews House, 48 Princess Street East, Leicester LE1 7DR, tel 0116 254 9568 and the British Confederation of Psychotherapists, 37a Mapesbury Road, London NW2 4HJ, tel 0181 830 5173, also keep lists of recognized practitioners.

The British Association of Counselling, 1 Regent Place, Rugby, Warwickshire CV21 2PJ, has a list of counsellors who have a recognized training.

Insurance Recognition

Private medical insurance schemes do not usually cover the cost of psychotherapy and counselling, unless you are referred by a psychiatrist.

What to Expect at a Consultation

Your first consultation may be with an assessor, who will talk to you about your problem, explain the process of psychotherapy and what it involves, and refer you to a therapist if they think that treatment will be helpful. Psychotherapy sessions take about 50 minutes, but follow no set pattern. Through your discussions the therapist will help you to become more self-aware and establish insight into the reasons for the particular problem. The process can be quite an emotional upheaval and it is important that you feel you can talk openly and freely to the therapist. This is not passive therapy – you have to have a willingness to change to benefit from it, although your therapist will help you identify anxieties and blocks to change.

Continuity is important because you are in essence re-educating your emotional reflexes. Your therapist might suggest you have sessions more than once a week if necessary. Psychotherapy open-ended, continuing for as long as it seems to be helpful.

Counselling is generally a shorter process, since it does not involve a fundamental change in your thinking or behaviour. It provides support while you come to terms with what has happened.

Contraindications

None. But psychotherapy does not suit everyone – you have to be prepared to 'open up' in order to make progress.

Compatibility with Other Therapies

Psychotherapy and counselling are compatible with all other therapies.

Hypnotherapy

Hypnotherapy is a technique for achieving deep relaxation and enabling the subconscious part of the mind to express itself and receive messages in order to bring about change in your feelings and actions.

Hypnosis, the inducing of a trance-like state in which the body's reactions are slowed down, has been used therapeutically in many cultures. In Europe it was developed by a Viennese doctor, Anton Mesmer (who gave his name to the term 'mesmerized'), whose rather theatrical approach to patient treatment gave hypnosis a poor reputation. In the 19th century a British doctor working in India developed hypnosis as a successful method of pain relief during surgery.

Nowadays hypnotherapy, which is a combination of hypnosis and counselling, is used to treat a wide range of stress-related disorders, addictions and phobias. It does not involve any mind manipulation or control, but depends on establishing a relationship of trust and co-operation between patient and therapist. It works by helping the patient uncover and talk about particular events, ideas or feelings that may lie behind psychological or even physical symptoms. The therapist can then try to replace those fears and feelings with more positive images and thoughts. In some cases the patient may be taught simple self-hypnosis techniques to help them overcome situations and feelings that trigger the problem in daily life.

Conditions Treated

Addictions such as cigarette smoking can respond quickly to hypnotherapy provided there is a real desire to stop the habit. Therapy may involve helping the patient feel indifferent to smoking and concentrating on the health benefits of giving up. Eating disorders may stem from a poor self-image which needs to be changed by boosting self-confidence. Phobias and irrational fears may be related to a specific event in the past and the patient will be helped by reliving it to

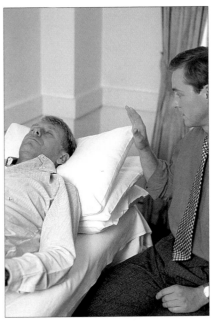

understand that the experience is over. Physical problems such as asthma, migraines, skin complaints and digestive disorders may be a symptom of stress if no medical reason can be established. The therapist will try and find out what idea or incident lies behind the pattern of stress and help the patient come to terms with it. Self-hypnosis techniques may be taught to help you relax in certain situations. Asthma sufferers, for instance, can be helped to deal with an impending attack and self-hypnosis can help deal with pain during labour.

Infants and Children

Children can benefit from hypnotherapy from about the age of five.

How to Choose a Practitioner

Anyone can claim to be a hypnotherapist, but many practitioners have qualifications in another therapy or a medical training. The National Council for Hypnotherapy, Woodbury House, Woodchurch Road, Tenterden, Kent TH30 7AE, tel 01590 644913 has a register of about 1,000 reputable hypnotherapists. The National Society for Hypnotherapists and

Psychotherapists, 28 Finsbury Park Road, London N4 2JX, tel 0171 226 6963, has a register of members who have undertaken a recognized training.

Insurance Recognition

Private medical schemes do not normally cover the cost of hypnotherapy.

What to Expect at a Consultation

The therapist will want to know about your health, your complaint and your likes and dislikes. Getting you really relaxed is the important first step. A number of techniques may be used to focus your conscious mind in order to achieve this. You may be asked to visualize a place or scene or imagine you are going down in a lift; alternatively a counting technique may be used. The idea is that in this deeply relaxed state you will find it easier to investigate and express your true feelings, which will give the therapist a guide to the cause of your problem. Once that is established the therapist will work on changing your emotional responses by suggesting a series of positive rather than negative thoughts and images.

Habits such as cigarette smoking usually respond quickly if they are going to be helped at all. Eating disorders will take longer. Sessions take about an hour, and one a week is recommended. Hypnotherapy should, however, be regarded as a short-term treatment. If you have not felt substantial benefits after ten sessions it may not be the therapy for you.

Contraindications

Anyone with a serious long-standing psychological disorder should not have hypnotherapy.

Compatibility with Other Therapies

Hypnotherapy can be used with all other treatments but is particularly effective if the patient has learned to relax through yoga or meditation.

Healing

Most people who visit healers do so only as a last resort, in cases of terminal illness. In such cases healing can relieve pain and discomfort, and in some cases patients find themselves in total remission. Healing is an effective way both of stopping pain and of reducing inflammation, as well as sometimes being an instrumental factor in eliminating the need for surgery.

Healing works with electro-magnetic energy (the aura). The healer acts as a channel for a much higher, limitless source of this energy and transfers it via his or her hands to the patient, re-aligning their aura and rebalancing the particular frequencies that are generated by the individual's internal organs

Many scientific and medical papers have been written proving the efficacy of healing and the benefits that individuals can derive from this energy transference.

Conditions Treated
Healing can treat any condition from back pain and migraine to stomach disorders, cancers, joint pain, depression and stress.

Infants and Children
People of any age may respond to healing, including babies and very young children.

How to Choose a Practitioner
Anyone can claim to be a healer and, as always, recommendation is the best policy here. Ask friends and family if they know of a good, effective healer who has helped someone they know personally.

If you are unable to find a healer through word of mouth, the National Federation of Spiritual Healers runs a referral service which can can be contacted on 0891 616 080.

Insurance Recognition
Few private medical schemes will cover

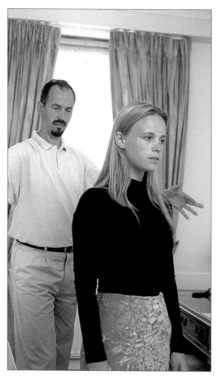

the cost of healing therapy. However, in the UK healers are allowed by the National Health Service to visit patients in hospital, and some general practitioners provide the services of healers in their surgeries.

What to Expect at a Consultation
Most healers will ask for a brief medical history at the initial visit. An experienced healer should be able to scan the patient and tell which parts of the body are 'out of synch'; if necessary he or she will advise the patient to see a specialist or consultant.

Healers work in one of two ways: either hands-on healing, in which the practitioner will actually lay his or her hands on the patient's body; or distance healing, in which the healer's hands are 30cm (12in) or more above the patient's body.

Most patients report sensations of hot, cold, electrical impulses or pins and needles. You should expect to leave a

session feeling lighter, relaxed, de-stressed and happier.

After the initial, more lengthy consultation, most sessions last for 30 minutes.

Contraindications
It is highly likely that a very good healer will channel such strong energy that patients with pacemakers will suffer arrhythmia or fibrillation as a result. Healing is therefore not recommended in these cases.

Compatibility with Other Therapies
Healing is compatible with all other therapies, including chemotherapy and all allopathic remedies. Patients must *never* stop taking any medication or therapy prescribed by their doctor or specialist without his or her approval. If in doubt, they should tell their doctor that they are having healing as a complementary therapy.

Colonic Hydrotherapy

Colonic hydrotherapy should be an important part of any detoxification programme. It is a gentle water treatment that spring-cleans the colon and the rest of the large intestine, clearing out accumulated waste matter. Colonic hydrotherapy is both popular and controversial. Many doctors and complementary practitioners dispute its therapeutic benefits. Others regard it as a sensible and entirely safe way to help cleanse the system.

Colonic hydrotherapists believe that many illnesses are caused or aggravated by problems in the gut. Faecal matter containing toxins and bacteria may have putrefied and set hard, disrupting bowel function and in effect slowly poisoning the body, which is unable to get rid of it. Therapists maintain that conventional medicine has paid insufficient attention to the role of the colon in protecting the body from disease.

Eating processed food and over-consumption of meat and even dairy products over time may lead to the build-up of toxins and mucus and encourage sluggishness in the system. Taking laxatives to deal with constipation can irritate the lining of the gut and damage the bowel muscles, which become unable to work properly. Even habits like eating too fast and not chewing food well can contribute to bloating and irritation.

Colonic hydrotherapy is much more effective than an enema, since cleansing extends beyond the natural expulsion area. It can help improve bowel muscle tone and it can be used to administer oxygen and any supplements recommended by a doctor. Problems such as infestation by parasites or failure of the system to break down certain food can also be identified from the waste matter.

Conditions Treated
Colonic hydrotherapy is a direct treatment for serious constipation, offering immediate relief. But longer-term treatment of this and other

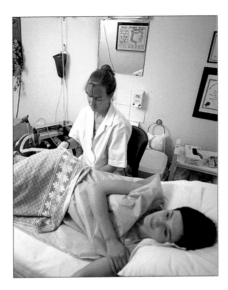

digestive complaints will certainly involve changes in diet as well. Cleaning out the bowel helps treat irritable bowel syndrome (IBS), candida and yeast infections, which may be caused by an imbalance of the micro-organisms in the gut Colonic hydrotherapy enables the bowel to be repopulated with 'friendly' bacteria which help control those bacteria that cause intestinal ailments.

Allergies can be helped, since many of these originate from particles of undigested food leaked through the gut wall. The treatment can also help detoxify the body in preparation for conception, and can help problems of infertility.

Infants and Children
Not recommended.

How to Choose a Practitioner
The Colonic International Association, 16 England Lane, London NW3 4TG, tel 0171 483 1595, has a list of qualified practitioners. All therapists on its register must have either a medical training or a diploma in anatomy and physiology or a recognized qualification in another complementary therapy.

What to Expect at a Consultation
At your first session the therapist will take a case history and make a clear assessment of whether this treatment can help your problem. Therapists are very wary of people who want colonic hydrotherapy purely for weight loss.

A disposable speculum with tube attached will be inserted into your back passage while you lie on your side and some 45-68l (10-15 gallons) of warm filtered water will be slowly flushed through your large intestine and out through a larger tube. The process takes about 45 minutes and may feel a little uncomfortable – as if you were permanently on the toilet – but it is not painful in any way. You change position a couple of times during the treatment and the therapist may also give you an abdominal massage to help things along.

Afterwards you will be given organic herbs to replace the essential bacteria in the gut. You will also be advised on diet. Therapists recommend six to eight treatments,one or two weeks apart, with follow-up sessions two or three times a year.

Insurance Recognition
Health insurance does not normally cover the cost of this treatment.

Contraindications
Anyone who has a heart problem or who is severely overweight is not advised to have colonic hydrotherapy. Nor is anyone who has inflamed or bleeding piles or kidney problems, high blood pressure, bowel cancer or severe diabetes, or who has had recent bowel surgery. Colonic hydrotherapy is also not suitable for women in the first three months or the last three months of pregnancy.

Compatibility with Other Therapies
Colonic hydrotherapy is most effective in combination with nutritional, herbal or homeopathic therapy that suggests changes in diet and lifestyle. For detoxification it is most effective with massage therapy.

Trichology

Trichos is the Greek word for hair, but trichology therapy is concerned with scalp as well as hair conditions and practitioners really see themselves as experts in a specialized branch of dermatology. Trichology addresses itself to three main areas. Firstly, the condition of the hair itself, which may be damaged by various treatments - colouring, perming and straightening treatments over a period of time can result in dry, brittle and lifeless hair and permanent damage to the scalp. Excessive exposure to sun, over-strong shampoos, conditioners and other hair products, and even overuse of heated rollers and hairdryers can all damage the hair and sometimes cause allergic reactions.

Secondly, hair condition and growth are very much affected by our general health and wellbeing. Illness, hormonal changes, certain medical treatments and an insufficiency of certain nutrients in our diet can all have a direct impact on hair-growth pattern, causing actual loss or noticeable thinning.

Finally skin disorders may affect the scalp, requiring specialist treatment and advice. Trichology therapy also involves identifying and treating allergies to various substances in hair products that can upset the scalp. Patients may be referred for nutritional therapy where a lack of essential minerals or an inappropriate diet is believed to be affecting the condition of the hair.

Conditions Treated

Hormonal changes are the main cause of the hair loss and thinning that many women experience, typically on the crown and at the sides of the head, after they have had a baby or during menopause. In both cases falling oestrogen levels cause a higher percentage of normal hairs to go into their resting phase prematurely. Normally there will be a balance of growing and resting hairs, so the 'turnover' is not noticed. Infra-red, ultra-

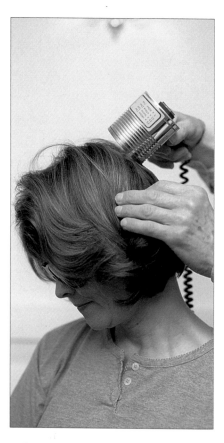

violet and low-level laser therapy may be used to stimulate the activity of the hair follicles to resume a normal growth pattern. This improves the circulation in the scalp and increases nutritional uptake.

Skin disorders such as psoriasis and eczema can also affect the scalp, but topical treatments for the rest of the body may not be practical for use on the head. Special creams can be used to remove scale and counter inflammation.

Problems with dandruff and with dry, damaged and oily hair can also be treated. Damaged hair will be improved by using topical products such as moisturizers, synthesized protein and restructurants.

Insurance Recognition

No.

Infants and Children

Topical preparations may be used for young children, but not the other trichological therapies.

How to Choose a Practitioner

The Institute of Trichologists, 20-22 Queensbury Place, London SW7 2DZ, tel 0171 733 2056, has a register of practitioners. The initials AIT after a practitioner's name mean he or she is an Associate of the Institute of Trichologists and has completed a three-year course. MIT means he or she is a Member of the Institute of Trichologists and has three years' clinical experience in addition.

What to Expect at a Consultation

At a first appointment you will be asked details about your medical history, diet and lifestyle. There may be a referral for blood tests to check for any iron and ferritin deficiencies and a hair analysis to check mineral levels. Trichology treatment may be combined with nutritional therapy.

Depending on the problem there may be treatment with low-power laser therapy or infra-red or ultra-violet ray therapy as well as steaming treatment (for dry and damaged hair) and topical preparations. Each session takes about 50 minutes and 8-12 weekly sessions are recommended, particularly for hair loss and damage problems. Products may also be suggested for use at home in between sessions.

Contraindications

Electro and laser therapy are not suitable for pregnant women.

Compatibility with Other Therapies

Trichology is compatible with all other therapies but is frequently used alongside nutritional therapy because of the close relationship between hair condition and our overall diet and health.

Sensory Integration Training

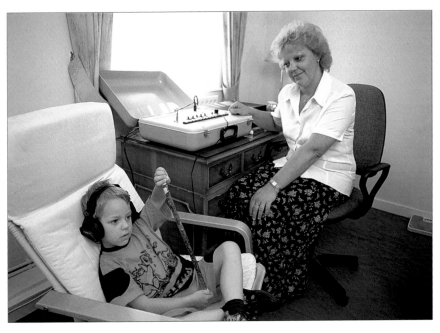

Sensory Integration Training for Communication (SITC) is a music-listening therapy designed to integrate the sensory processing systems in the brain. Through a variety of therapy techniques, including modulated music, SITC retrains individuals with communication and auditory processing difficulties to hear and listen in a more balanced manner. It was adapted by speech/language pathologist Aditi E. Silverstein from the principles of Auditory Integration Training, other sound therapies and Sensory Integration Training.

Acute sensitivity to certain sound frequencies or poor auditory processing abilities may distort the way everyday sound and speech are registered. We learn to communicate through hearing the world around us. If what we hear makes no sense, we may respond by blocking it out or by overreacting to it. Autistic children may cut themselves off from confusing outside stimulation, and therefore fail to develop normal language and communication skills.

During SITC, a variety of sound therapies and traditional speech therapy may be used. Electronic sound equipment is often used to modify and filter music, increasing and decreasing sound levels in an unpredictable pattern. These treatments are believed to stimulate the brain to listen in a new way and improve awareness of sound, thereby improving the capacity to process and rationalize what is heard in daily life.

Conditions Treated

This specially designed programme has been successful with people suffering from a variety of communication and learning problems which are linked to auditory processing difficulties. SITC has helped people suffering from autism to 'open up' to the world around them and begin to communicate with others. Improved communication abilities and reduced sound sensitivities help to reduce frustration and irritability, which

then enables people to focus and learn more effectively. People with dyslexia may be helped when the integration between hearing and the brain is stimulated, improving the capacity for relating sounds to letters. People with tinnitus are often relieved of the distress of the perception of constant sound.

Infants and Children

Children from the age of two or three, when problems may first be noticed, as well as adults with a variety of problems, can benefit from SITC.

How to Choose a Practitioner

SITC is available in the UK through the Hale Clinic, 7 Park Crescent, London W1N 3HE, tel 0171 631 0156.

Insurance Recognition

Not usually.

What to Expect at a Consultation

Audio-perceptual testing may be used to determine if there are specific areas of hypersensitivity, although many young or disabled children do not respond to this type of testing. A variety of question-

naires are completed by parents. Music-listening usually occurs over a ten-day period with daily hour-long listening sessions. The music is played through specially designed equipment that modulates sound frequencies randomly and to which the patient listens through headphones. Sometimes treatment is recommended using specially recorded therapeutic CDs which can be used at home. An essential element of SITC is group and individual family counselling.

Therapy can bring about immediate improvements, but the major benefits are noted over several months. Follow-up treatments or evaluations every three months are often recommended.

Contraindications

SITC may not be suitable for those suffering from severe hearing loss, and may not be as beneficial for anyone who is mentally retarded.

Compatibility with Other Therapies

Many other complementary therapies, including cranial osteopathy, homeopathy or naturopathy, may be recommended following SITC.

Oxypeel

Oxypeel is a remedial therapy for damaged skin. It evolved in the mid-1980s when a cosmetic scientist, Sujata Jolly, started to develop her own treatments for improving the appearance of skin affected by conditions such as acne, which can often leave unsightly scars and blemishes. Oxypeel can also be used to correct discoloration and uneven pigmentation, to rejuvenate tired, ageing skin and to treat scars left by surgery, burns and infections such as chicken pox. It can also help fade the brown marks that sometimes appear during pregnancy or the menopause.

Oxypeel therapy is based on biological exfoliation, which works only on damaged skin cells, not the healthy cells, gradually removing the blemished layers which are then replaced by healthy skin. Part of the process is increasing the supply of oxygen to the skin, enabling it to repair itself. Oxypeel treatment is non-abrasive and much gentler than conventional skin-peeling techniques. There are a variety of treatments containing therapeutic chemicals and natural plant extracts such as ivy, rosemary and horse chestnut which are applied as face masks. Products are also available so that you can continue treatments at home.

Oxypeel can improve eczema and soothe the discomfort of psoriasis, though it is not a treatment for either of these conditions.

Conditions Treated

Acne and its effects can be treated very successfully with Oxypeel therapy. Active acne – where the skin is inflamed – requires a minimum of six once-a-week treatments, possibly more in very severe cases. The treatment cleanses and unblocks the skin ducts, destroys micro-organisms by introducing oxygen and initiates the healing process. After six to eight treatments there will be a break before any more consultations to re-educate the skin and reduce its

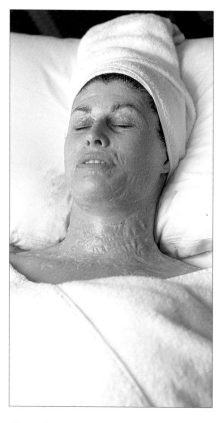

dependence on treatment.

Soft scarring resulting from past acne infection is treated with an enzyme peel which works by degrading damaged cells and releasing substances which stimulate growth and skin repair. Enzyme peel can be used to dissolve keloid scars left after surgery, to even out pigmentation and to reduce scars left by burns. It is particularly effective for dark skins which have post-acne scarring.

Deep pitting resulting from scratching spots is treated with a localized application of alkaline peel.

Tired and dry skin can be given a 'lift' with a mineral and herb corrective facial. This works by improving the flow of blood and nutrients to the skin, aiding the removal of waste products. It eases out fine lines and reduces any blotchiness and small scars on the skin. It is particularly recommended for

ageing skin. For best results you should have four treatments in the same week, followed by regular maintenance.

Infants and Children

Oxypeel is a very effective treatment for teenage acne.

How to Choose a Practitioner

There are trained therapists licensed to use Oxypeel products. Contact Depeche Mode Laboratories, 8 Chestnut Close, Maidenhead, Berks SL6 8SY, tel 01628 74644 and 0181 904 9594.

Insurance Recognition

No.

What to Expect at a Consultation

Unless you are having an alkaline peel your skin will be cleaned with a foaming milk applied with a brush before the mask is put on. Some masks give you a mild tingly feeling. Others harden on the skin and you will notice a throbbing of blood vessels in the face which can feel a little uncomfortable. The mask will remain on for between 30 and 45 minutes. Sometimes the treatment may involve using two different masks for shorter periods. There may be a gentle massage afterwards. You are advised not to wear any make-up for 24 hours after a treatment.

Your therapist will show you how to use products at home in between sessions, which is an important part of the treatment.

Contraindications

You should have an allergy test before having an enzyme peel or an alkaline peel. Allergic reaction to Oxypeel treatment is rare, but it is better to be safe. While you are having treatment no other products or medication should be used for treating the same problem.

Compatibility with Other Therapies

Oxypeel is complementary to all natural therapies.

Moor Therapy

The Moor is 6.5 hectares (150 acres) of boggy lake and marshland in Austria, created during the Ice Age and home to a rich inheritance of plants and herbs, some of which are unique and have no botanical name. The harvest from the Moor, which has never dried up or been contaminated, contains some 300 medicinal herbs, lipids, enzymes, essential oils, minerals and vitamins that correspond to the body's own pH levels. It has been regarded as having therapeutic properties from ancient times - Celtic and Roman bathing equipment has been found in the lake and its waters were used for healing by generations of monks in the nearby monastery.

Some 50 years ago Professor Otto Stober bought the lake and created a spa and health centre there, which is highly regarded by European health professionals for its treatments. More recently a processing plant has been established, enabling the products of the Moor and its therapies to be more widely available. Moor treatments include a pasteurized herbal drink, body oil, Moor paste and Moor bath for body therapy.

Conditions Treated

Acne, eczema, psoriasis and other skin disorders are treated with Moor facials, baths and body creams, which contain healing properties of the Moor. The Moor is naturally anti-inflammatory. Patients with rheumatism and arthritis can be treated with poultices or body wraps. The herbal drink, taken three times daily, helps to detoxify the body and reduce acidity in the system - this can also be given as part of a treatment for stomach ulcers.

Moor body wraps can be helpful in breaking down cellulite around the hips and thighs by stimulating the circulation and lymphatic system.

The Moor can also be used to treat thinning hair, by stimulating the circulation to the scalp. Moor baths and the herbal drink are also effective therapies for menopausal problems such as broken sleep, insomnia and hot flushes.

Infants and Children

Anyone can benefit from Moor therapy.

How to Choose a Practitioner

For a list of Moor therapists write to Unit 2, 6 Albany Villas, Hove, East Sussex BN3 2RU, tel 01273 739463. Moor therapists are required to have a recognized diploma in anatomy and physiology.

Insurance Recognition

No.

What to Expect at a Consultation

Moor therapy may involve a facial mask, baths, the application of a body cream, a massage with the Moor oil, the application of poultices to inflamed joints or a full or half body wrap depending on the therapist's recommendations. You may also be recommended to take the herbal drink and use other products at home in between sessions as part of the treatment. Six weekly sessions are usually recommended for skin disorders and for rheumatism and arthritis.

Contraindications

Pregnant women are not advised to have Moor therapy.

Compatibility with Other Therapies

Moor treatment can be used with all other therapies, but may be particularly effective in conjunction with aromatherapy and acupuncture.

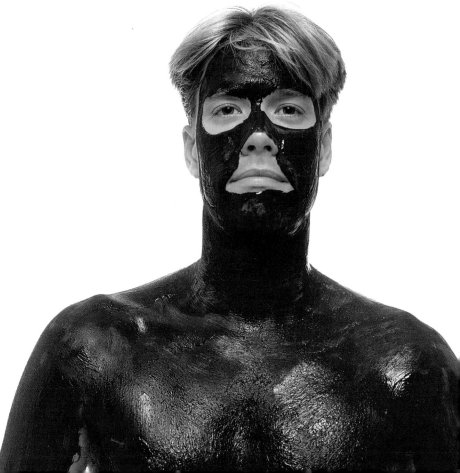

Yoga & Chi Kung

Yoga originated in India some 3,000-5,000 years ago as a way of bringing the mind, spirit and body together, leading to a higher level of self-realization. The word yoga means unity or oneness. There is only one yoga, but there are many different paths within it. Hatha yoga, probably the most widely known form in the West, involves learning control through the body and breath using the focus of the mind. The physical aspect consists of postures (*asanas*) that strengthen and free the body, and breathing exercises (*pranayama*) designed to promote concentration, balance and the flow of energy through the body.

Asanas are not exercises. They are slow, considered movement into positions which are then held for as long as is comfortable. The effect is to increase flexibility, self-awareness and control over our minds and bodies.

Chi Kung is an even more ancient system than yoga and often described as its Chinese equivalent, although as yet it is scarcely known in the West. Like yoga it is a series of exercises, positions and breathing techniques aimed at integrating the mind and body. Chi Kung is based on the traditional Chinese theory that the *chi* or life energy must flow freely round the body if health is to be maintained. The exercises, which relate to the acupuncture points on the body, are designed to stimulate the meridians or channels through which the energy flows and restore the balance of the body. There are hundreds of variations to seven basic Chi Kung exercises and all are suitable for health and relaxation.

Conditions Treated

Both yoga and Chi Kung breathing exercises can be used to relieve asthma, hyperventilation and other breathing disorders. Learning to control breathing enables the patient to pick up their natural breathing rhythm and control asthma spasms. The exercises can also

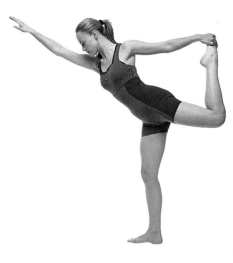

strengthen the back muscles without putting the muscles themselves under strain. If you have sports injuries, or have suffered an illness that has resulted in some physical limitations, yoga and Chi Kung can help you regain and retain movement and strength.

Both yoga and Chi Kung exercises can be used as a specific remedial therapy for circulation problems, digestive and skin disorders and menstrual problems. Each discipline has sets of movements that concentrate on each of the body's main organs and systems. The meditative aspects of yoga and Chi Kung make them ideal general treatments for stress and they help those suffering from ME and rheumatoid arthritis.

Infants and Children

Yoga and Chi Kung are safe for any age group, but children under 12 will probably lack sufficient concentration to benefit fully.

How to Choose a Practitioner

Yoga teachers should have a recognized training at one of three main organizations. Contact the British Wheel of Yoga, 1 Hamilton Place, Boston Road, Sleaford, Lincs NG34 7ES, tel 01529 306 851; the Yoga For Health Foundation, Ickwell Bury, Biggleswade, Beds SG18 9EF, tel 01767 627 271; or the Iyengar

Yoga Institute, 223a Randolph Ave London W9 1NL, tel 0171 624 308

There are very few Chi Kung practitioners in the UK. Contact P Chin at the Hale Clinic, 7 Park Cre London W1N 3HE, tel 0171 631 0

What to Expect at a Consultati

Remedial yoga and Chi Kung are taught on a one-to-one basis in one-and-a-half-hour sessions. Exercises will be selected with reference to the particular problem, but the sessions will all involve general body work, breathing exercises and relaxation. You will be expected to practise techniques at home in between weekly or fortnightly sessions. Ten sessions are usually recommended to get to grips with the fundamental principles and learn the exercises.

Insurance Recognition

No.

Contraindications

Mothers-to-be are not recommended to start yoga or Chi Kung in the first three months of pregnancy.

Compatibility with Other Therapies

Yoga and Chi Kung can be used alongside all other therapies, but are particularly compatible with osteopathy and psychotherapy.

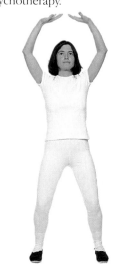

Aromatherapy

Aromatic essential oils extracted from parts of plants or trees have been used for thousands of years in many different parts of the world for healing, medicinal value and promoting a general feeling of relaxation and wellbeing. Contemporary medical interest in their healing powers dates from the 1920s.

There are some 400 of these highly concentrated natural plant oils, all with their individual fragrance and therapeutic properties, whose potency is now beginning to be scientifically investigated and appreciated. Aromatherapists use the oils singly or blended together diluted with carrier oils for massage, inhalation or bathing.

Aromatherapy massage is a most popular and effective form of therapy. The massage itself stimulates the acupoints and the blood and lymphatic circulation, and calms the nervous system. It is well established that oils applied directly to the skin are absorbed easily into the bloodstream and efficiently metabolized in the body. Their physiological effects are gentler and slower-acting than those of synthetic drugs, many of which are also plant-based. But each essential oil has a highly complex pharmacological structure with a wide variety of uses. Some are sedative and anti-inflammatory, others stimulate the circulation or have antiviral and immune-stimulating properties.

Fragrance is a key element of aromatherapy – smell has a direct effect on the brain and central nervous system, influencing our moods and feelings, relaxing the body and mind and promoting self-healing.

Conditions Treated
All stress-related problems and disorders respond well to aromatherapy, which has proved successful in treating flu, colds, asthma, bronchitis, digestive disorders, chronic fatigue, ME, migraines, depression, menopausal and menstrual complaints, infertility, neck

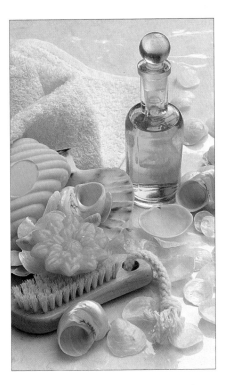

and back pain, RSI, rheumatic disorders, insomnia, anxiety, panic attacks and skin conditions where deep relaxation is essential for improvement.

Aromatherapy massage is also helpful for controlling chronic conditions such as arthritis, where it can help maintain mobility, and improving the quality of life for cancer and AIDS sufferers.

Infants and Children
Babies and young children can have aromatherapy provided only very dilute oils are used. If you use them at home be very careful to keep them well beyond the reach of tiny hands.

How to Choose a Practitioner
There are 13 recognized aromatherapy organizations in the UK and they all require their members to have a recognized training and qualification to standards laid down by the Aromatherapy Organizations Council (AOC), as well as professional insurance. Make sure that your aromatherapist is a member of one of these organizations. Further information, including lists of aromatherapists in your area, can be obtained from AOC, 3 Latymer Close, Braybrooke, Market Harborough, Leics LE16 8LN, tel 01858 434242.

Insurance Recognition
Some private insurance schemes will cover the cost of treatment if your doctor recommends it.

What to Expect at a Consultation
The first consultation will take about an hour and the therapist will ask very detailed questions about your medical history, general health, diet and lifestyle, as well as the particular complaint. This helps him or her decide which essential oils are appropriate for you. An aromatherapy massage from head to toe takes between one and one and a half hours – initially at least the therapist will want to massage the whole body and this should be a very relaxing, pleasurable experience. The therapist will probably want to inform your doctor that you are having aromatherapy treatment.

Contraindications
Essential oils contain powerful active ingredients, some of which may be harmful in combination with some medical treatments or conditions. Certain oils – including such popular ones as cedarwood, peppermint and rosemary – are not recommended during the early months of pregnancy, while others – including clary sage and cypress – should be avoided altogether by pregnant women. Diabetics, epileptics and people with heart conditions must also avoid certain oils.

Compatibility with Other Therapies
Aromatherapy is compatible with other therapies. But if you are having homeopathic or herbal medicine your therapist should first consult with the practitioner.

Flower Remedies

Flower remedies work on your state of mind, addressing a whole range of negative thoughts, fears and anxieties rather than any specific complaint. The theory is that flower essences have a vibrational energy of their own which helps guard against sickness and disease by balancing the emotions that cause or aggravate so many chronic disorders and prevent the body healing.

Flower essence remedies have been used for thousands of years in many different cultures. The best known system, however, is that of the Bach flower remedies, developed some 60 years ago by a London physician, Dr Edward Bach, who became convinced that his patients' state of mind had a direct effect on health. He found that his own emotions responded in certain ways to particular flowers, and so did those of his patients when he treated them with flower essences which he originally garnered from the dew on the flower heads. He identified 38 different remedies based on the flowers of domestic plants, trees and herbs – each one, he believed, had the ability to change and heal a particular emotional problem. His system categorized seven broad categories or personalities ranging from those who suffer uncertainty to those who feel loneliness or fear. There are, of course, many types of fear. The fears of everyday life would be treated with mimulus, while unspecified fears might be treated with aspen. Within the broad categories there are remedies for all the varieties of outlook and feelings Dr Bach defined in developing what he regarded primarily as a self-help system.

The Bach flower essences are obtained by putting the flower heads in spring water and leaving them in the sun, then preserving and bottling the residue in an alcohol solution. The resulting essence is taken in drinks or diluted in water.

Other systems such as Californian, Hawaiian and Australian Bush Flower

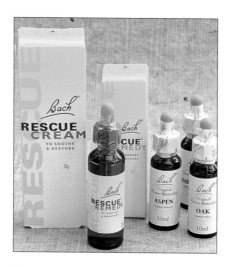

Essences work on similar principles and address themselves to a range of modern stresses and preoccupations. Some flower essences are also believed to have a physical impact on the body, such as on the nervous and immune systems, with some having an anti-viral effect as well.

Conditions Treated

Bach flower essence therapy deals with your emotions – how you feel about your life and any physical problems – rather than specific symptoms. If you are stressed, the therapist will try and work out how that stress affects you. Perhaps you are always in a hurry – impatiens may be prescribed. Perhaps it makes you rigid in your attitudes – rockwater would be prescribed. If you suffer from skin problems and feel self-conscious about your appearance, crab apple, the cleansing remedy, might be suggested. Loofah is another good cleanser for skin problems with an underlying emotional cause.

Menstrual problems, hay fever, arthritis, infertility and morning sickness have all been known to respond to flower essence therapy.

The Bach Rescue Remedy, a mix of five essences, is used for any kind of sudden shock or panic. It is also available as a cream.

Infants and Children

Even babies can safely be given flower essences.

How to Choose a Practitioner

A list of trained Bach therapists is available from the Bach Centre, Mount Vernon, Sotwell, Wallingford, Oxon OX10 0QZ, tel 01491 834678. The International Federation of Vibrational Medicine, Middle Piccadilly, Holwell, Sherborne, Dorset DT9 5LW, tel 01963 23468 has a list of trained therapists who use the whole range of flower essence therapies. Bach Flower remedies are widely available over the counter. Other ranges may be obtained by mail order from International Flower Essence Repertoire, tel 01428 741572.

Insurance Recognition

No.

What to Expect at a Consultation

The therapist will want to know everything about you as well as your symptoms before selecting the appropriate mix of remedies.

The consultation will take about an hour and you will be given a combination of remedies to take two or three times a day mixed with water or directly on the tongue. You will be given at least two months' supply, but if you feel that nothing has changed after a couple of weeks you should go back to the therapist, who may change the mix. Some therapists are also healers and will apply flower essences to the acupoints on the body during consultation.

Contraindications

None. Pregnant women and babies can safely take flower remedies.

Compatibility with Other Therapies

Flower essence therapy is compatible with all other treatments and is regarded as a valuable psychological aid to healing and promoting a sense of wellbeing.

Iridology

Iridology is frequently used for health analysis by complementary practitioners such as osteopaths and homeopaths as well as an increasing number of medical doctors. It is extremely useful in helping to pinpoint the cause of chronic complaints which conventional medicine often has difficulty in establishing.

Iridologists believe that the iris (the coloured part of the eye) holds vital clues to our health. The system was developed by a Hungarian doctor, Ignatz von Peczely. As a boy he had rescued an owl with a broken leg. He noticed that a black mark appeared in its eye the moment it had been injured. His studies of patients convinced him that their illnesses were also reflected in the iris.

The iris is made of connective tissue linked to the central nervous system – the eye is the only place on the body where the system is visible. Iridologists believe each part of the iris relates to a different part of the body, and that strengths and weaknesses are reflected in the appearance of the relevant zone. Iridologists use a 'map' of the iris – the brain is at the top of the circle, the legs at the bottom – to divide the body and its organs up into sections. Then they study the colour, texture and markings on the iris, which tell them the condition of each part of the body. White indicates inflammation, for instance, while toxicity is registered as yellow or brown. Iridology is an important part of preventive medicine. It can show changes in tissues or organs before symptoms develop.

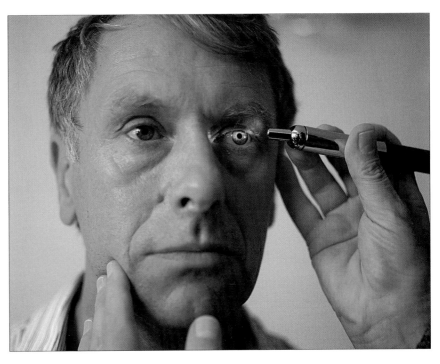

Conditions Treated

Iridology is not a treatment. But by identifying weaknesses it can help you find the correct therapy for complaints that seem to have no particular cause. Headaches, skin disorders, fatigue, ME, back problems and a wide range of other complaints may be linked to unsuspected dysfunction in other parts of the body, and the appropriate therapy and lifestyle changes can then be suggested. The colour and condition of the iris can also indicate a predisposition to various health problems.

Infants and Children

Iridology procedures are non-invasive and entirely safe.

How to Choose a Practitioner

Many complementary practitioners such as osteopaths and homeopaths, naturopaths and chiropractors now have a training in iridology as well. The National Council and Register of Iridologists, 998 Wimborne Road, Bournemouth BH9 2DE, tel 01202 518078, has a list of trained practitioners.

Insurance Recognition

No.

What to Expect at a Consultation

Analysis is done before any case history is taken. The practitioner will examine both eyes with a torch and magnifying glass and make a 'map' of the iris. Some practitioners will use a camera to photograph the iris and project the image on to a large screen.

After notes are taken and the analysis is completed the practitioner will discuss the findings with you, indicating areas which appear to be weak and explaining why and how this may be related to your particular complaint. You may be given advice on diet changes, or referred to another practitioner or doctor. The session will take an hour or less. Some people like to have a check-up once a year to monitor any changes in their bodies.

Contraindications

None. But iridology should not be viewed as a substitute for X-rays, blood tests, mammograms or other conventional diagnostic tests.

Compatibility with Other Therapies

Iridology is used as a diagnostic aid by many complementary therapists.

Other Therapies

The Tangent Method treats stress-related issues such as back problems, increasing the patient's ability to relax and improving posture, self-esteem, lifestyle and focus. This enhances general health and wellbeing. Using a variety of different techniques, including aromatherapy, pressure-point work along meridians, breathing methods, holistic healing, food herbs, corrective exercise and movement, the tangent method addresses physical and emotional problems on many levels.

The Tangent therapist uses her hands skilfully, breaking down habitual patterns to establish balance of both body energy and mind energy, to promote optimum performance.

Simple energy-building and corrective exercises with breathing are individually programmed to maintain the balance of the shoulders, hips and feet, allowing the method to permeate the nervous system. When the body is well aligned, the joints move freely and stress-related pain is alleviated. The mind relaxes and mental performance is greatly enhanced.

The first session begins with an in-depth health and lifestyle questionnaire, which determines how the rest of the treatment progresses. Sometimes the focus will be on specific areas of the body; for others, movement and exercise will play a greater part.

With the patient's input, the Tangent method gives a complete health maintenance programme which provides lasting effects.

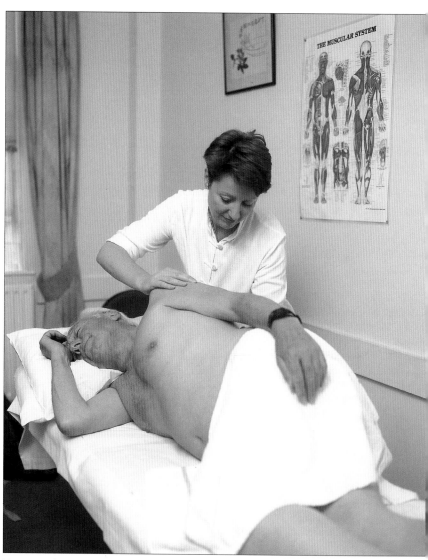

Tangent Therapy

Eye Movement Desensitization and Reprocessing (EMDR) is based on the workings of our mental information process, which is geared to absorbing disturbing information and integrating it through our minds. This normally allows the negative component to be discharged and enables the newly filtered interpretation to be stored for future learning. However, when a person perceives an event as highly traumatic, there is a disruption of this process, which may be said to 'freeze' the information in its original anxiety-producing state. This information cannot then be processed in the normal way, but continues to be sparked by intrusive thoughts, uncomfortable feelings, flashbacks or nightmares, often giving rise to fears, phobias and panic attacks.

EMDR involves restimulating the information channels via rapid image exercises which re-establish the mind's balance, allowing locked or 'frozen' information to be reprocessed down to its logical conclusion, through the gentle expert guidance of a trained therapist. Once this reprocessing has been completed, negative images, feelings and emotions and their associated fears fall away. New and positive outlooks are subsequently formed, enabling the patient to resume a more peaceful life.

The technique was developed through work with veterans of the Vietnam War and can help people with a wide range of problems such as post-traumatic stress disorder, obsessive compulsive behaviour or panic disorders. It has been especially beneficial for concerns resulting from sexual, physical and mental abuse; traumas, fears and phobias; burn, accidents and violence victims; for those suffering from loss or grief; and previously resistant combat veterans.

EMDR is suitable for adults and children with the ability to communicate (i.e. from about the age of five), although patients with certain symptoms such as epilepsy and heart conditions may need to have their sessions conducted in a suitably equipped medical centre where their progress can be monitored.

Patients should ensure that they undertake this therapy only under the guidance of a practitioner fully trained through the EMDR Institute. A list of UK practitioners can be obtained from EMDR UK, 123 Dukes Avenue, Muswell Hill, London N10 2QD.

One of the most welcome benefits of EMDR is that positive results are often achieved in a few sessions.

GDS Method

GDS Method is based on the work of Godlieve Denys-Struyf, a Belgian physiotherapist and osteopath who developed her own form of 'body therapy' in the 1960s, formulating her theory of the 'muscular and articular chains' after many years of observation, experience and scientific research. She discovered that all the muscles of the body, when working in harmony, are connected together in six families, but under certain conditions they can develop into what she called 'chains' which limit the joints and affect the body. These 'chains' may be caused by injury, mental strain or underlying problems, but they are also influenced by the individual character, which determines individual body shape, and ways of misusing the body.

Godlieve Denys-Struyf developed a method of clinical observation and analysis of the body combined with preventive techniques and treatment for optimal body use in relation to the patient's character. Therefore no two people will receive exactly the same treatment, even if they appear to have identical problems.

A consultation begins with a comprehensive assessment. Adapted treatment will be given for specific problems related to the 'chains' that may be involved in the body. Patients will also be educated in self-awareness so that they can help themselves to prevent a recurrence of the problem, or to live better in their body.

GDS Method can encourage babies and children to the fullest development of their potential, particularly those who have undergone a difficult birth or who have physical problems which may be affecting their ability to concentrate. It can also help adults with a variety of problems, all of which may be the result of poor body use: surgery, accident, stress, sports injuries, rheumatic pains, spine problems, pregnancy, breathing difficulties and underlying problems.

A future GDS practitioner should initially be trained in a medical or para-medical profession or in any body therapy; a three-year course of GDS training follows.

BioEnergetic Medicine

BioEnergetic Medicine is a modern system of diagnosis which uses a computer to measure electromagnetic energy in the brain. Sensors attached to the patient's body measure the physical reaction to over 3,000 conditions, treatments and compounds, including homeopathies, viruses, chemical toxins, fungi, amino acids and vitamins. Through identification of the substances to which the immune system has an allergic response, BioEnergetics has had success in treating a range of conditions including autism, food allergies, food cravings and other eating disorders, smoking addiction, hyperactivity, learning difficulties, toxicity, irritable bowel syndrome, RSI, migraine, arthritis, gout, pre-menstrual syndrome, ME, chronic fatigue, emotional problems and depression.

Poor metabolism and a stressed endocrine system cause weight problems. Blood sugar levels fluctuate and food cravings result. Using selected homeopathic remedies, BioEnergetics diagnosis and NLP (neuro-linguistic programming) repositioning of attitudes to certain foods, the London Bio-Dynamics Centre at the Hale Clinic has created a dynamic solution to this

problem. The metabolism is supported and improved, thus ensuring a safe, effective and revolutionary method of reversing this condition.

BioEnergetics treatment is perfectly safe for babies and children. A practitioner should have a Certificate in Bio-Electric Therapy in Complex Homeopathy, which homeopaths or other recognized practitioners could obtain after a year's additional training. It would not be appropriate for a non-qualified student simply to take the on-year course and no reputable college would accept a non-qualified practitioner for this training.

Art Therapy

Art Therapy has been used in the UK since the 1940s and is now a state registered practice, rapidly gaining recognition for its efficacy in working with imagery as a means of self-expression. It may be difficult for people in distress to find words to express what is it they need or for which they are searching. Troubling questions can often be addressed through the non-verbal medium of art, and words will ensue when the images, often symbolic, have been released into a picture.

Art therapy has been found to be particularly valuable with children, who by nature find it difficult to articulate their feelings and inner needs – even more so a child in distress. Art therapy can also be a beneficial palliative when applied to those with life-threatening illnesses or suffering as a result of bereavement. The emotional impact of being diagnosed with a terminal illness is considerable, but many people are unable or unwilling to burden those around them with their feelings. Art therapy offers an opportunity to express their anxieties. Art is able to cut through the taboos that surround death and can be of great therapeutic value for those facing the end of their own life.

Art therapy often has a healing effect when treating psychosomatic and emotional disorders and phobias, particularly when phobias result from childhood traumas. The therapist helps the patient make sense of the inner feelings and experiences that have been expressed, allowing them to regain their capacity to relax and lead a normal, creative life.

Useful Addresses

Australia

Maharishi Ayur-Veda Health Centre
P O Box 81
Bundoora
Victoria 3083

Acupuncture Education Council Australia Inc
P O Box 126
Hurstbridge
Victoria 3099

Chiropractors' Association of Australia
P O Box 241
Springwood
NSW 2777

Australian Association of Practitioners of
Homeopathy
(617) 2026917

Australian Osteopathic Association
P O Box 699
Turramurra
ACT 2074

Reflexology Association of Australia
15 Kedumba Crescent
Turramurra 2074
NSW

National Herbalists' Association of Australia
P O Box 65
Kingsgrave
NSW 2208

Buteyko Australia
Suite 7
Specialist Medical Centre
235 New South Head Road
Edgecliff
Sydney
NSW 2010

Shiatsu Therapy Association of Australia
P O Box 1
Balaclava 3183

Shiatsu Australia
26 Wellington Street
St Kilda 3182

Australian Shiatsu College
P O Box 1188
Collingwood 3066

Veronica Urquhart
Yoga for Health
P O Box 313
Marville
Queensland 4560

Living Essences of Australia
Box 355
Scarborough
Perth
Western Australia 6019

Australian Bush Flower Essences
8a Oaks Avenue
Dee Why
NSW 2099

Canada

Canadian Medical Acupuncture Society
9904 106 Street
Edmonton
Alberta T5K 1C4

Canadian Chiropractic Association
1396 Eglinton Avenue West
Toronto
Ontario M6C 2E4

Canadian Osteopathic Association
575 Waterloo Street
London
Ontario N63 2R2

Shiatsu School of Canada Inc
547 College Street
Toronto
Ontario M6G 1A9

Canadian Society of Teachers of the Alexander
Technique
2181 Avenue Road
Toronto
Ontario M5M 4B8

Association of Physiotherapists & Massage
Practitioners of BC
Suite 103, 1089 West Broadway
Vancouver
BC V6H 0V3

Fédération Québécoise des Masseurs and
Massothérapeutes
Suite 204
1265 Mont-royal Est
Montreal
Quebec H2J 1Y4

Reflexology Association of Canada
11 Glen Cameron Road
Unit 4
Thornhill
Ontario L8T 4NB

Canadian Society of Homeopathy
87 Meadowland Drive West
Nepean
Ontario K2G 2R9

The Beharry Medical Centre
567 Bathurst Street
Toronto
Ontario M5S 2P8
(naturopathy)

National Institute of Nutrition
Suite 302
265 Carling Avenue
Ottawa
Ontario K1S 2E1

Canadian Guidance and Counselling Association
55 Parkdale Avenue
Ottawa
Ontario K1Y 4G1

Canadian Institute of Hypnotism
110 rue Greystone
Montreal
Quebec H9R 5T6

Ontario Society of Clinical Hypnosis
Suite 402
200 St Clair Avenue West
Toronto
Ontario M4V 1R1

Pacific Essences Victoria
Box 8317
Victoria
BC V8W 3R9

New Zealand

Maharishi Foundation of New Zealand (Inc)
5 Adam Street
Greenlane
Auckland
(Ayurveda)

New Zealand Chiropractors' Association
P O Box 7144
Wellesley Street
Auckland

Homeopathic Society (NZ) Inc
P O Box 67095
Mount Eden
Auckland

New Zealand Register of Osteopathy
707 W Frederick Street
Hastings

The Holistic Centre (for acupuncture and
osteopathy)
21 Taharoto Road
Takapuna
Auckland

Shiatsu College Aotearoa
68 View Road
Mount Eden
Auckland 3

Alexander Technique Associates
69 Wellpark Avenue
Grey Lynn
Auckland

New Zealand College of Massage
23 Domain Road
Panmure
Auckland

International School of Natural Health Sciences
c/o Waikuku Post Office
Main Road
Waikuku
North Canterbury

New Zealand Reflexology Association
P O Box 31 084
Auckland 4

Merivale Health Centre
232 Papanui Road
Christchurch
(naturopathy)

South Pacific College of Natural Therapeutics
(NZ) Inc
Box 11-311
Auckland

Bibliography

New Zealand Hypnotherapists Associaion
P O Box 90314
Auckland

The Psychotherapy Centre
7B Union Street
Dunedin

Terri Walsh
Yoga for Health
37 Te Henga Road
Henderson
RD1
Auckland

New Zealand School of Yoga
201 Hobson Street
Auckland

and 120 Cuba Mall
Wellington

Aromatherapy New Zealand Ltd
P O Box 47470
Ponsonby
Auckland

New Perception Flower Essences
P O Box 160-127
Titirangi
Auckland 7

South Africa

Maharishi Ayur-Veda Health Centre
P O Box 5155
Halfway House 1685

Chiropractic Association of South Africa
8a Marlowe Avenue
Westville 3630

South African Reflexology Society
P O Box 201858
Durban North 4016

Mari Fondue
P O Box 115
Voelklip 7203
(for addresses of remedial yoga practitioners)

Waratah Eagle Foundation
P O Box 259
Tableview 7439
(flower essences)

Roger Golten at the Hale Clinic, 7 Park Crescent,
London W1N 3HE, tel 0171 631 0156, has the
names of recognized Hellerwork practitioners in
New Zealand.

The British Acupuncture Council, Park House,
206-208 Latimer House, London W10 6RE, tel
0181 964 0222 has the names of recognized
acupuncturists in New Zealand and South Africa.

The Shiatsu Society, 31 Pullman Lane,
Godalming, Surrey GU7 1XY, tel 01483 860771,
has the names of recognized practitioners in
Australia, Canada and New Zealand.

There are far too many books on complementary
medicine and health for it to be possible to
provide a comprehensive list here. The following
are a few suggestions for those wanting to find
out more about some of the general. Over 60,000
are available from the Nutri Centre at the Hale
Clinic which runs a mail order hotline, tel 0171
436 5122, fax 0171 436 5171

Adamson, Suzanne & Harris, Ailish
The Reflexology Partnership (Kyle Cathie)

Aihara, Cornellia
Natural Healing from Head to Toe (Avery)

Belshaw, Chris
Osteopathy – Is It for You? (Element)

Bradley, Dinah
Hyperventilation: A Guide to Better Breathing
(Kyle Cathie)

Chaitow, Leon
Acupuncture Treatment of Pain (Thorsons)

Downer, Jane
Shiatsu (Hodder & Stoughton)

Fox, Brian A, & Cameron, Allan G,
Food Science, Nutrition and Health (Edward
Arnold)

Godagama, Dr Shantha
Handbook of Ayurveda (Kyle Cathie, 1997)

Gray, Robert
*Colon Health Book – New Health Through Colon
Rejuvenation* (Emerald)

Harvey, Clare G & Cochrane, Amanda
Encyclopaedia of Flower Remedies (Thorsons)

Hodgkinson, Liz
Alexander Technique (Piatkus)

Hunter, Alan
Allergies Make You Fat (Ashgrove)

Lawless, Julia
Home Aromatherapy (Kyle Cathie)

Lockie, Dr Andrew
Family Guide to Homeopathy (Hamish
Hamilton)

Mabey, Richard & McIntyre, Michael
New Age Herbalist (Gaia)

Maisner, Paulette with Turner, Rosemary
*Consuming Passions – What to Do when Food
Rules Your Life* (Thorsons)

Mason, Keith
Medicine for the 21st Century (Element)

Mills, Simon Y
Essential Book of Herbal Medicine (Arkana)

Morrison, Judith
Book of Ayurveda (Gaia Books)

Murray, Michael, & Pizzorno, Joseph,
Encyclopaedia of Natural Medicine
(Little Brown)

Nagendra, Dr, Nagarathna, Dr, & Monro, Dr
Robin *Yoga for Common Ailments* (Gaia)

Null, Gary
*Healing Your Body Naturally: Alternative
Treatments to Illness* (Fours Walls, Eight
Windows)

Peck, Alan *Introduction to T'ai Chi* (Optima)

Ryman, Daniele
Aromatherapy (Piatkus)

Scott, Julian & Susan
Natural Medicine for Women (Gaia)

Starck, Marcia
Complete Handbook of Natural Healing
(Llewellyn)

Tebbetts, Charles
Dreamer's Guide to Mastering Self-Hypnosis
(Breese)

Whitaker, Julian
Dr Whitaker's Guide to Health and Healing
(Prima)

Wilson, Michael B Howitt
Introductory Guide to Chiropractic (Thorsons)

Research

The following are a few of the many published papers dealing with the therapies and conditions in this book.

Allison DB. Kreibich K. Heshka S. Heymsfield SB. *A randomised placebo-controlled clinical trial of an acupressure device for weight loss.* Int J of Obesity & Related Metabolic Disorders. 1995; 19(9):653-8

Andrade LEC, Berraz MB, Atra E, Castro A, Silva MSM *A randomized controlled trial toevaluate the effectiveness of homeopathy in rheumatoid arthritis* Scand J Rheumatol 1991; 20: 204-8

Barabasz M; Spiegel D*Hypnotizability and weight loss in obese subjects* Int J Eating-Disord 1989;8(3): 335-341

Becker-Carus C. Heyden T. Kelle A. *Effectiveness of acupuncture and attitude-relaxation training in the treatment of primary sleep disorders.* Zeitschrift fur Klinische Psychologie Psychopathologie und Psychotherapie 1985;33(2): 161-72

Bittiner SB, Tucker WFG, Cartwright I, Bleehen SS *A double-blind, randomised, placebo-controlled trial of fish oil in psoriasis* Lancet 1988 Feb 20;1(8582):378-80

Boline PD, Kassak K, Bronfort G, Nelson C, Anderson AV *Spinal manipulation vs. amitriptyline for the treatment of chronic tension-type headaches: a randomized clinical trial* J Manipulative Physiol Ther 1995 Mar-Apr;18(3): 148-54

Brigo B, Serpelloni G *Homeopathic treatment of migraines: a randomized double-blind controlled study of sixty cases (homeopathic remedy versus placebo)* Berlin J Res Homoeopath 1991 Mar;1(2)98-106

Budde J. Tronnier H. Rahlfs VW. Frei-Kleiner S. [Systemic therapy of diffuse effluvium and hair structure damage]. [German] Hautarzt. 1993;44(6):380-4

Buguet A. Sartre M. Le Kerneau J.*[Continuous nocturnal automassage of an acupuncture point modifies sleep in healthy subjects].* [French] Neurophysiologie Clinique. 1995; 25(2):78-83

Chapman EH, Angelica J, Spitalny G, Strauss M *Results of a study of homeopathic treatment of PMS* J Am Inst Homeopath 1994 Spring;87(1):14-21

Chou CT, Kuo SC *The anti-inflammatory and anti-hyperuricemic effects of Chinese herbal formula Danggui-Nian-Tong-Tang on acute gouty arthritis: a comparative study with indomethacin and allopurinol* Am J Chin Med 1995;23(3-4):261-7

Christensen BV, Iuhl IU, Vilbek H, Bulow HH, Dreijer NC, Rasmussen HF *Acupuncture treatment of severe knee osteoarthrosis. A long-term study* Acta Anaesthesiol Scandinavica 1992 Aug;36(6): 519-25

Colgan SM, Faragher EB, Whorwell PJ *Controlled trial of hypnotherapy in relapse prevention of duodenal ulceration* Lancet 1988 Jun 11;1(8598):1299-300

Cox IM, Campbell MJ, Dowson D *Red blood cell magnesium and chronic fatigue syndrome* Lancet 1991; 337 (8744) 757-60

Dadkar VN. Tahiliani RR. Jaguste VS. Damle VB. Dhar HL. *Double blind comparative trial of Abana and methyldopa for monotherapy of hypertension in Indian patients.* Japanese Heart Journal. 1990;31(2):193-9

Dale A, Cornwell S *The role of lavender oil in relieving perineal discomfort following childbirth: a blind, randomised clinical trial* Journal of Advanced Nursing 1994;19:89-96

de Lange de Klerk ES. Blommers J. Kuik DJ. Bezemer PD. Feenstra L. *Effect of homoeopathic medicines on daily burden of symptoms in children with recurrent upper respiratory tract infections.* BMJ. 1994; 309(6965):1329-32

Diakow PR, Gadsby TA, Gadsby JB, Gleddie JG, Leprich DJ, Scales AM *Back pain during pregnancy and labor* J Manipulative Physiol Ther 1991 Feb;14(2):116-8

Dunn PA, Rogers D, Halford K *Transcutaneous electrical nerve stimulation at acupuncture points in the induction of uterine contractions* Obstet Gynecol 1989 Feb;73(2):286-90

Egashira Y. Nagano H. *A multicenter clinical trial of TJ-96 in patients with steroid-dependent bronchial asthma. A comparison of groups allocated by the envelope method.* Annals of the New York Academy of Sciences. 1993;685:580-3

Egger J, Carter CM, Soothill JF, Wilson J *Oligoantigenic diet treatment of children with epilepsy and migraine* J Pediatr 1989; 114(1): 51-8

Egger J, Carter CM, Wilson J, Turner MW, Soothill JF *Is migraine food allergy?: A double-blind controlled trial of oligoantigenic diet treatment* Lancet 1983; 2: 865-9

Ehrlich D, Haber P *Influence of acupuncture on physical performance capacity and haemodynamic parameters* International Journal of Sports Medicine August 1992;13(6): 486-91

Ewer TC, Stewart DE *Improvement in bronchial hyper-responsiveness in patients with moderate asthma after treatment with a hypnotic technique: a randomised controlled trial* Br Med J (Clin Res) 1986 Nov 1;293(6555): 1129-32

Freeman RM, Macaulay AJ, Eve L et al.*Randomised trial of self hypnosis for analgesia in labour* Br Med J 1986; 292: 657-8

Geirsson G, Wang YH, Lindstrom S, Fall M *Traditional acupuncture and electrical stimulation of the posterior tibial nerve. A trial in chronic interstitial cystitis.* Scandinavian Journal of Urology & Nephrology 1993;27(1):67-70

Goodale IL. Domar AD. Benson H. *Alleviation of premenstrual syndrome symptoms with the relaxation response.* Obstetrics & Gynecology. 1990;75(4):649-55

Greer S, Moorey S, Baruch JDR, Watson M et al.*Adjuvant psychosocial therapy for patients with cancer: a prospective randomised trial* Br Med J 1992; 304(14 Mar): 675-80

Griffiths RA, Channon-Little L *The hypnotizability of patients with bulimia nervosa & partial syndromes participating in a controlled treat ment outcome study* Contemp Hypn 1993;10(2):81-7

Griffiths RA; Hadzi Pavlovic D; Channon Little L *A controlled evaluation of hypno-behavioural treatment for bulimia nervosa: Immediate pre post treatment effects* Eur Eating Disord Rev 1994;2(4):202-220

Haanen HC, Hoenderdos HT, van Romunde LK, Hop WC, Mallee C, Terwiel JP, Hekster GB *Controlled trial of hypnotherapy in the treatment of refractory fibromyalgia* J Rheumatol 1991;18(1):72-5

Helms JM *Acupuncture for the management of primary dysmenorrhea* Obstet Gynecol 1987 Jan;69(1):51-6

Jacobs GD. Rosenberg PA. Friedman R. Matheson J. Peavy GM. Domar AD. Benson H. *Multifactor behavioral treatment of chronic sleep-onset insomnia using stimulus control and the relaxation response. A preliminary study.* Behavior Modification. 1993;17(4):498-509

Jobst K, McPherson K, Brown V, Fletcher HJ, Mole P, Chen JH, Arrowsmith J, Efthimiou J, Maciocia G, Lane DJ *Controlled trial of acupuncture for disabling breathlessness* Lancet 1986 Dec 20-27;2(8521-2):1416-8

Johansson K. Lindgren I. Widner H. Wiklund I. Johansson BB. *Can sensory stimulation improve the functional outcome in stroke patients?* Neurology. 1993 Nov;43(11):2189-92

Khoo SK. Munro C. Battistutta D. *Evening primrose oil& treatment of premenstrual syndrome* Med. J Australia. 1990;153(4):189-92

Klauser AG, Flaschentrager J, Gehrke A, Muller-Lissner SA *Abdominal wall massage: effect on colonic function in healthy volunteers and in patients with chronic constipation* Zeitschrift Fur Gastroenterologie 1992 Apr; 30(4):247-51

Klauser AG, Rubach A, Bertsche O, Muller-Lissner SA *Body acupuncture: effect on colonic function in chronic constipation* Z Gastroenterol 1993 Oct;31(10):605-8

Kleber RJ; Brom D *Psycho-therapy and pathological grief controlled outcome study* ISR J Psychiatry Relat Sci. 1987;24(1):-(99 109

Kleijnen J, Ter Riet G, Knipschild P *Acupuncture and asthma: a review of controlled trials* Thorax 1991 Nov;46(11):799-802

Koes BW, Bouter LM, van Mameren H, Essers AHM, Verstegen GMJR, Hofhuizen DM, Houben JP, Knipschild PG *Randomised clinical trial of manipulative therapy and physiotherapy for persistent back and neck complaints: results of one year follow up* British Medical Journal1992; 304: 601-5

Kulkarni RR, Patki PS, Jog VP, Gandage SG, Patwardhan B *Treatment of osteoarthritis with a herbomineral formulation: a double-blind, placebo-controlled, cross-over study* J Ethnopharmacol 1991 May-Jun;33(1-2):91-5

Kunze M, Seidel HJ, Stuebe G Vergleichende [*Comparative studies of the effectiveness of brief psychotherapy, acupuncture and papaverin therapy in patients with irritable bowel syndrome*] Zeitschrift für die Gesamte Innere Medizin und ihre Grenzgebiete 1990; 45(20):625-7

Labrecque M, Audet D, Latulippe LG, Drouin J *Homeopathic treatment of plantar warts* Can Med Assoc J 1992 May 15;146(10): 1749-53

Lecoyte T, Owen D, Shepherd H, Letchworth A, Mullee M *An investigation into the homeopathic treatment of patients with irritable bowel syndrome* Proceedings of the 48th Congress of the LMHI 1993:251-258

Lewith GT, Field J, Machin D *Acupuncture compared with placebo in post-herpetic pain* Pain 1983; 17: 361-8

McEwen LM *A double-blind controlled trial of enzyme potentiated hyposensitization for the treatment of ulcerative colitis* Clin Ecology 1987; 5(2):47-51

McGlynn FD. Moore PM. Rose MP. Lazarte A. *Effects of relaxation training on fear and arousal during in vivo exposure to a caged snake among DSM-III-R simple (snake) phobics.* Journal of Behavior Therapy & Experimental Psychiatry. 1995; 26(1):1-8

McGuinness TP *Hypnosis in the treatment of phobias: a review of the literature* Am J Clin Hypn 1984 Apr;26(4):261-72

McKee AM, Prior A, Whorwell PJ *Exclusion diets in irritable bowel syndrome: are they worthwhile?* J Clin Gastroenterol 1987 Oct; 9(5): 526-8

Meade TW. Dyer S. Browne W. Frank AO. *Randomised comparison of chiropractic and hospital outpatient management for low back pain: results from extended follow up.* BMJ.199 ; 311(7001):349-51

Meade TW, Dyer S, Browne W, Townsend J, Frank AO*Low back pain of mechanical origin: randomised comparison of chiropractic and hospital outpatient treatment* BMJ 1990 Jun 2;300(6737):1431-7

Mok MS. Parker LN. Voina S. Bray GA. *Treatment of obesity by acupuncture.* American Journal of Clinical Nutrition. 1976;29(8):832-5

Murphy JJ, Heptinstall S, Mitchell JR *Randomised double-blind placebo-controlled trial of feverfew in migraine prevention* Lancet 1988 Jul 23;2(8604):189-92

O'Morain C, Segal AW, Levi AJ *Elemental diet as primary treatment of acute Crohn's disease: a controlled trial* Br Med J 1984; 288: 1859-62

Oleson T. Flocco W. *Randomized controlled study of premenstrual symptoms treated with ear, hand, and foot reflexology.* Obstetrics & Gynecology. 1993;82(6):906-11

Panjwani U. Gupta HL. Singh SH. Selvamurthy W. Rai UC. *Effect of Sahaja yoga practice on stress management in patients of epilepsy.* Indian Journal of Physiology & Pharmacology. 1995; 39(2):111-6

Paranjpe P, Kulkarni PH *Comparative efficacy of four Ayurvedic formulations in the treatment of acne vulgaris: a double-blind randomised placebo-controlled clinical evaluation* J Ethnopharmacol 1995 Dec 15;49(3):127-32

Paranjpe P, Patki P, Patwardhan B *Ayurvedic treatment of obesity: a randomised double-blind, placebo-controlled clinical trial* J Ethnopharmacol 1990 Apr;29(1):1-11

Reilly D, Taylor M, Beattie NGM et al *Is evidence for homoeopathy reproducible?* Lancet 10 Dec 1994; 344: 1601-6

Sheehan MP, Atherton DJ *A controlled trial of traditional Chinese medicinal plants in widespread non-exudative atopic eczema* Br J Dermatol 1992;126:179-84

Spiegel D, Bloom JR *Group therapy and hypnosis reduce metastatic breast carcinoma pain* Psychosom Med 1983; 45: 333-9

Spiegel D, Bloom JR, Kraemer HC, Gottheil E *Effect of psychosocial treatment on survival of patients with metastatic breast cancer* Lancet 1989; 2: 888-91

Takeda W. Wessel J. *Acupuncture for the treatment of pain of osteoarthritic knees.* Arthritis Care & Research. 1994 ;7(3):118-22

van de Laar MA, van der Korst JK *Food intolerance in rheumatoid arthritis I: a double-blind, controlled trial of the clinical effects of the elimination of milk allergens and azo dyes* Ann Rheum Dis 1992; 51(3): 298-302

Whorwell PJ, Prior A, Faragher EB *Controlled trial of hypnotherapy in the treatment of severe refractory irritable bowel syndrome* Lancet 1984 Dec 1;2(8414):1232-4

Wilkinson S *Aromatherapy and massage in palliative care* Int Journal of Palliative Nursing 1995;1(1):21-30

Williams T, Mueller K, Cornwall MW *Effect of acupuncture-point stimulation on diastolic blood pressure in hypertensive subjects; a preliminary study* Phys Ther 1991; 71(7); 523-9

Demonstration nad treatment of hyperventilation, causing asthma? British Journal of Psychiatry 1988; 153; 687-689

Index